# 麻醉医师面试病例集锦

## Cases for Anesthesia Exam

### （英汉对照）

U0397828

主　　编　童传耀　俞卫锋
副主编　孟令忠　王振猛

世界图书出版公司

上海·西安·北京·广州

**图书在版编目(CIP)数据**

麻醉医师面试病例集锦：英汉对照 / 童传耀，俞卫锋主编. —上海：上海世界图书出版公司，2018.10
ISBN 978-7-5192-5127-7

Ⅰ. ①麻… Ⅱ. ①童… ②俞… Ⅲ. ①麻醉学—病案—英、汉 Ⅳ. ①R614

中国版本图书馆 CIP 数据核字(2018)第 212871 号

| | |
|---|---|
| 书　名 | 麻醉医师面试病例集锦(英汉对照) |
| | Mazui Yishi Mianshi Bingli Jijin（Yinghan Duizhao) |
| 主　编 | 童传耀　俞卫锋 |
| 副主编 | 孟令忠　王振猛 |
| 责任编辑 | 胡　青 |
| 装帧设计 | 南京展望文化发展有限公司 |
| 出版发行 | 上海世界图书出版公司 |
| 地　址 | 上海市广中路 88 号 9-10 楼 |
| 邮　编 | 200083 |
| 网　址 | http://www.wpcsh.com |
| 经　销 | 新华书店 |
| 印　刷 | 上海景条印刷有限公司 |
| 开　本 | 787mm×1092mm　1/16 |
| 印　张 | 25.75 |
| 字　数 | 420 千字 |
| 版　次 | 2018 年 10 月第 1 版　2018 年 10 月第 1 次印刷 |
| 书　号 | ISBN 978-7-5192-5127-7/ R·462 |
| 定　价 | 100.00 元 |

# 主编简介

■**童传耀**

医学博士,威克大学(Wake Forest University)麻醉学教授。1983 年毕业于上海医科大学医学系。在上海市第一人民医院外科工作 2 年后,于 1985～1989 年学习临床麻醉和麻醉实验室研究(硬膜外麻醉对全身和内脏血流动力学的影响——获中国自然科学基金 1986—1990)。1989 年于威克大学做博士后,1991 年被聘为威克大学麻醉科实验室研究员;1996 年于威克大学做麻醉住院医生。2000 年任威克大学麻醉主治医

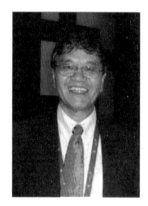

生,2005 年任威克大学麻醉副教授,2012 年为威克大学麻醉学教授。基础研究为脊髓疼痛的神经解剖通路和药理,内脏疼痛的神经解剖生理;建立了鼠的分娩疼痛动物模型。主导的研究课题受到 ASA 的 FAER(Training 2002—2003)和 NIH - RO1 2003—2008 的资助。临床麻醉主要在于神经外科、泌尿科和妇科的麻醉尤其是机器人手术的麻醉管理、创伤外科麻醉和麻醉教育。2016—2017 年任国际华人麻醉学院(ICAA)的院长。

## ■俞卫锋

　　博士，主任医师、教授。中华医学会麻醉学分会副主任委员、中国医师协会麻醉学医师分会前任会长、上海交通大学医学院附属仁济医院麻醉科主任。1985年毕业于第二军医大学医疗系，1989年师从于著名麻醉学家王景阳教授和著名的肝胆外科学家、国家最高科技奖获得者吴孟超院士，分别攻读硕士和博士学位。

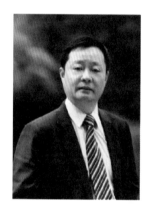

　　任硕士生导师17年，博士生导师12年来，共培养研究生100多名，本人及领导团队承担20多项国家自然科学基金的科研任务，主编专著4部。共发表论文近200篇，SCI收录50余篇，有3篇在世界最著名的麻醉学杂志《Anesthesiology》上发表。研究方向包括吸入麻醉药肝毒性机制研究、围术期肝保护与黄疸麻醉的基础临床研究、慢性疼痛的信号转导与基因治疗等。获国家军队科技进步二等奖一项，另获总后勤部"科技新星"、上海市卫生系统"银蛇奖"、军队院校"育才奖"银奖、上海市优秀学科带头人等各种奖励。

# 副主编简介

## ■孟令忠

医学博士。现任耶鲁大学医学院麻醉学正教授，神经外科兼职正教授，神经麻醉主任。他是国际华人麻醉学院（ICAA）执行董事会董事，国际华人麻醉学院会员委员会主席。于1997年获中国协和医科大学医学博士学位。先后在美国范比尔德大学（Vanderbilt University）外科、迈阿密大学（University of Miami）麻醉科、加利福尼亚大学洛杉矶分校（UCLA）麻醉科接受住院医生培训。在耶鲁大学之前，先后任职于加州大学欧文分校（UC Irvine）麻醉学助理教授、杜克大学 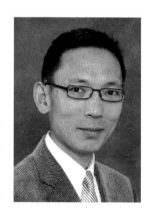 （Duke）和加州大学旧金山分校（UCSF）麻醉学副教授。于1996年获华瑞医学奖学金，2013年获国际华人麻醉学院杰出贡献奖，2014年获 UCSF 学术参议院旅游讲学奖，2015年获 UCSF 麻醉科临床科研种子资金奖，2017年荣获耶鲁大学荣誉艺术硕士。发表了60余篇同行审阅的 SCI 文章。科研兴趣有围术期神经科学、应用血流动力学、脑血流调节和组织氧监测。热衷于中美医学交流合作，目前担任潍坊医学院、潍坊人民医院、西安交通大学医学部、首都医科大学宣武医院和中南大学湘雅医院的客座教授。多次在中国参加学术交流活动，并在美国接受培养了30余名中国进修医生。

## ■王振猛

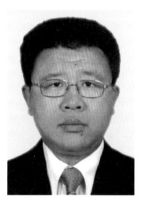

医学博士，第二军医大学附属东方肝胆外科医院麻醉科副主任医师、副教授。

2000年毕业于第二军医大学，后师从俞卫锋教授攻读硕士和博士学位。2014年由国学留学基金委公派赴美国威克大学（Wake Forest University）医学院麻醉科访学，师从童传耀教授。2016年入选上海市杰出青年医学人才培养资助计划。

早期主要从事吸入麻醉药肝损害与肝保护的相关研究，近期主要从事梗阻性黄疸的病理生理改变及其对临床麻醉的影响，对这一领域的相关知识和最新进展有深入全面的了解，具有较强的科研工作能力。近5年来以第一申请人累计申请科研经费100万元，其中国家自然科学基金2项。以第一作者或共同第一作者发表论文16篇，其中SCI论文7篇。

# 编者名单

Peishan Zhao，MD，PhD

Associate Professor

Department of Anesthesiology

Tufts University School of Medicine

赵培山，医学博士

副教授

塔夫斯大学麻醉科


Jianzhong Sun，MD，PhD

Professor and Director of Clinical
　　Outcomes Research

Department of Anesthesiology

Thomas Jefferson University
　　and Hospitals

Philadelphia，Pennsylvania

孙健中，医学博士

教授、临床转归研究主任

托马斯杰斐逊大学和医院麻醉科

费城，宾夕法尼亚州

Chuanyao Tong，MD

President-elected of ICAA

Professor

Department of Anesthesiology

Wake Forest University

Winston Salem，North Carolina

童传耀，医学博士

国际华人麻醉学院院长

教授

维克森林大学麻醉科

温斯顿塞勒姆，北卡罗莱纳州


Ming Xiong，MD，PhD

Associate Professor

Department of Anesthesiology

New Jersey Medical School of
　　Rutgers University

Newark，New Jersey

熊铭，医学博士

副教授

罗格斯大学新泽西医学院麻醉科
纽瓦克,新泽西州

Dongdong Yao, MD, PhD
Assistant Professor
Department of Anesthesiology
Brigham & Women's Hospital of Harvard
　Medical School
Boston, Massachusetts
姚东东,医学博士
助理教授
哈佛医学院布列根和妇女医院麻醉科
波士顿,马萨诸塞州

Renyu Liu, MD
President-elected of ICAA
Associate Professor
Department of Anesthesiology
University of Pennsylvania
Philadelphia, Pennsylvania
刘仁玉,医学博士
国际华人麻醉学院候任院长
副教授
宾夕法尼亚大学麻醉科
费城,宾夕法尼亚州

Chris C. Lee, MD, PhD
Associate Professor

Department of Anesthesiology
Washington University School
　of Medicine
St. Louis, Missouri
李成付,博士
副教授
圣路易斯华盛顿大学医学院麻醉科
圣路易斯,密苏里州

Zhongcong Xie, MD, PhD
Henry K. Beecher Professor
Professor and Director of Geriatric
　Anesthesia Research Unit
Department of Anesthesia, Critical Care
　and Pain Medicine
Massachusetts General Hospital and
　Harvard Medical School
谢仲淙,博士
Henry K. Beecher 荣誉教授
教授、老年麻醉研究室主任
麻醉、重症监护和疼痛医学科
哈佛大学医学院附属麻省总医院

Sunny Chiao, MD
Assistant Professor
Department of Anesthesiology
University of Virginia
Charlottesville, Virginia

Sunny Chiao,博士
助理教授
弗吉尼亚大学麻醉科
夏洛茨维尔,弗吉尼亚州

Zhiyi Zuo,MD,PhD
Robert M. Epstein Professor
Professor and Director of
　　Research Committee
Department of Anesthesiology
University of Virginia
Charlottesville,Virginia
左志义,博士
Robert M. Epstein 荣誉教授
教授、科研委员会主任
弗吉尼亚大学麻醉科
夏洛茨维尔,弗吉尼亚州

Yong G. Peng,MD,PhD,FASE
Professor and Chief of
　　Cardiothoracic Anesthesia
Department of Anesthesiology
University of Florida Shands Hospital
Gainesville,Florida
彭勇刚,博士
教授、心胸麻醉主任
佛罗里达大学尚兹医院麻醉科
盖恩斯维尔,佛罗里达州

Lingzhong Meng,MD
Professor of Anesthesiology
　　and Neurosurgery
Chief,Division of Clinical and
　　Investigational Neuroanesthesia
Department of Anesthesiology
Yale University School of Medicine
New Haven,Connecticut
孟令忠,博士
麻醉科和神经外科教授
神经麻醉临床研究部主任
耶鲁大学医学院麻醉科
纽黑文,康涅狄格州

Yun Xia,MD,PhD
Associate Professor
Department of Anesthesiology
Ohio State University
Columbus,Ohio
夏云,博士
副教授
俄亥俄州立大学麻醉科
哥伦布,俄亥俄州

Lingqun Hu,MD
Associate Professor
Department of Anesthesiology
Northwestern University Feinberg School

of Medicine

Chicago，Illinois

胡灵群，博士

副教授

西北大学范伯格医院麻醉科

芝加哥，伊利诺伊州


Hong Liu，MD

Professor and Acting Vice Chair
of Research

Department of Anesthesiology and
Pain Medicine

University of California Davis
Health System

Sacramento，California

刘虹，博士

教授、研究部执行副主席

麻醉和疼痛医学科

加州大学戴维斯健康系统

萨克拉门托，加利福尼亚州


Shaofeng Zhou，MD

Associate Professor

Department of Anesthesiology

University of Texas Health
Science Center

Houston，Texas

周少凤，博士

副教授

德州大学健康科学中心麻醉科

休斯顿，得克萨斯州


Yanfu Shao，MD

Associate Professor

Department of Anesthesiology

Lewis Katz School of Medicine at
Temple University

Philadelphia，Pennsylvania

邵燕夫，博士

副教授

天普大学路易斯卡茨医学院麻醉科

费城，宾夕法尼亚州


Weifeng Yu，MD

Professor，Director

Vice Chairman of Chinese Society
of Anesthsiology

Department of Anesthesiology

Shanghai Renji Hospital

Shanghai

俞卫锋，博士

教授、主任

中华医学会麻醉学分会副主任委员

上海交通大学附属仁济医院麻醉科

上海

Jing Zhao，MD
Professor，Director
Department of Anesthesiology
Beijing China-Japan Friendship Hospital
Beijing
赵晶，博士
教授、主任
北京中日友好医院麻醉科
北京

Yi Zhou，MD
Attending
Department of Anesthesiology
Henan Cancer Hospital
Zhengzhou，Henan
周一，博士
主治医师
郑州大学附属肿瘤医院麻醉科
郑州，河南

Bo Zhu，MD
Attending
Department of Anesthesiology
Peking Union Medical College Hospital
Beijing
朱波，博士

主治医师
中国医学科学院北京协和医院麻醉科
北京

Wenjuan Guo，MD
Associate Professor
Department of Anesthesiology
Peking Union Medical College Hospital
Beijing
郭文娟，博士
副教授
中国医学科学院北京协和医院麻醉科
北京

Zhenmeng Wang，MD
Associate Professor
Department of Anesthesiology
Shanghai Eastern Hepatobiliary
　　Surgery Hospital
Shanghai
王振猛，博士
副教授
第二军医大学附属东方肝胆外科医院麻
　　醉科
上海

# 序 一

随着科技的飞速发展,我国的麻醉学在过去的 20 年里取得了长足的进步。我国在麻醉机、麻醉监护设备、辅助设备和麻醉药等方面的发展与欧美发达国家相比已相差无几。然而人是决定性因素,做好麻醉最重要的是麻醉医师的水平。

麻醉医师不仅要熟悉掌握临床麻醉的理论和技术,各种麻醉药和相关药物的药效学和药物动力学,还要了解各种疾病的病理生理改变以及手术操作对患者的影响。麻醉医师要掌握产科、儿科、脑外科、心胸外科、耳鼻喉科等各专科的基本知识。麻醉医师面临的患者,包括新生儿、高危产妇及心肺功能减退的老年人等。只有通过日积月累,麻醉医师才能掌握相关知识,独立处理各种复杂困难病例。

中国医师协会麻醉学医师分会(CAA)和国际华人麻醉学院(ICAA)近年来广泛合作,尝试共同促进麻醉学科的发展和住院医生培养。2015～2017 年,连续 3 年举办麻醉教育研讨会,介绍并推广美国麻醉住院医生口试。这本由 CAA 和 ICAA 联合主编的麻醉面试病例集锦,通过真实的病例分析突出相关的知识要点,内容涵盖了全面的相关学科,贴近临床麻醉工作。本书有助于让更多的麻醉医师了解麻醉面试的形式和作用,提高麻醉医师,特别是住院医师的应变能力和临床水平。该书由美国各大医学院的一线麻醉学专家编写,英中对照的形式,还有助于麻醉医师对专业英语的学习,促进年轻医师间的国际交流。我推荐各年资麻醉医师,尤其是麻醉住院医师认真学习本书的病例,从中获得启发,提高为患者服务的能力。

作为 CAA 会长以及 ICAA 多年的合作者,我很高兴看到本书的出版并为本书作序。

2017 年 8 月

# 序 二

国际华人麻醉学院(ICAA)的主要宗旨在于建立国际麻醉学领域的学术交流和人才培养平台,与世界各地尤其是中国麻醉学专家学者们互相学习、交流,共同提高,为祖国的麻醉事业进步和发展贡献一份力量,并在一些领域里引领世界麻醉学发展的方向。

2015年以来,ICAA在其院长童传耀教授的组织和领导下,在中国医师协会麻醉医师分会(CAA)会长、上海交通大学俞卫锋教授及北京协和医院赵晶教授等的协助下,一直致力于在中国推广麻醉口试的交流和学习。之后,童传耀教授、孟令忠教授、赵晶教授和俞卫锋教授积极协作,发表了相关文章并出版这本麻醉面试病例集锦。而现在,我很高兴地看到这本麻醉口试病例集锦要再版了。

众所周知,麻醉口试可以更好地评估麻醉医师的知识面、判断力、交流的能力以及适应性和专业性,这是笔试所不能替代的。2017年4月份的《Anesthesiology》上刊登了美国梅奥诊所和哈佛大学医学院等共同完成的一项科研成果,这项研究收集了美国从1971～2011年,所有通过美国麻醉医师资格考试并拿到行医执照的医师资料,追踪到2014年,检查这些医生中有多少医生其执照被吊销或者受到其他纪律处理。他们的研究发现:比起那些一次就通过笔试和口试的医师来说,第一次口试和笔试都没有通过的医师,其受到这些处理的风险要高出3.6倍,而只通过笔试没有通过口试的医师也要高出3.51倍。这些研究结果表明,和麻醉笔试相比,口试的通过与否能更好地预示一个麻醉医师以后是否能成为一个优秀的麻醉医师。

我希望ICAA开展的麻醉口试交流和学习,能对中美两国的麻醉医师的教育和培养起到良好的推动及促进作用。美国和其他国家现行的麻醉口试有很多需要改进的地方，我相信中美的麻醉学教育专家们会很好地完善目前的麻醉口试方法，找到适合中国国情并可以引领世界麻醉学教育的方法。

ICAA 与中国麻醉学界的专家、教授们有着长期广泛的合作和交流，这期间大家结下了深厚的友谊。我期待着在今后的日子里，我们互相学习、互相帮助、互相交流，能够为中国的麻醉学发展略尽绵薄之力。

2017 年 8 月

# 目　录

1 Geriatric anesthesia-anesthesia management for colectomy in an elderly patient with significant cardiac disease
老年手术麻醉——心脏病患者非心脏手术麻醉 / 1

2 Abdominal surgery-Whipple resection
腹部外科手术病例——胰十二指肠切除手术麻醉 / 46

3 Anesthesia management for total thyroidectomy
普外科手术病例——甲状腺手术麻醉 / 61

4 Ambulatory endoscopic surgery-ureteroscopic stone manipulation
日间内窥镜手术病例——输尿管镜碎石术 / 73

5 Anesthesia for total laryngectomy
耳鼻喉手术病例——全喉切除麻醉 / 106

6 Anesthesia management for left adrenalectomy of pheochromocytoma
嗜铬细胞瘤患者左肾上腺切除术的麻醉管理 / 137

7 Anesthesia for hip surgery in elderly
老年患者髋关节手术的麻醉 / 150

8 Anesthesia consideration for pneumonectomy
普胸手术病例——肺叶切除手术麻醉 / 162

9 Anesthesia management for pituitary tumor
脑外科手术病例——垂体瘤手术麻醉 / 172

10　Anesthesia management for left carotid artery stent placement
置入颈动脉内支架的麻醉管理 / 188

11　Anesthetic management for complex posterior spinal fusion and instrumentation
复杂后路脊柱融合术及脊柱矫形器械置入术的麻醉管理 / 209

12　Perioperative care for intracranial aneurysm clipping
颅内动脉瘤夹闭术的围术期管理 / 251

13　Perioperative care for carotid endarterectomy
颈动脉内膜剥脱术的围术期管理 / 264

14　Complicated obstetric case
合并多种疾病的临产妇的麻醉管理 / 279

15　Elective C-section for a term pregnancy with placenta previa
足月妊娠合并前置胎盘的剖宫产麻醉 / 299

16　Anesthesia management for aortic valve replacement
主动脉瓣置换术的麻醉管理 / 307

17　Anesthesia management for ascending aortic aneurysm surgery
升主动脉瘤手术麻醉管理 / 319

18　Anesthetic management of coronary artery bypass graft
冠状动脉搭桥术的麻醉 / 332

19　Pediatric anesthesia-anesthesia for tonsillectomy
小儿手术麻醉——扁桃体切除术的麻醉 / 352

20　Anesthesia management for MVA trauma victim
车祸/多发伤手术麻醉 / 379

# 1 Geriatric anesthesia-anesthesia management for colectomy in an elderly patient with significant cardiac disease

## 老年手术麻醉——心脏病患者非心脏手术麻醉

> **Basic information** <

A 70 years old woman with bloody stool and constipation for 2 months was scheduled for laparoscopic right hemicolectomy.

Past medical history: She has a long list of comorbidities, which include: hypothyroidism, chronic obstructive pulmonary disease (COPD) on 2 L/min home O₂ for 2 years (mainly used during the night). She quitted smoking 3 weeks ago. Diabetes mellitus (DM) type 2, hyperlipidemia, hypertension (HTN), peripheral vascular disease (PVD) with a fem-fem bypass surgery 6 years ago, coronary artery disease (CAD) for 10 years, myocardial infarction (MI) 2 times in the past. She had CABG with 3 vessels graft 6 years ago, and 3 drug eluting stents (DES) 2 years ago. She has angina two to three times a month, usually resolved by taking nitroglycerine or rest.

Medications: metoprolol 50 mg bid, Diovan (Valsartan) 160 mg, atorvastatin, metformin, Lasix, synthroid, Aspirin 81 mg, albuterol inhaler, atrovent (ipratropium), Symbicort (budesonide and formoterol) inhaler, Neurontin (gabapentin), Plavix, nitroglycerine.

Physical exam：166 cm，89 kg，BMI 32.3，BP 145/89，HR 88，RR 16，Temperature 36.2℃.

ECG：SR 80，ST - T changes in lateral and inferior leads, old infarction can't be ruled out.

ECHO：LVH with mild decreased LV function，EF 45%；mild mitral regurgitation. Sclerotic trileaves aortic valve without stenosis. Normal RV and RA in size and function.

Labs：Hb 10.4；WBC 8.0；Plat 210；Na 136，K 3.1，Cl 109，$HCO_3$ 29，Glu 145，BUN 35，Cr. 1.9（calculated GFR 35），HbA1c 8.4. ABG pH 7.42，$PaO_2$ 86，$PaCO_2$ 55，$HCO_3$ 34，BE 2.

## > 基 本 信 息 <

70 岁女性,大便带血和便秘 2 个月。计划腹腔镜右半结肠切除术。

病史:患者有很多的并发症,包括甲状腺功能低下、慢性阻塞性肺疾病;在家使用 2 L/min 的氧气已经有 2 年(主要在夜间使用)。3 周前戒烟。2 型糖尿病、高脂血症、高血压、外周血管疾病,6 年前做过股动脉-股动脉搭桥术。冠状动脉疾病10 年,心肌梗死 2 次。在 6 年前接受了 3 次血管移植冠状动脉搭桥术,2 年前接受了 3 个药物洗脱支架。目前,她每个月发生 2～3 次心绞痛,通常通过服用硝酸甘油或休息缓解。

目前用药:美托洛尔 50 mg 每天 2 次、缬沙坦、阿托伐他汀、二甲双胍、呋塞米、甲状腺素、阿司匹林 81 mg、沙丁胺醇吸入剂、异丙托铵吸入剂、布地奈德和福莫特罗吸入剂、加巴喷丁、波立维和硝酸甘油。

体检:身高 166 cm,体重 89 kg,BMI 指数 32.3,血压 145/89 mmHg,心率88 次/ min,呼吸 16 次/min,体温 36.2℃ 。

心电图:窦性心律 80 次/min,侧壁和下壁导联非特异性 ST - T 改变,陈旧性心肌梗死不除外。

心动超声:左心室肥大伴轻度左心室功能减退,心脏射血分数 45%;轻度二尖瓣反流。主动脉瓣为三瓣膜,硬化但没有狭窄。右心房、右心室的大小和功能正常。

实验室检查:血红蛋白 104 g/L,白细胞 $8.0 \times 10^9$/L,血小板 $210 \times 10^9$/L,钠 136 mmol/L,钾 3.1 mmol/L,氯 109 mmol/L,碳酸氢盐 29 mmol/L,血糖 8.06 mmol/L,尿素 6.23 mmol/L(尿素氮 12.46 mmol/L),肌酐 167.96 $\mu$mmol/L(计算肾小球滤过率 35),糖化血红蛋白 8.4%。血气分析 pH 7.42,血氧分压 86 mmHg,二氧化碳分压 55 mmHg,碳酸氢根 34 mmol/L,剩余碱 2 mmol/L。

## > **Preoperative management** <

### Assessment

1. Do you think the patient is ready for surgery,why/why not? (1 - Patient care; 6 - System-based practice)

I need more information to decide if this patient is ready or not for the surgery. She has a lot of comorbidities; my question is if these conditions are stable.

1) I need to know her functional status and will ask the patient what kind of physical activities she can do.

If Mets>4, which is unlikely, I will proceed with surgery.

If Mets<4, I will ask cardiology for pharmacological stress test and to optimize her cardiac condition.

2) I need to know if she took her inhalers today or not and will listen to her lungs to see if she is actively wheezing.

Wheezing relieved by albuterol inhaler is ok to proceed. Otherwise, delay the case.

2. If, this patient cannot climb to the 2nd floor. Would you consider a

cardiac stress test, which one would be your choice, exercise or drug induced stress test? (1 - Patient care)

The patient cannot do strenuous activities. So, I think pharmacological stress test is reasonable to evaluate her cardiac function and possible ischemia.

3. How about Cardiac catheterization? Why/why not? (1 - Patient care; 6 - System based practice)

Depending on the result of stress test, I will consult cardiologist and even cardiac surgeon to decide if the patient will be benefit from preoperative cardiac catheterization and revascularization. I think the patient will need cardiac catheterization if her stress test showed ischemia (controversial).

4. What would be this patient's cardiac risks? explain. (2 - Medical Knowledge)

Patient's cardiac risks are very high.

1) Hypertension: poorly controlled chronic HTN can cause end organ diseases including LV hypertrophy, heart failure and cardiac ischemia. Others include PVD, cerebral vascular disease, stroke, renal insufficiency.

2) History of CAD/PVD and current anginas:

* Major adverse cardiac events after noncardiac surgery is often associated with prior CAD events (History of cardiac ischemia is one of the independent risk factors for postoperative major cardiac complications).

* Preoperative troponin T value of $\geqslant 0.02$ is associated with 2% of the 30 - day mortality.

3) DM: diabetic dyslipidemia, increased vascular inflammation, vascular endothelial dysfunction, impaired coronary microcirculation and decreased coronary collateral circulation will all contribute to cardiac risks. In fact, more than 70% of DM patient have HTN and cardiovascular disease, which is the major cause of death in DM patients.

4) Hyperlipidemia: is a strong risk factor for CVD demonstrated by many

studies. Hyperlipidemia causes atherosclerosis with consequences of CAD，PVD and cerebral vascular disease.

5）COPD：chronic hypoxemia and hypercarbia may cause cor pulmonale and RV dysfunction. COPD patient has long history of smoking.

6）Smoking history：major cause of COPD，PVD and CAD. Carbon monoxide decreases oxygen delivery and increases myocardial work. Catecholamine released by smoking may cause coronary vasoconstriction.

7）Obesity：often complicated with HTN and DM.

5. Should her metformin to be stopped before the surgery，explain?（2 - medical knowledge）

1）She should stop her metformin at least in the morning of the surgery because of NPO after midnight.

2）The risk of lactic acidosis is low if the patient has normal renal functions，but her Cr 1.9 and GFR 35，meaning she has stage Ⅲ renal insufficiency and may have higher risk for perioperative lactic acidosis. Some guidelines recommend to stop metformin 48 h before the surgery. I will ask her to stop metformin 48 h prior to surgery.（The candidate can also continue metformin to get survival benefit for cancer patient，which published recently）

6. What about the beta blocker? Do you have any evidence support your decision?（5 - Practice-based learning and improvement）

1）Based on AHA and ASA guidelines，patient who has been on beta blocker should continue beta blocker during perioperative period because many studies have shown that preoperative use of beta blockers was associated with a reduction in perioperative cardiac events. So，she should continue her beta blocker.

2）Having said that. I know that preoperative beta blockers do not reduce the risk of postoperative mortality. Some studies also demonstrated increased postoperative stroke with perioperative beta blocker use.

7. If she was not on beta blocker, would you start it on the day of surgery? Why? (5 - Practice-based learning and improvement)

1) No. It is not recommended to start beta blockers ≤1 day before surgery or on the day of surgery since it would not be effective and may be harmful. Such as severe bradycardia and hypotension.

2) Beta blockers should be started 2 to 7 days before surgery or even> 30 days is preferred. This allows preoperative dose titration and clinical assessments for patient's tolerability.

## Enhanced Recovery After Surgery (ERAS)

8. What is ERAS? Has it been demonstrated to improve postoperative recovery in colon surgery?

1) ERAS is a multidisciplinary program that aims to optimize perioperative management in order to reduce postoperative complications and achieve early recovery.

2) Several meta-analyses have demonstrated that ERAS reduced surgical complications and length of hospital stay in colorectal surgery.

9. Do you consider ERAS for this patient? If yes, what do you plan to do regarding NPO, bowel preparation, pain management, iv fluid, etc.?

1) I will definitely consider ERAS for this patient.

2) There are several ERAS guidelines published for colorectal surgery and surgery in other specialties. To be specific to colorectal surgery. Assume the patient nutrition is fine,

a) I will let the patient have solid food up to 8 h and clear fluids up to 2 h prior to induction of anesthesia.

Preoperative oral carbohydrate fluids should be used routinely.

For this diabetic patient, the carbohydrate treatment can be given along with the blood sugar monitoring and insulin treatment.

b) I will recommend surgery not to do mechanical bowel preparation (MBP) because MBP will cause dehydration, distress for the patient and is associated with prolonged ileus after colonic surgery.

c) If the patient is not extremely anxious, I will not give preoperative sedation since it may delay immediate recovery from surgery.

d) I will give preoperative SQ heparin to prevent venous thromboembolism (VTE) formation and ask surgeon to continue VTE prophylaxis for 4 more weeks after surgery. The patient should have well-fitting compression stockings and intermittent pneumatic compression during the surgery as well.

e) I will give antibiotics within one hour before incision and repeat doses during the surgery based on the half-life of the medications.

f) I will use multimodal approach to manage intraoperative and postoperative pain. Considering preoperative thoracic epidural placement.

g) Intraoperative fluid management will aim patient to normovolemic and not over hydrate the patient and cause possible intestinal edema and even heart failure in this patient.

h) I will pull the OGT (oral gastric tubing) out at the end of surgery after consulting the surgeon and give antiemetics to prevent postoperative nausea and vomiting (PONV).


10. Would you ask this patient to stop smoking before the surgery if she did not quit smoking? Why?

1) Although study showed one month of smoking secession is needed to reduce the incidence of complications, I will still ask the patient to stop smoking because education of patient is our responsibility and surgery time is the perfect time to educate the patient.

2) Smoking cessation is also part of ERAS.

11. You need one month to reduce the postoperative complications. Except for the best time to educate the patient, any other benefits to ask her to stop smoking right before the surgery?

1) The half-life of carboxyhemoglobin is about $4 \sim 6$ hours when patient breaths room air. So, the patient's serum carboxyhemoglobin level will decrease after $12 \sim 24$ hour cessation of smoking.

2) This will make P50 (the arterial oxygen pressure at which hemoglobin is 50% saturated with $O_2$) of oxyhemoglobin dissociation curve back to normal and may improve oxygen delivery.

3) Carbon monoxide may have negative inotropic effect on cardiac contractility, decreased plasma level of carbon monoxide may improve cardiac function.

## Hyperglycemia

12. What is HbA1c?

1) HbA1c is referred to the glycated haemoglobin. Blood glucose normally attaches to haemoglobin. The amount of glucose that binds to Hb is directly proportional to the total amount of sugar in someone's body at that time.

2) Because the life time of red blood cells in the human is $8 \sim 12$ weeks before renewal, measuring HbA1c can be used to reflect average blood glucose levels over that duration.

3) The ideal level is $<6.5\%$ for diabetic patient.

13. Hers is 8.4, would it have any impact on the intraoperative management?

1) HbA1c 8.4 is higher than normal, meaning her DM is NOT well controlled.

2) The problems with uncontrolled DM are:

a) Increased risk of wound infection, surgical site infection increases perioperative morbidity and mortality;

b) Osmotic diuresis, dehydration and electrolytes disturbance;

c）Hyper viscous blood and thrombogensis;

d）Diabetic ketone acidosis（DKA）;

e）Because this patient may have chronic hyperglycemia, which may cause endothelial dysfunction and impair coronary microcirculation and cardiac ischemia.

14. What is your goal of managing her glucose during surgery and why?

Traditional intraoperative glucose control is$<220\sim250$ mg/dL. Recently, very strict control, the glucose$<110$ mg/dL, which could result in more often in hypoglycemia. My target is moderate strict$<150$ mg/dL, which minimizes the chance of hypoglycemia and still decreases surgical site infection without increase in the incidences of post-operative stroke and death.

## Chronic obstructive pulmonary disease （COPD）

15. Explain your concerns of her COPD and being on home $O_2$?

Her COPD is very severe since home $O_2$ means her $PaO_2$ is most likely$<$55 mmHg on room air and under general anesthesia she will need more $O_2$ and may need to continue mechanical ventilation after surgery. She may also have cor pulmonale and right heart dysfunction from chronic hypoxemia and hypercarbia.

16. What is the purpose of oxygen therapy?

1）To treat hypoxia;

2）To decrease pulmonary vascular resistance;

3）To prevent erythrocytosis.

17. Do you need a pulmonary function test （PFTs）, why/why not?

1）I don't think it is necessary unless patient feels her breathing is getting worse recently. If her COPD is not stable, I will order PFTs as a tool to monitor if her pulmonary function improved after treatment.

2）If her pulmonary condition is stable, the PFTs only tell me she has COPD and how severe her COPD is that I have already known from her history and my physical exam.

3）PFTs may be more useful for predicting postoperative pulmonary functions after lung resection, but not for non-thoracic surgery.

18. The surgeon ordered PFTs anyway. Her PFT results came back with FEV1/FEV<40%, FVC 1,000 mL, concerned?

1）These results confirm my diagnosis that she has severe COPD demonstrated by FEV1/FEV < 40%. Most patient with FEV1 < 40% has dyspnea during daily life activities. This is consistent with her home $O_2$ use.

2）Normal FVC is more than 10 mL/kg. It also depends on the patient's effort. FVC 1,000 mL is normal for this patient, which is consistent with her COPD, an obstructive, not a restrictive lung disease which has a decreased FVC.

19. Could you do anything to improve her pulmonary status?

1）It depends on her history and my physical exam. If she has signs of infection, such as copious purulent sputum or even fever, I can give her antibiotics treatment to improve her pulmonary condition.

2）If she is actively whizzing, I can treat her with beta - 2 agonist, such as albuterol to relieve bronchospasm.

20. How does the anesthesia affect the pulmonary function?

All inhalational agents have bronchodilation effect which is good for this patient. But inhalational agents also inhibit hypoxic pulmonary vasoconstriction （HPV） and increase V/Q mismatch. They impair ciliary function and mucus clearance as well.

21. Does epidural maintain pulmonary functions?

Yes，if the level is below T6. Above T6，regional anesthesia may impair active expiration and cough.

22. The patient asked you about her chance to be ventilated postoperatively，your response?（3 - Professnioalism；4 - Interpersonal and communication skills）

I will explain that is a real possibility based on her respiratory disease. And this is for her safety.

## ＞ 术 前 管 理 ＜

### 评估

1. 你认为患者准备好手术了吗？为什么？（1 - 患者护理；6 - 基于系统的实践）

我需要更多的信息来决定是否准备好对患者进行手术。她有很多并发症，我的问题是，这些并发症的病情是否稳定？

1）我需要知道她的身体功能状况，我会问患者可以做什么样的体力活动。

如果 Mets＞4，我会进行手术。虽然，这种可能性不大。

如果 Mets＜4，我会请心脏科进行药理学应激试验，并优化她的心脏状况。

2）我需要知道她今天是否用了吸入剂，并且会听诊她的肺，看看她是否有哮鸣音。

如果有哮鸣音，但吸入沙丁胺醇后可以缓解，我可以进行手术。否则，我会延迟手术。

2. 假如，这个患者不能爬到二楼。你会考虑一个心脏应激试验吗？运动或药物诱导的你会选择哪一个？（1 - 患者护理）

患者不能进行剧烈的活动。所以，我认为用药物诱导的应激试验来评价她的心脏功能和可能的缺血是合理的。

3. 你会要求做心导管吗？为什么？（1-患者护理；6-基于系统的实践）

这要根据应激试验的结果来定。我会咨询心脏病学家，甚至心脏外科医师，以决定患者是否将受益于术前心导管和血管重建。我认为如果她的应激试验显示心脏有缺血改变，患者需要做心导管（有争议）。

4. 这个患者的心脏病风险是什么？请解释。（2-医学知识）

患者的心脏病风险非常高。

1）高血压：控制不佳的慢性高血压可引起各系统器官的疾病，包括左心室肥大、心力衰竭和心脏缺血。其他包括外周血管病变、脑血管疾病、卒中和肾功能不全。

2）冠心病、外周血管病病史和当前心绞痛的病史：

＊非心脏手术后的严重心脏并发症常与先前的冠心病有关（心脏缺血史是术后严重心脏并发症的独立危险因素之一）。

＊术前肌钙蛋白 T 值≥0.02 的患者，术后 30 天死亡率为 2%。

3）糖尿病：糖尿病患者常有血脂异常、血管炎症、血管内皮功能障碍、冠状动脉微循环受损和冠状动脉侧支循环减少等，这些都是导致心脏并发症的危险因素。事实上，超过 70% 的糖尿病患者有高血压和心血管疾病，这是导致糖尿病患者死亡的主要原因。

4）高脂血症：许多研究都显示，高血脂是心血管疾病的危险因素。高脂血症导致动脉粥样硬化，因此造成冠心病、外周血管病变和脑血管疾病等后果。

5）慢性阻塞性肺病：慢性低氧血症和高碳酸血症可引起肺心病、右心室功能障碍。慢性阻塞性肺病患者常有长期吸烟史。

6）吸烟史：是慢性阻塞性肺病、冠心病和外周血管病的主要原因。一氧化碳减少氧气传送并增加心脏工作负荷。吸烟引起的儿茶酚胺释放可能导致冠状动脉血管痉挛。

7）肥胖：通常合并有高血压和糖尿病。

5. 她的二甲双胍在手术前应该停止服用吗？请解释。（2-医学知识）

1）至少在手术当天的早晨，她应该停止服用二甲双胍，因为午夜后她禁食。

2）如果患者的肾功能正常，二甲双胍导致乳酸性酸中毒的风险很低。但是她的肌酐是167.96 μmmol/L，肾小球滤过率为35，这意味着她患有Ⅲ期肾功能不全，可能有较高的围术期乳酸性酸中毒的风险。一些临床指南建议在手术前48个小时停止服用二甲双胍。我会建议她在手术前48个小时停止服用二甲双胍。（考试人也可以回答继续使用二甲双胍，因为最近发表的文献显示，二甲双胍能改善癌症患者预后）

6. 对β受体阻滞剂有何建议？你有任何证据支持你的决定吗？（5-基于实践的学习和改进）

1）根据美国心脏病协会和麻醉医师协会的临床指南，已经在服用β受体阻滞剂的患者应在围术期期间继续使用β受体阻滞剂，因为许多研究显示术前使用β受体阻滞剂可以减少围术期心脏并发症。所以，她应该继续服用β受体阻滞剂。

2）虽然这样说，我知道术前β受体阻滞剂不能降低手术后死亡的风险。一些研究还证实了使用β受体阻滞剂的患者，术后卒中发生率增加。

7. 如果她术前没有使用β受体阻滞剂，你会在手术当天开始给她用吗？为什么？（5-基于实践的学习和改进）

1）不会。一般不建议在手术前一天或手术当天开始使用β受体阻滞剂，因为它对降低术后心脏并发症不仅没有效果，还可能有害。比如严重的心动过缓和低血压。

2）β受体阻滞剂应在手术前2～7天开始，最好是前30天开始。这样可以在术前评估患者是否能够耐受，并调整剂量。

## 加速康复外科

8. 什么是加速康复外科？这种做法对改善结肠手术的术后恢复有证据吗？

1）加速康复外科是一个多学科计划，旨在优化围术期管理，减少术后并发症以实现患者早期恢复、出院为目的。

2）几项荟萃分析表明，加速康复外科计划确实减少了肛肠手术并发症和患者住院时间。

9. 你会考虑给这个患者实施加速康复外科计划吗？如果考虑，关于术前禁食、肠道准备、疼痛管理、静脉给液等，你打算怎么做？

1）我肯定会考虑给这个患者做术后加速康复计划。

2）针对肠道外科手术和其他专科手术，已经有几个临床指南颁布。具体到肛肠外科，假如这个患者营养状况良好，

a）我将让患者在麻醉诱导之前禁食固体食物 8 个小时以上，透明饮料可以在麻醉诱导前 2 个小时禁用。术前应常规饮用含碳水化合物的液体。糖尿病患者，也可以饮用含碳水化合物的液体，但要监测血糖，在需要时给予胰岛素治疗。

b）我会建议不做术前灌肠准备，因为术前灌肠准备会导致患者脱水，感觉难受，并且在结肠手术后延长肠功能恢复的时间。

c）如果患者不是非常焦虑，我不会给她术前镇静药，因为有可能会延迟术后麻醉的快速苏醒。

d）术前我会给予皮下注射肝素，预防静脉血栓栓塞形成，并要求外科医师在术后 4 周继续进行静脉血栓栓塞预防。在手术过程中，患者应该穿合体的弹力袜，并有间歇性气压按摩。

e）我将在切皮前 1 个小时内给予抗生素，并在手术期间根据药物的半衰期重复给药。

f）我将使用多模式方法来管理术中和术后疼痛。考虑术前放置胸段硬膜外导管。

g）术中输液以保持患者正常血容量为目的。避免过度输液，造成肠水肿，对这个患者来说，甚至导致心力衰竭。

h）在咨询外科医师后，我将在手术结束时拔出胃管，并给予止吐药以防止术后恶心和呕吐。

10. 如果这个患者没有戒烟，你会要求患者在手术前戒烟吗？为什么？

1）虽然研究显示，需要戒烟 1 个月以上才能减少并发症的发生率，但我仍然会要求患者戒烟，因为对患者的教育是我们的责任，手术时期是教育患者的最佳时机。

2）戒烟也是加速康复外科计划的一部分。

11. 如果需要戒烟 1 个月以上才能减少术后并发症,除了你说的患者教育,术前短时间内戒烟有其他好处吗?

1)在患者呼吸空气,也就是不吸氧时,碳氧血红蛋白的半衰期 4～6 个小时。因此,在停止吸烟 12～24 个小时后,患者血液中的碳氧血红蛋白水平将会降低。

2)这将使氧合血红蛋白解离曲线的 P50(50%的血红蛋白被氧饱和时的动脉氧分压)回到正常,从而改善氧的传送。

3)一氧化碳可能对心脏收缩有负性肌力作用,血浆一氧化碳水平降低可能改善心脏功能。

## 高血糖

12. 什么是 HbA1c?

1)HbA1c 是指糖化血红蛋白。血糖通常附着于血红蛋白,与血红蛋白结合的葡萄糖的量与当时人身体中的糖的总量成正比。

2)由于人体红细胞的寿命是 8～12 周,测量 HbA1c 可用于反映该段时间内的平均血糖水平。

3)糖尿病患者糖化血红蛋白的理想水平<6.5%。

13. 她的糖化血红蛋白是 8.4,这会对术中管理有什么影响吗?

1)糖化血红蛋白(8.4)高于正常,意味着她的糖尿病没有得到很好的控制。

2)糖尿病血糖控制不好可能导致:

a)增加(伤口)感染的风险,手术部位感染增加围术期并发症和死亡率。

b)渗透性利尿、脱水和电解质紊乱。

c)血液黏稠性增加和血栓栓塞形成。

d)糖尿病酮症酸中毒(DKA)。

e)因为该患者可能患有慢性高血糖,这可以引起血管内皮功能障碍并损害冠状动脉微循环,导致心脏缺血。

14. 术中管理中,你对她的血糖控制目标是什么? 为什么?

传统上,术中血糖控制在<12.22～13.89 mmol/L。最近,非常严格的控制建议

为<6.11 mmol/L,但这导致更多的低血糖。我的目标是中度严格为<8.33 mmol/L,这既能最大限度地减少低血糖的概率,也能减少手术部位感染,而不增加术后卒中和死亡的发生率。

## 慢性阻塞性肺病

15. 请解释一下你对她的慢性阻塞性肺病及在家中用氧的情况的理解?

她的慢性阻塞性肺病非常严重,因为家中用氧意味着,她的氧分压在呼吸空气时很可能<55 mmHg。在全身麻醉下她需要更多的氧气,可能在术后需要继续机械通气。她还可能患有慢性低氧血症和高碳酸血症引起的肺血管病和右心功能障碍。

16. 氧气治疗的目的是什么?
1) 治疗缺氧。
2) 降低肺血管阻力。
3) 防止红细胞增多症。

17. 你需要术前让患者做肺功能测试吗? 为什么?
1) 我觉得不需要,除非患者感到她的肺病最近又加重了。如果她的慢性阻塞性肺病不稳定,我会要求做肺功能测试,来监测治疗后她的肺功能是否改善。
2) 如果她的慢性阻塞性肺病病情稳定,肺功能测试只告诉我她患有严重的慢性阻塞性肺病,这个从她的病史和体检,我已经知道了。
3) 肺功能测试可能更适用于预测肺切除后的术后肺功能,但对非胸外科手术意义不大。

18. 外科医师要求做了肺功能测试。她的结果回来是 FEV1/FEV<40%,FVC 1 000 mL,你担心吗?
1) 这些结果证实了我的诊断,她有严重的慢性阻塞性肺病。FEV1/FEV<40%可以说明这点。大多数 FEV1<40%的患者在日常生活活动中会有呼吸困难。这与她在家中使用氧气是一致的。

2）正常 FVC>10 mL/kg。当然,这个值的测定也取决于患者是否用力呼出。该患者的 FVC 为 1 000 mL 是正常的,这与她的诊断一致。慢性阻塞性肺病是阻塞性而非限制性肺病,限制性肺病的 FVC 是降低的。

19. 你能做什么事情来改善她的肺部状况吗?

1）这取决于她的病史和我的体检。如果她有感染的迹象,如很多的脓性痰或甚至发热。我可以给她抗生素治疗,以改善她的肺部感染。

2）如果她有哮喘,我可以给她吸入 $\beta_2$ 激动剂,如沙丁胺醇来缓解支气管痉挛。

20. 麻醉会影响肺功能吗?

所有吸入麻醉剂都有支气管扩张作用,对患者有益。但吸入麻醉剂也抑制缺氧性肺血管收缩(HPV)和增加通气/血流(V/Q)失调。吸入麻醉剂也损害纤毛功能和黏液清除。

21. 硬膜外会影响肺功能吗?

如果硬膜外平面低于 T6 不会。在 T6 以上,可能会损害有效的呼气和咳嗽。

22. 患者问你术后继续使用呼吸机的概率有多大,你怎么回答?（3 - 职业道德；4 - 人际和沟通技巧）

我会解释说,根据她的肺病病史,这非常可能。但这是为了她的安全。

> **Intraoperative management** <

**Monitoring**

1. Would you place an arterial line，why/why not? (1 - patient care；2 - knowledge)

Yes，definitely. A line is for 2 purposes for this patient. First，her cardiac history needs a close monitoring of BP to make sure her heart, brain, and kidneys and other vital organs perfused. Second, I need frequent blood drawn during the surgery to check her blood sugar, CBC, electrolytes etc.

2. What is your goal of intraoperative hemodynamics and how do you achieve it? (1 – patient care; 2 – knowledge)

1) The goal of intraoperative hemodynamics is to maintain adequate perfusion and oxygen delivery to the heart and other organs, and to minimize the oxygen consumption.

2) I will keep patient's BP ±20% of her preoperative level (high enough) to maintain organ perfusion and (not too high) to prevent target organ damage, such as stroke or myocardial ischemia or infarction.

3) Avoid tachycardia to decrease myocardial work and oxygen demand.

3. Would you consider any other monitoring, CVP, PAC, or TEE?

1) If I cannot maintain her hemodynamic stability, I may (ask one of my cardiac colleagues to) do (if the candidate know how to do) TEE to evaluate her cardiac function and volume status.

2) Since I will put A-line in, I can use FlowTrac and pulse pressure variation (PPV) to guide my fluid management.

3) CVP is the least accurate to estimate intravascular volume and wedge pressure may not be accurate in COPD patient. Central line is invasive and not without complications. So, I will not do CVP and PAC.

4. When you were placing the arterial line, the surgeon walked in and commented that this is a minimal invasive surgery, why you make the anesthesia so complicated, your response? ( 3 – Professnism; 4 – Interpersonal and communication skills)

I will say: "understand what you are saying. The surgery is MINIMAL invasive, but anesthesia is always BIG and never minimal, especially for this patient. Please give me some time to line her up". (The candidates may have their own answers depending on their experience)

## Induction of anesthesia

5. What is your choice of induction agent, propofol or etomidate or ketamine, why?

1) It does not matter which medication to use. It does matter how to use the medication.

Personally, I will use propofol if her preoperative BP is normal or on the higher side. The effect of propofol is more predictable. It will lower the patient's BP, but duration is short and I can treat with vasoconstrictor like Neo-Synephrine (Phenylephrine) if her BP is too low after induction.

2) Etomidate and ketamine are good induction agents for hypovolemic and hypotensive patient, but they tend to cause hypertension in normotensive patient, the effect is dose-dependent.

6. How would you achieve a smooth induction?

I will titrate medication to effect and watch her BP closely and treat accordingly.

7. Assuming etomidate, fentanyl, and rocuronium were given, how would you know the patient was ready to be intubated?

1) When patient is in sleep and totally paralyzed, she is ready for intubation.

2) I will check her eyelash reflex to make sure it is disappeared before intubation. I can also use BIS monitor to make sure the BIS number is below 60, in the general anesthesia range. Normally patient's BP drops 20% form baseline when in sleep.

3) I will use twitch monitor to make sure she doesn't have any twitches

before intubation.

8. The blood pressure is 70/43 before intubation, what would you do? Intubate or treat?

I will intubate that will increase the patient's BP by sympathetic stimulation. If the patient's BP is still low after intubation, I will treat with vasopressors.

9. Her blood pressure became 210/135 after intubation, would you treat it, why?

Definitely. I will treat immediately. Diastolic BP > 120 mmHg is a hypertensive crisis by definition. BP like this high, if left untreated, may cause myocardial infarction, heart failure, pulmonary edema, stroke or other organ damage.

10. What are your choice of agents and explain why?

1）I will use 30 mg of propofol first because it works fast and the duration is short.

2）In the meantime, I will make sure she has enough inhalational agent on board.

3）If light anesthesia is not the reason of her hypertension. I will use labetalol or metoprolol because the patient has been on beta blocker and should continue it perioperatively.

4）I can also use nitroglycerin, nicardipine or nitroprusside (nipride) drip if needed.

## Bronchospasm

11. Assuming the resident did the intubation, but there was no $etCO_2$, and no breath sound could be auscultated, what would you do? What might be the

causes?

1）I will see if the patient's $O_2$ saturation is still good. If it is, let's say$>$ 95%, I will do direct laryngoscopy to see if the tube is in the trachea. If it is not, I will take the tube out, ventilate and re-intubate. If it is, I will turn up the inhalational agent and bag ventilate the patient.

2）The possible reasons of "no breath sound and no $etCO_2$" are esophageal intubation and bronchospasm.

12. If this is a severe bronchospasm, what are your steps of treatment?

1）I will deepen the anesthesia with inhalational agent first. All inhalational agents are bronchodilator.

2）I will also give albuterol through endotracheal tube.

3）If these treatments are not working, I will give i.v. epinephrine $0.1\sim$ 0.3 mg and then start a drip at $5\sim10$ mcg/min. I will titrate it up until bronchospasm is relieved.

4）I will also give steroid to prevent recurrence.

## Bradycardia

13. During the placement of trocar, a several episodes of bradycardia HR 40 showed on ECG monitor, treat it or not, and how? Explain the possible cause and mechanism of this bradycardia.

1）It depends on patient's BP. If her BP is stable, I will not treat, but I will inform surgeon and let him stop what he is doing.

2）If hypotension happens with bradycardia or if the bradycardia persists after surgeon stopped putting trocar, I will treat with 0.5 mg of atropine.

3）The possible mechanism is vagal nerve stimulation from peritoneal stretching by the trocar (celiac plexus reflex).

14. After all ports are placed, you noticed her blood pressure increased to

160/95 and heart rate 120, what would be the cause? How would you treat, fentanyl or labetalol, or nitroglycerine? Why are you concerned?

1) BP can increase when $CO_2$ insufflation. Because increased intra-abdominal pressure can compress the aorta and increase in SVR. Compression on SVC will transiently increase in venous return and decrease venous return subsequently. HR should not change too much or maybe decrease due to baroreceptor reflex.

2) This patient's BP and HR both increased, looks like a sympathetic response. So, first I will make sure the patient is getting enough inhalational anesthetic. Second, if the inhalational agent is enough, patient may be responding to pain. I will give fentanyl. If patient's BP is still high after these treatments. I will consider labetalol or nitroglycerin.

3) Hypertension and tachycardia will increase cardiac work and oxygen demand and cause cardiac ischemia or infarct. That's why I am concerned.

## Ventilation

15. How would you ventilate differently in severe COPD and normal lung patient?

1) For normal patient, traditionally we give the tidal volume (TV) $10 \sim 12$ mL/kg based on ideal body weight to prevent atelectasis. Recently, studies have demonstrated that lower TV $6 \sim 8$ mL/kg decreased lung injury and postoperative pulmonary complications in ICU patients and in surgical patients.

2) For COPD patient. I will use higher end of TV, 8 mL/kg ideal body weight and lower rate ($8 \sim 12$ bpm) to minimize the turbulent flow and overcome resistance of constricted airway and give more time for trapped air to come out.

3) I will use I : E ratio 1 : 3 to increase exhalation time as well.

16. What is the difference between volume controlled and pressure

controlled ventilation?

1) In volume controlled ventilation, the ventilator delivers preset TV. Inspiration stops when preset TV is reached. Airway pressure changes with the patient's condition, such as airway resistance and pulmonary compliance.

2) In pressure controlled ventilation, the airway pressure is preset and inspiration stops when preset airway pressure is reached. TV varies with the patient's condition, such as airway resistance and pulmonary compliance.

17. Explain the concept of ventilator induced lung injury (VILI), would this patient be in risk for lung injury?

1) VILI is the diffuse alveolar damage similar to the pathologic changes seen in the acute respiratory distress syndrome (ARDS) caused by large TV (conventional $10 \sim 15$ mL/kg ideal body weight) and/or high inflation pressures (inspiratory plateau pressures $> 30$ cmH$_2$O). It is also called volutrauma and barotrauma, respectively.

2) Because the risk factors for VILI is large TV and high airway pressure. I think COPD patient is at higher risk than other patient because they may have air trapping and over-distended alveoli, which increases the chance of volutrauma. They also have obstruction of small airway which may increase the chance of barotrauma.

18. What is intrinsic PEEP and how to prevent? Would this patient be high risk for intrinsic PEEP?

1) PEEP is the elevated positive end-expiratory pressures (PEEP) when COPD patient has respiratory insufficiency or failure. They are too weak to exhale the air and return to their normal lung volume, called "air trapping" and produce intrinsic PEEP. This patient is definitely at a higher risk for PEEP.

2) PEEP is directly proportional to TV and reversely proportional to expiratory time. So, during mechanical ventilation, I will use slow respiratory

rate and small I : E ratio to make expiration phase longer and prevent PEEP. I will use small TV too.

19. Would you use $N_2O$, why/why not?

No. I will not. Because:

1) This patient may need higher oxygen concentration during the surgery and nitrous will decrease the oxygen flow.

2) This patient may have pulmonary bullae and pulmonary hypertension. Nitrous could make the bullae bigger and even rupture, resulting in pneumothorax. Nitrous also cause pulmonary vasoconstriction.

20. Why do you think this patient may need higher oxygen flow?

1) She has severe COPD and already used home oxygen to correct her hypoxemia.

2) Inhalational agents inhibit hypoxic pulmonary vasoconstriction and produce more intrapulmonary shunt and hypoxemia. Higher oxygen will offset this effect.

21. 30 min into surgery, the $PaCO_2$ was 65 mmHg, will you treat it and how?

I will not do anything as long as her $O_2$ saturation is above 90% ($PaO_2 >$ 60 mmHg) and $pH > 7.2$.

22. What is permissive hypercapnia? What would be the acceptable highest $PaCO_2$ for this patient, why?

1) The goal of conventional ventilator setting tidal volumes at $10 \sim 12$ mL/ kg is to achieve "normal values for acid base status, $PaO_2$, and $PaCO_2$ and to prevent atelectasis".

2) With the "lung protective strategy", the goal is to maintain adequate

oxygenation while accepting an increase in $PaCO_2$ and respiratory acidosis, so called "permissive hypercapnia".

3) There is no cut off $PaCO_2$ number for COPD patient. I will monitor her ABGs to make sure increased $PaCO_2$ does not cause pH$<$7.2. The biological enzymes do not work properly at pH$<$7.2.

## Transfusion

23. 90 min into surgery, due to extensive adhesion from previous hysterectomy and cholecystectomy, there was a significant blood loss, about 700~900 mL, would you go ahead to transfuse?

No. I will see if the patient is hemodynamically stable and send CBC to check her Hgb/HCT. I will not transfuse if the patient is hemodynamically stable.

24. What is your transfusion threshold? Hgb came back 8.3, would give RBC, why/why not?

1) Yes. I will transfuse this patient, especially if I need to use pressors to maintain her BP.

2) There are 2 transfusion strategies: restrictive and liberal. Criterion for restrictive transfusion is Hgb less than $7\sim8$ g/dL and hematocrit values less than 25%. Liberal strategy is to keep Hgb level$>$9~10 g/dL.

3) Although RCTs have not confirmed benefit of restrictive transfusion on mortality, cardiac, neurologic or pulmonary complications, many studies demonstrated that there is no difference in cardiac or surgical complications between restrictive and liberal transfusion, even in patient with preexisting cardiac disease. Considering the complications of blood transfusion, many guidelines recommended restrictive transfusion strategy, i.e., do not transfuse if the patient's Hgb$>7\sim8$ g/dL. Clinical symptoms and signs should also be considered when thinking about transfusion.

4）This patient has extensive cardiac history and surgical bleeding may be ongoing. Plus，some studies suggested patient with underlying cardiovascular disease and the Hb level of less than 10 g/dL had a higher mortality than patients without cardiovascular disease. Although her Hgb is above 8 g/dL，I will transfuse her to help her BP and to optimize oxygen delivery.

（It is ok if the candidate does not transfuse the patient and stick strictly with the guidelines，but should mention to call for blood sent to the room，watch BP and ECG carefully and check another Hgb soon depending surgical bleeding and patient's hemodynamics）

25. Would the transfusion affect the patient's survive?

1）Some studies did suggest that perioperative blood transfusion is associated with worse survival rate. But it is hard to claim a causal relationship.

2）While there is no high quality studies on this topic，meta-analysis of current literature indicated that restrictive strategy appears to decrease blood utilization without increasing morbidity or mortality in oncology patient.

26. How does transfusion affect cancer recurrence?

Same thing with blood transfusion and mortality. Meta-analysis confirms the association between perioperative blood transfusion and the recurrence of curable colorectal cancers.

However，a causal relationship cannot still be claimed due to other confounders.

27. At which point，would you consider to advice the surgeon to convert to open?

If the surgeon has difficulty in stopping bleeding and the patient's BP needs more pressor support. I will ask the surgeon to open.

28. Do you think anesthesiologist also has a role in the patient's surgical management?

Yes, the best medical care should be a team work.

29. If so, how would you talk to the surgeon?

I will tell the surgeon that the patient's BP is dropping even I increased pressor support and gave blood transfusion. Ask him if he consider open or call for help.

## Cardiac ischemia

30. Another 30 min later, heart rate was from 85 to 115, MAP from 80 trending to 65, are you concerned? Would you treat? If so, how would decide for volume vs. vasopressor? What might the cause?

1) Yes, I am very concerned (as a rule on the board exam, always reply "concerned" when asked). Whatever reasons, I will open up the intravenous fluid, start or bump up neosynephrine to bring the BP up. Her tachycardia is the baroreceptor reflex to her hypotension.

2) The most likely reason of sudden drop BP is acute bleeding. Other causes may include compression of SVC by surgeons, vagal stimulation, or drug errors if the circulator or I gave some drugs before the BP dropped.

31. Would you have a preference to treat HR or MAP, which would be the first, why?

1) I think neosynphrine will treat both at the same time. If I have to treat one first, I will treat hypotension first because her tachycardia is most likely the result of baroreceptor reflex to her hypotension.

2) Although the other way around is possible, tachycardia, by decreasing the left ventricular filling, causes hypotension, I do not think tachycardia is the primary reason of hypotension in the situation of bleeding. It is more likely that

hypotension results from loss of intravascular volume.

32. Assumed the patient did not respond to 500 mL crystalloid and neosynephrine infusion at 100 mcg/min, and ECG monitor showed ST elevation in lead V, was the patient having MI? Would you call for TEE or emergent cardiology consult?

1) Yes. ST elevation indicates that the patient may have ST elevation myocardial infarction (STEMI). Lead V suggests the ischemia is in the left ventricle.

2) TEE is a good tool to diagnose if patient has a hypovolemia, cardiac ischemia or heart failure. I will call for it.

3) I may ask for cardiology consult if the patient's condition does not improve after treatment with fluid, vasopressors and coronary dilator.

33. When would you ask the surgeon to stop surgery?

If I have trouble to maintain her BP and her heart rate does not improve after I treated her cardiac ischemia. I will ask the surgeon to wrap up the surgery as soon as possible.

34. Explain what could be done to prevent it? Would you get the blood sample for troponin T?

1) Preoperatively, we should have cardiology consult if we did not.

2) Intraoperatively, we should keep her MAP$>$75 and HR$<$80 to optimize cardiac perfusion and oxygen deliver and minimize oxygen consumption.

3) Although keeping balance of oxygen delivery and consumption may prevent her cardiac ischemia. There is no guaranty for this since every patient is different and needs different MAP to perfuse end organs. Even the patient's medical condition was optimized before the surgery, the cardiac complication can still occur. We need to prepare to treat what happened.

4）Yes. I will get troponin checked. Troponin is not only for diagnosis but also for prediction of recurrence of cardiac events and mortality.

**Emergence**

35. Assuming the patient's hemodynamics were stabilized with neosynephrine and low dose epinephrine infusion，ST elevation resolved，would you consider to extubate in OR，why/why not?

No. I will keep her intubated because of her severe COPD and intraoperative episode of cardiac ischemia. I want her condition stabilized postoperatively before extubation.

36. What are your criteria to extubate for a patient without significant cardiopulmonary disease?

1）Patient is awake and can follow commands.

2）Muscle relaxant is fully reversed.

3）Hemodynamically stable and no significant electrolyte/acid base disturbances.

4）Mechanic criteria include：TV＞5 mL/kg；VC＞10 mL/kg；RR＜25 bpm；negative inspiratory pressure＞25 cmH$_2$O.

> 术 中 管 理 <

## 监护

1. 你会放置动脉导管吗？为什么？（1-患者护理；2-知识）

当然会。为这个患者放置动脉导管有两个目的。首先，她的心脏病史需要密切监测血压，以确保她的心脏、脑、肾脏和其他重要脏器灌注。第二，我需要在手术期间频繁抽血，以检查她的血糖、血常规、电解质等。

2. 你的术中血流动力学目标是什么？你将如何实现你的目标？（1-患者护理；2-知识）

1）术中血流动力学的目标是，维持心脏和其他器官的血流灌注和氧气输送，并尽量降低耗氧量。

2）我将保持患者的血压在术前水平的 ±20%。这样，血压足以维持器官灌注，又不太高以防止靶器官损伤，例如卒中、心肌缺血或梗死。

3）避免心动过速减少心脏做功和氧需求量。

3. 你会考虑其他监测，像中心静脉压、肺动脉导管或经食道心动超声吗？

1）如果我不能维持她的血流动力学稳定，我会（请我的一个心脏麻醉专业的同事）做（如果候选人知道如何做）经食道心动超声，评估她的心脏功能和血管容量状态。

2）因为我已经放了动脉导管，我可以使用 FlowTrac（一种可以监测心脏每搏输出量、外周血管阻力等的仪器，需要和动脉导管连接使用）和脉压变化（PPV）来指导我的液体管理。

3）中心静脉压是估计血管容量最不准确的方法。肺动脉导管测定楔压（Wedge pressure）在慢性阻塞性肺病患者中可能不准确。放置中心导管是有创性的，不是没有并发症。所以，我不会做中心静脉压、肺动脉导管。（如果考试者说做，是因为没有 FlowTrac 和 PPV，或是可以观察变化趋势来参考，也可以。）

4. 当你放置动脉导管时，外科医师走进来，他说这是一个微创手术，为什么你使麻醉这么复杂，你的反应？（3-专业精神；4-人际和沟通技巧）

我会说："我明白你说的。手术是微创性的，但麻醉从来没有微创或简单麻醉特别是对于这个患者来说。请给我一些时间把她需要的各种通路做好。"（考试人可能有自己的答案，取决于他们的经历）

## 麻醉诱导

5. 你会选择哪个诱导剂，丙泊酚、依托咪酯或氯胺酮，为什么？

1）使用哪种药物无关紧要，重要的是如何使用药物。

就我个人而言,如果她的术前血压正常或偏高,我会使用丙泊酚。丙泊酚的作用更可预测。它会降低患者的血压,但持续时间短。如果她的血压在诱导后过低,我可以用血管收缩药,比如去氧肾上腺素来治疗。

2)依托咪酯和氯胺酮是低血容量和低血压患者的良好诱导剂,但它们往往在血压正常的患者中引起高血压。

**6. 你怎样使诱导平稳?**

我会慢慢给药,观察药物作用,同时密切观察她的血压,并做相应处理。

**7. 假设给予依托咪酯、芬太尼和罗库溴铵,如何得知可以给患者气管插管了?**

1)当患者处于睡眠并完全肌松状态时,就可以给她插管了。

2)我会检查她的睫毛反射,以确保它在插管前消失。还可以使用 BIS 监视器,以确保 BIS 数值低于 60,在全麻范围内。通常在睡眠时,患者的血压从基础水平下降 20% 左右。

3)我会使用肌松监测仪,以确保她在插管前没有任何肌颤。

**8. 在插管前血压为 70/43 mmHg,你会做什么?插管还是给升压药?**

我会插管,通过交感神经刺激使患者的血压升高。如果患者的血压在插管后仍然低,我将用血管升压药治疗。

**9. 插管后她的血压变成 210/135 mmHg,你会治疗吗?为什么?**

绝对会,我会立即治疗。舒张压＞120 mmHg 是高血压危象。这样高的血压如果不治疗,可能会导致心肌梗死、心力衰竭、肺水肿、卒中或其他器官损伤。

**10. 你会选择什么药物?为什么?**

1)我将首先使用 30 mg 丙泊酚,因为它起效快,持续时间短。

2)与此同时,我将确保患者有足够的吸入麻醉剂。

3)如果浅麻醉不是其高血压的原因。我将使用拉贝洛尔或美托洛尔,因为患者术前已经使用 β 受体阻滞剂,应该在围术期继续使用。

4)如果需要,我也会使用硝酸甘油、尼卡地平或硝普钠持续静脉滴注。

## 支气管痉挛

11. 假设住院医做了插管,但没有呼气末二氧化碳,也没听到呼吸音,你会怎么做?可能是什么原因?

1)我会先看患者的血氧饱和度是否仍然良好。如果是,比如说>95%,我会做直接喉镜检查,看看导管是否在气管里。如果不是,我会拔出管子,重新插管。如果是,我会加大吸入麻醉剂浓度,并用手控方式给患者通气。

2)"没有呼吸音,也没有呼气末二氧化碳"的可能原因是食管插管和支气管痉挛。

12. 如果这是严重的支气管痉挛,你的治疗步骤是什么?

1)我将首先用吸入麻醉剂加深麻醉,所有的吸入麻醉剂都是支气管扩张剂。

2)我也会通过气管插管给予沙丁胺醇吸入剂。

3)如果这些治疗不见效,我会静注肾上腺素 0.1~0.3 mg,然后以 5~10 μg/min 开始滴注,并逐渐加大剂量,直至支气管痉挛缓解。

4)我也会给予激素以预防复发。

## 心动过缓

13. 在放置套管针时,有几次心动过缓,心电图监视显示心率 40 次/min,治疗或不治疗,如何治疗?请解释这种心动过缓的可能原因和机制。

1)这要取决于患者的血压。如果她的血压平稳,我不会治疗,但我会通知外科医师,让他停止正在做的事情。

2)如果血压伴随心动过缓降低,或者如果外科医师停止放置套管针后心动过缓持续存在,我会给 0.5 mg 阿托品治疗。

3)可能的机制是通过套管针对腹膜的牵拉,造成迷走神经刺激而引起的心动过缓。

14. 所有的套管放好后,你注意到她的血压升高到 160/95 mmHg 和心率

120 次/min,原因是什么? 你如何治疗,芬太尼或拉贝洛尔,或硝酸甘油? 为什么你会担心?

1）当腹腔内充入二氧化碳时,血压可升高。因为增加的腹内压力可压迫主动脉并使得外周血管阻力增加。下腔静脉受压后,有短暂的静脉回流增加,但很快静脉回流会减少。心率不会改变太多或可能由于压力感受器反射而降低。

2）该患者的血压和心率都增加,看起来像交感刺激反应。所以,首先我将确保患者得到足够的吸入麻醉。其次,如果吸入麻醉剂足够,患者可能对疼痛有反应,我会给芬太尼。如果患者的血压在这些治疗后仍然很高。我会考虑拉贝洛尔或硝酸甘油。

3）高血压和心动过速将增加心脏做功和氧需求量,并引起心脏缺血或梗死。这就是为什么我很担心。

## 通气

15. 给重度慢性阻塞性肺疾病和肺部正常患者通气有何不同?

1）对于肺部正常患者,传统上,给予每千克理想体重 10～12 mL 的潮气量,以预防肺不张。最近的研究表明,较低的潮气量,6～8 mL/kg 可以减少 ICU 患者和手术患者肺损伤和术后肺部并发症。

2）对于慢性阻塞性肺疾病的患者,我将使用每千克理想体重 8 mL 的潮气量和较低的呼吸频率 8～12 次/min,以使气道内湍流最小化,并克服气道的阻力。这样能给患者更多的时间把滞留在肺里的气体呼出来。

3）我将使用吸呼比率(I∶E)1∶3 来增加呼气时间。

16. 容量控制和压力控制通气有什么区别?

1）在容量控制通气中,呼吸机提供预设的潮气量。当达到预设潮气量时,吸气停止。气道压力随着患者的状况,如气道阻力和肺顺应性而变化。

2）在压力控制通气中,气道压力是预设的。当达到预设气道压力时,吸气停止。潮气量随患者情况,如气道阻力和肺顺应性而变化。

17. 请解释呼吸机诱导的肺损伤(VILI)的概念,这个患者是否有肺损伤的风险?

1) 呼吸机诱导的肺损伤是和急性呼吸窘迫综合征患者中观察到的病理变化类似的弥漫性肺泡损伤。这是由大潮气量(传统上 10～15 mL/kg 理想体重)和/或高充气压力(吸气平台压力＞30 cmH$_2$O)引起的,分别称为容量损伤和气压损伤。

2) 因为呼吸机诱导的肺损伤的风险因素是大潮气量和高气道压力。我认为慢性阻塞性肺疾病的患者比其他患者有更高的风险,因为他们可能有肺内气体滞留和过度膨胀的肺泡,这增加了容量损伤的机会。他们同时有阻塞的小气道,这可能增加气压损伤的机会。

18. 什么是内源性呼气末呼气正压,如何预防? 这个患者是否有内源性呼气末呼气正压的高风险?

1) 内源性呼气末呼气正压(PEEP)是慢性阻塞性肺疾病的患者,在呼吸功能不全或衰竭时呼气末呼气压升高。患者太虚弱而不能呼出肺里的气体,气体积返回到他们的正常肺容积,这个现象称为"空气滞留",从而产生内源性呼气末正压。这个患者肯定有较高风险。

2) 内源性呼气末呼正压与潮气量成正比,与呼气时间成反比。因此,在机械通气时,我会使用较慢的呼吸频率和小的吸呼比率,使得呼气期更长来防止内源性呼气末呼正压。我也会使用小的潮气量。

19. 你会使用氧化亚氮吗? 为什么?

我不会。因为:

1) 该患者在手术期间可能需要更高的氧浓度,使用氧化亚氮会降低氧流量。

2) 该患者可能患有肺大泡和肺动脉高压。氧化亚氮可能使肺大泡变大,甚至破裂,导致气胸。氧化亚氮还会引起肺血管收缩。

20. 为什么你认为这个患者可能需要更高的氧气流量?

1) 她患有严重的慢性阻塞性肺疾病,并且已经在家使用氧气来纠正其低氧血症。

2）吸入麻醉剂抑制缺氧性肺血管收缩，从而产生更多的肺内分流和低氧血症。较高的氧气将抵消这种效应。

21. 手术进行 30 min 后，二氧化碳分压是 65 mmHg，你会治疗它吗？怎么治疗？

只要她的血氧饱和度高于 90%（血氧分压＞60 mmHg）和 pH＞7.2，我就不会做任何事情。

22. 什么是允许性高碳酸血症？对于这个患者，什么是可接受的最高二氧化碳分压，为什么？

1）以往呼吸机设置潮气量在 10～12 mL/kg，目的是维持"酸碱平衡，血氧分压和二氧化碳分压的正常值，并防止肺不张"。

2）对于"肺保护策略"来说，目标是保持足够的氧合，同时接受二氧化碳分压升高和呼吸性酸中毒，所谓的"允许性高碳酸血症"。

3）对慢性阻塞性肺疾病患者，没有明确的二氧化碳分压最高值的共识。我会监测她的动脉血气分析，以确保增加的二氧化碳分压不会导致 pH＜7.2。因为生物酶在 pH＜7.2 时不能正常工作。

## 输血

23. 手术进行了 90 min 时，由于以前的子宫切除术和胆囊切除术引起的广泛粘连，患者失血 700～900 mL，你会马上输血吗？

不会。我要看患者血流动力学是否稳定，并查血红蛋白水平和血细胞比容。如果患者血压稳定，我不会输血。

24. 你的输血阈值是多少？血红蛋白结果是 83 g/L，你会输红细胞吗？为什么？

1）会的。我会给这个患者输血，特别是如果我需要使用升压药来维持她的血压。

2）有 2 种输血策略：限制性和自由性。限制性输血的标准是血红蛋白＜

80 g/L和血细胞比容<25%。自由性策略是保持血红蛋白>90～100 g/L。

3)虽然随机分组对照研究尚未证实限制性输血对死亡率、心脏、神经系统或肺部并发症的益处,但许多研究表明限制性和自由性输血,在心脏或手术并发症方面没有差异,即使是在有心脏病病史的患者中也是一样。考虑到输血的并发症,许多临床指南推荐限制性输血策略,即如果患者的血红蛋白>70～80 g/L,则不输血。但是考虑输血时,也应考虑临床症状和体征。

4)该患者具有广泛的心脏病史,并且手术出血可能还没有止住。此外,一些研究表明,有心血管疾病的患者,血红蛋白<100 g/L的死亡率高于没有心血管疾病的患者。虽然她的血红蛋白高于80 g/L,我会输血来支持她的血压和优化氧气输送。

(如果考试人严格遵守指南,不予输血。则应提到要血库将血液送到手术室备用,并密切观察血压和心电图,根据手术出血情况和患者的血流动力学复查血红蛋白。)

25. 输血会影响患者的生存吗?

1)一些研究表明,围术期输血与生存率降低相关。但是很难说是因果关系。

2)虽然对这个问题没有高质量的研究,但目前文献的荟萃分析表明,限制性策略似乎降低了用血量,而且不增加肿瘤患者的并发症或死亡率。

26. 输血会影响癌症复发吗?

与输血和死亡率的关系一样,文献的荟萃分析证实了围术期输血与可治愈的大肠癌复发之间的关联。然而,由于其他诸多因素的影响,仍然无法说明两者是因果关系。

27. 在什么时候,你会考虑建议外科医师转换为开放式手术?

如果外科医师难以止血,并且患者的血压需要更多的升压药来维持。我会请外科医师开腹。

28. 你认为麻醉师也在外科医师处理患者中有一定的作用吗?

是的。最好的医疗服务应该是团队合作提供的。

29. 如果是这样,你怎么跟外科医师说?

我会告诉外科医师,患者的血压正在下降,即使我增加了升压药和输了血,也很难维持。问他是否考虑开腹或寻求帮助。

## 心肌缺血

30. 又过了 30 min,心率从 85 次/min 降到 115 次/min,平均动脉压从 80 mmHg 逐渐降到 65 mmHg,你担心吗? 你给予治疗吗? 如果是,你怎样决定是补充液体还是给血管加压药? 血压、心率变化的原因是什么?

1) 是的,我很担心(作为一个考试规则,在问到"你是否担心"时,总是回答"是,我很担心")。无论什么原因,我会先加快补液,同时加用或加大去氧肾上腺素剂量来升高血压。她的心动过速是压力感受器对低血压的反射造成。

2) 血压突然下降,最可能的原因是急性出血。其他原因包括外科医师压迫了下腔静脉,迷走神经刺激反射或给药错误,比如循回护士或我在血压下降之前给了一些药物。

31. 你先处理心率还是平均动脉压? 哪个第一? 为什么?

1) 我认为去氧肾上腺素会同时治疗这两个问题。如果非要选一个先治疗,我将首先治疗低血压,因为她的心动过速最有可能是压力感受器反射造成的,起因是低血压。

2) 虽然,反过来心率过速也可能导致心室充盈减少,而使血压下降,但在刚有出血的情况下,我不认为心率加快是低血压主要原因。血容量减少造成低血压的可能性更大。

32. 假设你给了 500 mL 晶体,同时用了 100 μg/min 的去氧肾上腺素,患者情况没有好转。并且心电图监测仪显示 V 导联中的 ST 升高。患者是否有心肌梗死发生? 你会叫人做经食道超声,或是紧急请心脏科会诊吗?

1) 是的。ST 段抬高表明患者可能有 ST 段抬高性心肌梗死(STEMI)。V 导联表明缺血是在左心室。

2) 经食道超声是诊断患者是否具有血容量不足、心脏缺血或心力衰竭的良好工具。我会叫人来做。

3)如果经过补液、升压和扩张冠状动脉治疗后,患者情况没有好转,我有可能请心脏科会诊。

**33. 你什么时候会要求外科医师停止手术?**

如果我用上述各种办法还不能维持她的血压,并且在治疗她的心肌缺血后,血压、心率仍不改善。我会请外科医师尽快结束手术。

**34. 请解释你可以做些什么来防止心肌缺血? 你会抽血测肌钙蛋白 T 吗?**

1)术前,如果没做的话,我们应该请心脏科会诊。

2)术中,我们应该保持她的平均动脉压>75 mmHg 和心率<80 次/min,以优化心脏灌注和氧气传送,并使耗氧量最小化。

3)尽管保持氧气传送和消耗的平衡可能预防她的心脏缺血,但并不是 100%有效。因为每个患者是不同的,需要不同的压力来灌注末端器官。即使患者的身体状况在手术前被优化,心脏并发症仍然可能发生。我们需要准备好,治疗任何可能发生的并发症。

4)是的。我会检测肌钙蛋白。肌钙蛋白不仅用于诊断,而且用于预测心脏并发症的复发和死亡率。

## 苏醒

**35. 如果经过去氧肾上腺素和低剂量肾上腺素治疗,患者的血流动力学稳定了,ST 段也正常了,你会考虑在手术室拔管吗? 为什么?**

不会。我将保留气管插管。因为她有严重慢性阻塞性肺病,加上术中心脏缺血发作,我希望她的病情稳定后再拔管。

**36. 对于没有心肺疾病的患者,你的拔管标准是什么?**

1)患者清醒,并能完成我要求做的动作。

2)肌松剂拮抗完全。

3)血流动力学稳定,无明显的电解质/酸碱紊乱。

4）机械标准包括：潮气量＞5 mL/kg；肺活量＞10 mL/kg；呼吸频率＜25 次/min；吸气负压＞25 cmH₂O。

> **Postoperative management** <

## Postoperative ventilation

1. Despite trying, your patient was remained intubated and admitted to ICU, how would you set up her mechanical ventilation? Would it be the same for a non-COPD patient, explain?

1) Same as intraoperative. Lung protection strategy with TV, 8 mL/kg ideal body weight and lower rate (8~12 bpm).

2) Since the current trend is to use lung protection strategy for every surgical patient, I would say the difference for this patient is I will use I : E ratio 1 : 3 to increase exhalation time to prevent PEEPi.

2. How often would you like to have ABG sample, why?

It depends on the patient's clinical status and purpose of blood drawn. There is no consensus on how often I need to check ABG. Too often blood drawn is one of the reasons of causing anemia in hospitalized patient.

## Atrial fibrillation

3. 8 hrs. in ICU, the nurse called you for a new onset of irregular heart rate on ECG monitor. Would you be surprised? Her blood pressure was stable despite HR of 125~140, what are you going to do?

1) I am not surprised. With her cardiac history and intraoperative event, arrhythmia can happen any time.

2) I will go and exam the patient, double check her vital signs and mental

status.

3) I will request for cardiology consult if the patient is hemodynamically stable and no symptoms.

4. 30 min later, HR 145 and MAP was less 55, the patient became diaphoretic, what are you going to do? When would you consider a cardioversion?

1) The patient is symptomatic and hemodynamically unstable. I will treat her tachycardia.

2) I assume this irregular heart rate is with narrow QRS complex, most likely is atrial fibrillation (A Fib) with rapid atrial response (RVR). Because the patient does not have history of A Fib, this is a new onset. Cardioversion is the first choice in unstable and symptomatic patient.

3) If the QRS complex is wide, irregular, I need to defibrillate the patient.

5. Would you order blood troponin T? How about brain natriuretic peptide (BNP)? Why/why not?

Yes. The underline reasons of arrhythmia can be multiple. Hypotension, cardiac ischemia, infarct, heart failure. I will order troponin and BNP. Troponin is not only for diagnosis of ischemia, but also for prediction of prognosis. BNP is used to diagnose heart failure. If BNP value $>400$ pg/mL, patient most likely has heart failure.

**Delirium vs. POCD**

6. Two days later, the patient was extubated, vitals were stable. However, her family member came to tell you that she has been changed, does not know where she is, nor does date and time, easily agitated. What is your diagnosis and treatment?

1) The diagnosis is mostly likely postoperative delirium which often happens within 3 days after surgery. It manifested as confusion and disturbance

of awareness and attention.

2）Management include nonpharmacological and pharmacologic. I will find and treat possible underline causes，such as poor pain control，sleep deprivation，pneumonia，urinary tract infection，etc.

3）If there is no other apparent cause，I will try low dose haloperidol (Haldol) or ketamine.

7. The patient was discharged on postoperative day 5，but the family member came to tell you that she became a different person，does not remember grandchildren's names，personality is different too，they were told by the surgeon "anesthesia always affect the brain，young and old"，agree，how would you respond to the family?

1）Another common postoperative complication in elderly patient is postoperative cognition dysfunction（POCD）. Although diagnosis of POCD needs pre- and postoperative formal neuropsychological testing，this usually is not feasible. Because POCD happens 1 week or long after surgery，this patient may have POCD.

2）Some recent studies suggested that anesthesia may have neurotoxicity on developing brain，but there has not been solid evidence to say anesthesia will harm the brain. Some studies also demonstrated protective effect of inhalational agent on human brain. There is no evidence that anesthesia cause the POCD either.

3）I will tell the family：

a）Anesthesia does work on human brain，but there is no evidence in medical research to confirm anesthesia will harm the brain. What the surgeon said probably meant anesthesia works on the brain.

b）The patient may have POCD and most POCD will resolve itself in weeks or months although some may last one year or longer. There is no specific treatment although the antidepressant，selective serotonin reuptake inhibitor

（SSRI） may help sometimes.

c）Age is one of the risk factors for POCD. I won't mention less years of prior education and lower preoperative cognitive test scores are also risk factors unless they ask me.

4）There is no evidence that postoperative delirium is related to POCD. The relationship of POCD and Alzheimer disease is not clear yet.

## ＞ 术 后 管 理 ＜

### 术后通气

1. 尽管你试了,患者仍然不能拔管,并要送入 ICU。你如何设置她的呼吸机? 是否和没有慢性阻塞性肺疾病的患者一样? 请解释一下。

1）对这个患者与术中相同。使用肺保护策略,8 mL/kg 理想体重的潮气量和较低的呼吸频率,8～12 次/min。

2）由于目前的趋势是对每个手术患者都使用肺保护策略,我觉得这个患者和没有慢性阻塞性肺疾病的患者的区别是,我将使用 1∶3 的吸呼比率来增加呼气时间,以防止内源性呼气末正压。

2. 你准备多长时间查一次血气分析? 为什么?

这取决于患者的临床状况和抽血的目的。对于血气分析的频率,没有共识。过频的抽血是引起住院患者贫血的原因之一。

### 房颤

3. 患者住进 ICU 后 8 个小时,护士呼叫你,说心电图监护仪上出现新发作的不规则心率。你会感到惊讶吗? 尽管心率是 125～140 次/min,患者的血压稳定,你打算怎么做?

1）我不感到惊讶。根据她的心脏病史和术中发生的心脏缺血,心律失常可以在任何时间发生。

2）我会去检查患者，复查她的生命体征和神志。

3）如果患者生命体征稳定，没有症状，我会请心脏科会诊。

4.30 min 后，患者心率 145 次/min，平均动脉压小于 55 mmHg，出虚汗，你怎么办？什么时候你会考虑电复律？

1）患者出现症状，并且血压下降，我会积极治疗她的心动过速。

2）假如这种不规则的心动过速是伴有窄的 QRS 复合波，最可能是心房颤动（A Fib）。因为患者没有房颤病史，也就是说是新发作的房颤，电复律是体征不稳定和有症状的患者的首选治疗。

3）如果 QRS 复合波是宽的，不规则，我需要对患者进行除颤。

5. 你会查血肌钙蛋白 T 吗？脑利钠肽（BNP）呢？为什么？

会的。心律失常的原因可以是多种的，低血压、心肌缺血、梗死和心力衰竭等。我会查肌钙蛋白和 BNP。肌钙蛋白不但用于诊断缺血，还能预测预后。BNP 用于诊断心力衰竭。如果 BNP 值 >400 pg/mL，患者可能患有心力衰竭。

## 谵妄与术后认知功能障碍

6.2 天后，患者拔管，生命体征稳定。可是她的家人告诉你，她变了一个人，不知道她在哪里，也不知道日期和时间了，还很容易着急。你的诊断和治疗是什么？

1）诊断很可能是谵妄，常在术后 3 天内发生。表现为糊涂、意识和注意力的异常。

2）治疗包括非药理学和药理学方法。我会先寻找并治疗可能的潜在原因，比如疼痛控制不好、睡眠不足、肺炎和尿道感染等。

3）如果没有明显原因，我将尝试小剂量的氟哌啶醇或氯胺酮。

7. 患者在术后第 5 天出院，但家庭成员回来告诉你，她整个变了一个人，不记得孙子的名字，性格也变了。外科医师告诉他们"不管年幼还是年老，麻醉总是影响大脑"，你同意吗？你会如何回答患者家属？

1）老年患者的另一种常见术后并发症是术后认知功能障碍（POCD）。虽然，术后认知功能障碍的诊断需要术前和术后的正式神经心理测试，但通常人们不这样做。由于术后认知功能障碍发生在手术后 1 周或更长时间，该患者可能患有此症。

2）一些最近的研究表明，麻醉可能对发育中的大脑有神经毒性，但没有确凿的证据证实麻醉会伤害大脑。一些研究还证明了吸入麻醉剂对人类大脑有保护作用。目前，没有证据表明麻醉导致术后认知功能障碍。

3）我会告诉家人：

a）麻醉药是作于人类大脑，但医学研究没有证据证实麻醉会损害大脑。外科医师说的可能是指麻醉作用于大脑。

b）患者可能患有术后认知功能障碍，大多数这样的患者将在数周或数月内自愈，尽管有些人的症状可能持续一年或更长时间。虽然抗抑郁药，选择性 5－羟色胺再摄取抑制剂可能有帮助，但目前对这个没有特异治疗。

c）年龄是术后认知功能障碍的危险因素之一。我不会提及以前受教育少和术前较低的认知水平也是危险因素，除非他们问我。

4）没有证据表明术后谵妄与术后认知功能障碍有关。术后认知功能障碍和阿尔茨海默病的关系尚不清楚。

**Reference**

［1］2014 ACC/AHA Guideline on perioperative cardiovascular evaluation and management of patients undergoing noncardiac aurgery. Circulation. 2014；130(24)：e278－333.

［2］Aldam P. Perioperative management of diabetic patients：new controversies. Br J Anaesth. 2014；113(6)：906－909.

［3］Hines RL and Marschall KE. Anesthesia and co-existing diseases，5th edition 2008；Chapter 9 COPD p168－174；Chapter 16 Diabetes Mellitus p365－378.

［4］Gustafsson UO. Guidelines for perioperative care in elective colonic surgery：Enhanced Recovery After Surgery (ERAS) Society recommendations. Clinical Nutrition. 2012；31：783－800.

［5］Neto AS. Association between use of lung-protective ventilation with lower tidal volumes and clinical outcomes among patients without acute respiratory distress syndrome：A meta-analysis. JAMA. 2012;308(16):1651-1659.

[6] Ferguson ND. Low tidal volumes for all? JAMA. 2012;308(16):1689-1690.

[7] Slinger P. Don't make things worse with your ventilator settings: How you manage the lungs during the perioperative period affects postoperative outcomes. IARS 2013 REVIEW COURSE LECTURES.

[8] Berger M. Postoperative cognitive dysfunction: Minding the gaps in our knowledge of acommon postoperative complication in the elderly. Anesthesiol Clin. 2015; 33 (3): 517-550.

[9] Isik B. Postoperative cognitive dysfunction and Alzheimer disease. Turk J Med Sci. 2015; 45: 1015-1019.

Peishan Zhao

赵培山

# 2 Abdominal surgery-Whipple resection

## 腹部外科手术病例——胰十二指肠切除手术麻醉

·········································> **Basic information** <·········································

64 years old male with progress jaundice for 6 weeks is scheduled for Whipple surgery. His co-morbidity includes CAD (coronary artery disease), previous myocardial infarction 4 years ago, in which he had a 4 - vessel CABG (coronary artery bypass surgery); DM type 2 (diabetes mellitus), COPD (chronic obstructive pulmonary disease). He tolerates normal daily life with walk, shopping, and frequent angina on exertion, relieved by take a rest and/or nitroglycerine.

PE: Wt 89 kg, BP 130/88, HR 83 bpm, RR 16, $SaO_2$ 92% on RA (room air).

Labs: WBC $8.6 \times 10^9$/L, Hgb 11.8 g/L, plt $232 \times 10^9$/L; Na 132 mmol/L, K 3.5 mmol/L, $Cl^-$ 96 mmol/L, $HCO_3^-$ 29, BUN 29, Cr 1.9, Glu 198; HbA1c 7.3; total bilirubin 7.8, direct bilirubin 5.2.

ECG: HR 82, PVCs, ST - T changes, old inferior infarct.

Echocardiography (Echo): LV size is normal, global mild hypoknesia, EF 45%, all valves are normal with some calcifications; normal RV and RA, no pulmonary hypertension.

Medications: metformin, ASA 81 mg, metoprolol, albuterol, Multi Vits, Diovan-HCTZ.

## 基 本 信 息

病史：64 岁男性，进展性黄疸 6 周，预定惠普尔手术（Whipple operation）。其他疾病包括冠心病、4 年以前的心肌梗死和四血管冠状动脉旁路移植术；2 型糖尿病，COPD（慢性阻塞性肺疾病）。能耐受日常生活的步行、购物，但有频繁劳累性心绞痛，通过休息或硝酸甘油缓解。

体检：体重 89 kg，血压 130/88 mmHg，HR 83 次/min，RR 16 次/min，血氧饱和度 92%（空气）。

实验室检查：白细胞 $8.6 \times 10^9$/L，血红蛋白 118 g/L，血小板 $232 \times 10^9$/L；钠 132 mmol/L，钾 3.5 mmol/L，氯 96 mmol/L，$HCO_3^-$ 29 mmol/L，尿素氮 10.32 mmol/L（尿素 5.16 mmol/L），肌酐 79.56 $\mu$mmol/L，谷氨酸 198 U/L；糖化血红蛋白 7.3%；总胆红素 33.38 mmol/L，直接胆红素 88.92 mmol/L。

心电图：心率 82 次/min，多发室早，ST-T 改变，陈旧性下壁心肌梗死。

超声心动图：左心室大小正常，全心轻度收缩无力，EF 45%，各瓣膜正常伴钙化；右室内径和右房内径正常，无肺动脉高压。

目前用药：二甲双胍、阿司匹林 81 mg、美托洛尔、沙丁胺醇、复合维生素和缬沙坦氢氯噻嗪。

## Preoperative management

1. Cardiac：can you interpreter his echo report? Does this patient need further cardiac work up? If so, will you recommend cardiac catheterization? Explain which type study and it may help the intraoperative management? May consider add a-fib（atria fibrillation）as another comorbidity and reassess his perioperative risk.

Keypoint：The keypoint for preoperative evaluation is obvious coronary artery disease and major non-cardiac surgery, how to prepare, including preoperative examination and drugs, et al. Echocardiography shows the cardiac function is mild decreased with the ejection fraction 45% (normal EF 50%~70%).

Recent clinical guidance (Circulation. 2014; 130: 2215 - 2245) discussed about this with lengthy speech, we should briefly illustrate what kind patients need extra cardiac examination and how does the results help.

2. Should you tell the patient to continue or stop his beta blocker, why/why not? Do you have any evidence to support your decision? Explain, how does beta block protective the cardiac? How would you know the patient has been beta blockaded? Will beta blocker protect the brain? How about his ASA, stop or continue?

Keypoint: This is another major issue. You should discuss the recent POISE trials (Lancet, 2008; 371: 183947; N Engl J Med. 2014; 370: 1494 - 1150) and clinical guicance (Circulation. 2014;130: 2215 - 2245).

3. Will you obtain a PFT preoperatively, why/why not? What would be a typical report for a COPD patient? How would his poor PFT affect your anesthesia plan?

Keypoint: This is to evaluate your understanding about pulmonary function. Pulmonary function test (PET) was introduced in the last 50s' to evaluate the risk of postoperative complications. PET includes vital capacity measurement, lung volume, pulmonary carbon monoxide diffusion (DLCO), blood oxygen saturation and arterial blood gas analysis, and all of this has been used to evaluate the postoperative risks of pulmonary resection. Additional measures include radionuclide lung scan, exercise test, invasive pulmonary hemodynamic measurement and risk stratification analysis. In patients with restrictive lung disease, one second forced expiratory volume (FEV1) and forced lung activity (FVC) are both decreased, but the lung volume decreased more than FEV1, resulting in a false FEV1/FVC ratio higher than 80%. As for obstructive pulmonary disease, the FEV1/FVC ratio is less than 0.7.

4. Will you recommend stopping his metformin? Why and why not? Explain the pharmacology of this drug? What is the target of perioperative glycemic control?

Keypoint: Perioperative blood sugar control is common question. Reviewing recent NICE Sugar study (N Engl J Med. 2009; 360: 1283 - 1297) is helpful to answer this question.

5. Could you estimate this patient's preoperative cardiac risk factors?

Keypoint: Come back to cardiac risk factors evaluation, and how do you do in your hospital? Reviewing recent clinical guidance (Circulation, 2014; 130: 2215 - 2245) is helpful to answer this question.

6. Severe jaundice with TB (total bilirubin) 7.8 and DB 5.2, would the elevated bilirubin (jaundice) affect the anesthetic choice? Explain?

Keypoint: Hepatic synthetic function can be measured by albumin, prothrombin time or cholinesterase, and its excretory function can be evaluated by bilirubin level. These changes affect the metabolism and secretion of drugs. These related changes will affect the metabolism and secretion of drugs.

7. The patient has a history of chronic alcoholism, and has been diagnosed with hepatic cirrhosis and portal hypertension, would this could affect your anesthesia?

Keypoint: Perioperative fatality rate is high in end stage hepatic disease patients. The pharmacokinetics and pharmacodynamics of anesthetics are significant changed in hepatic disease. Coagulation disorders, intravascular volume and extrahepatic effects of liver diseases must be resolved before operation. As for major operation in end stage hepatic disease，it is recommended to perform invasive monitoring，pay close attention to hepatic blood flow and renal function in case of encephalopathy and sepsis.

8. What is the patient's risk to DT（Delirium tremens）?

Keypoint：Around half patients with alcoholism may have abstinence symptoms. Among them，3%～5% had delirium tremensor epileptic attack.

9. GI preparation：What is the new guideline, fasting time, bowel preparation?

Keypoint：Minimum fasting time of intakes is as followed：clear liquids 2 h；breast milk 4 h；infant formula 6 h；nonhuman milk 6 h；light meal 6 h；fried foods，fatty foods or meat，8 h.

## > 术 前 管 理 <

1. 心脏：你能解释他的超声心动图报告吗？这个患者需要进一步的心脏检查吗？你推荐心脏导管检查吗？解释哪些类型的研究可能有助于术中管理？考虑如果合并房颤，重新评估围术期风险。

要点：术前评估的关键是要考虑患者的冠心病与大型非心脏手术的风险，如何准备，包括术前检查、药物等。该患者超声心动图报告显示心功能轻度降低，EF45%（正常 EF 50%～70%）。

新近的临床指南（Circulation. 2014；130：2215－2245）有长篇大论，需要用简洁的语言说明哪些患者需要进一步心脏检查，检查结果有何帮助。

2. 你应该告诉患者继续或停止β受体阻滞剂，为什么继续/为什么不？你有什么证据支持你的决定吗？解释一下β受体阻滞剂是如何保护心脏的？你怎么知道患者已经β受体化了？β受体阻滞剂会保护大脑吗？阿司匹林呢？是停下来还是继续？

要点：又是一个重要的大问题，需要提及新近的 POISE trials（Lancet，2008；371：183947；N Engl J Med. 2014；370：1494 - 1500）和新近的临床指南（Circulation. 2014；130：2215 - 2245）。

3. 你会要求术前做 PFT 检查吗，为什么是或不？慢性阻塞性肺病患者的典型 PFT 报告是什么？如果这个患者的 PFT 不好的话，将如何影响你的麻醉计划？

要点：这是检测你对肺功能知识的了解。肺功能测试（PFT）自 20 世纪 50 年代用来评估术后并发症的风险。PFT 包括肺活量测定、肺容积、肺一氧化碳弥散量（DLCO）、血氧饱和度和动脉血气分析，被用于评估肺切除术后风险。额外的评价可包括放射性核素肺扫描、运动试验、侵入性肺血流动力学测量和危险分层分析。限制性肺疾病，一秒钟用力呼气容积（FEV1）和用力肺活量（FVC）减少，但是肺活量下降大于 FEV1，导致在一个 FEV1/FVC 比值高于 80% 的假象。在阻塞性肺疾病，FEV1/FVC 小于 0.7。

4. 你建议停止二甲双胍吗？为什么是或不？解释这个药物的药理学？围术期血糖控制的目标？

要点：围术期血糖控制是常问的问题。复习一下新近的 NICE Sugar study（N Engl J Med. 2009；360：1283 - 1297）将有助回答这个问题。

5. 你将如何估计这个患者的术前的心脏危险因素？

要点：重新回到心脏危险因素的评估，你所在医院是怎么做的？复习一下新近的临床指南（Circulation，2014；130：2215 - 2245）将有助回答这个问题。

6. 严重的黄疸，如总胆红素 133.38 $\mu$mmol/L 和直接胆红素 88.92 $\mu$mmol/L 或胆红素升高（黄疸）会影响麻醉的选择吗？解释？

要点：评价肝脏合成功能可测定白蛋白、凝血酶原时间或胆碱酯酶，而肝排泄功能可由胆红素水平来评价。这些改变会影响药物的代谢和分泌。

7. 患者有慢性酒精中毒史,并已被诊断为肝硬化和门静脉高压症,这会影响你的麻醉吗?

要点:终末期肝病患者围术期病死率高。麻醉药物在肝脏疾病中的药动学和药效学显著改变。凝血障碍、血管内容量和肝脏疾病的肝外影响必须在外科手术之前得到解决。对终末期肝病患者的主要手术,建议进行侵入性监测,并密切关注肝血流量和肾功能,预防脑病及脓毒症。

8. 患者有震颤性谵妄风险?

要点:大约有一半的酒精中毒患者会出现戒断症状。其中,3%~5%发生震颤性谵妄或有癫痫发作。

9. 胃肠道准备:什么是新的指导方针,禁食时间,肠道准备?

要点:不同食物的最短禁食期:透明液体2个小时;母乳4个小时;婴儿配方奶粉6个小时;非人奶6个小时;少量饮食6个小时;油炸食品、脂肪食品或肉8个小时(Anesthesiology. 2017;126:376-393)。

## Intraoperative management

1. Regional anesthesia: will you recommend the epidural? The location of placement, thoracic or lumbar, why? Agent selection, why? Will you use it intraoperatively or solely for postoperative? Is there any evidence support that the epidural would improve the outcome?

Keypoint: Epidural anesthesia is eligible if there is no contraindication. It is available not only for perioprative demand, but also for postoperative analgesia. There is no evidence show epidural anesthesia could improve prognosis.

2. Induction of anesthesia: the choice of agents, does it matter? Would you

have some rescue medication ready, what are they?

Keypoint: Due to significant coronary artery disease, more attention should be paid to hemodynamic stability in choosing induction agents. Routine drugs should be prepared for emergency use.

3. Invasive monitoring: will you place an arterial line, why/why not? How about the central line? If so, which information would help your intraoperative management? Do all patients need invasive monitoring during Whipple surgery?

Keypoint: Whipple resection is major abdominal operation, so it is necessary for invasive monitoring, including invasive blood pressure and central venous catheter. The purposes are not only for monitoring, but also for possible treatment, including transfusion, blood transfusion and drug administration.

4. Fluid management strategy: your goal of fluid management? One and half hour into the surgery, EBL 750, HR 80 to 110, MAP 85 to 65, what would you do, fluid (crystalloid vs. colloid)? Vasopressor, which one and why? Your transfusion threshold?

Keypoint: The goal for fluid management is maintaining hemodynamic stability and protecting cardiac perfusion. The threshold for blood transfusion is 8 g/dL.

5. New ST - T depression appeared in the ECG monitor, is it any concerned? Explain how will you find out the causes and management plan?

Keypoint: New ST - T depression is meaningful if it exceeds 1 mm in V5 - V6 lead or exceeds 1.5 mm in AVF or Ⅲ lead. Usually it is sign for cardiac ischemia and the main cause is coronary insufficiency. The non-ischemic causes include side effect of digoxin, hypokalemia, hypertrophy of left and right ventricles, abnormal ventricular conduction (such as right or left bundle branch block, preexcitation, etc.), hypothermia, tachycardia, and mitral valve prolapse. The treatment for new ST‐T depression should be aimed at etiology. If it is due to cardiac ischemia, the cause, such as hypotension, tachycardia or hypovolemia should be corrected.

6. Preparation for emergence: will you extubated in OR or PACU, should the patient be admitted to ICU or CCU postoperatively? If the ST‐T changes were resolved by given phenylephrine raised MAP, will you insist the cardiologist to see him postoperatively, why/why not?

Keypoint: Extubation could be performed according to patient condition in OR, PACU or ICU. No matter where, you can extubate when patient meets the criteria. As for this patient, cardiac troponin should be monitored due to history of coronary artery disease and perioperative ST‐T change. Cardiologist is necessary for participation or consultation if the ST‐T change is continued or no improvement.

## > 术 中 管 理 <

1. 区域麻醉：你会推荐硬膜外吗？位置是胸还是腰，为什么？如何选择区域麻醉药物，为什么？你是术中用还是仅用于术后？是否有任何证据支持硬膜外会改善预后？

要点：如果无禁忌证，可以行硬膜外麻醉。术中可用，术后止痛也可用。没有证据支持硬膜外会改善预后。

2. 诱导麻醉：药物选择，为什么？你会准备一些急救药物吗，哪些？

要点：患者有严重冠心病，诱导麻醉药物选择应注意血流动力学的稳定。常规准备好急救药物。

3. 有创监测：你是否放置动脉导管，为什么/为什么不？中心静脉导管怎么样？如果是的话，哪些信息将有助于术中管理？惠普尔手术所有患者需要有创性监测吗？

要点：惠普尔手术是大型腹腔手术，一般需要有创性监测，包括有创动脉压和中心静脉导管。目的一是为了监测，二是为了可能的治疗，包括输液、输血和给药。

4. 液体管理策略：你的液体管理目标？1 个半小时后，估计出血 750 mL，HR 由 80 到 110 次/min，由 MAP 85 到 65 mmHg，你会做什么，晶体液还是胶体液？是否用升压药，选哪个，为什么？你的输血阈值？

要点：液体管理目标是血流动力的稳定，注意保护心脏的灌注。输血阈值 8 g/dL。

5. 在心电监护仪出现新的 ST－T 压低，有何意义？你将如何找出原因和你的处理计划？

要点：新的 ST－T 压低，如果是在 V5－V6 导联超过 1 mm 或在 AVF 或Ⅲ导联超过 1.5 mm，则是显著的。它常常是心肌缺血的标志，其中冠状动脉供血不足是一个重要原因。其他非缺血性原因包括：地高辛不良反应、低钾血症、左右心室肥大、心室内传导异常（例如右或左束支传导阻滞、预激等）、低温、心动过速和二尖瓣脱垂。新的 ST－T 压低的治疗应当针对原因，如果是心肌缺血，即应针对心肌缺血的原因，比如低血压、心动过速或低血容量。

6. 苏醒准备：你在 OR 还是 PACU 拔管？术后患者应该送至 ICU 或 CCU（心脏监护室）？如果给予苯肾上腺素提高 MAP 后解决了 ST－T 变化，你是否坚持术后请心脏内科医师会诊？为什么？

要点：在 OR，PACU 或 ICU 拔管，应当根据患者的情况；不论在哪里，符合拔管指标即可拔管。这类有明确冠心病史的患者，术中存在 ST－T 改变，应当监测心肌肌钙蛋白。如果 ST－T 持续变化或无改善，心脏内科医师的参与或会诊是需要的。

---------------- > **Postoperative management** < ----------------

1. At the end of the surgery, you were unable to extubate this patient, he was taken to ICU intubated, and the ICU nurse ask you for ventilator set up. What is difference between Volume Control vs. Pressure Control? Does it matter to support this patient's ventilation? Which mode would be your choice?

Keypoint: You should master the basic knowledge: volume control ventilation (VCV) and pressure control ventilation (PCV) are different ventilation mode, but the different control variables are in mode. The debate on optimal ventilation mode never stops, and the same with control variables. VCV provides pre-set tidal volume and minute volume to ensure safety, and requires the clinician to set inspiratory flow, flow waveform and inspiratory time. During VCV, due to compliance decreases, airway resistance increases or active exhalation, airway pressure increases, so that the risk of ventilator induced lung injury increases. PCV limits the maximum airway pressure to the lung through setting the restriction, but it may lead to changes in tidal volume and minute volume. During PCV, the clinician could adjust inspiratory pressure to get the proper tidal volume, but the inspiratory flow rate and the flow waveform are determined by the ventilator. The beneficial characteristics of VCV and PCV can be combined in dual control mode, including volume targeted, pressure limited and time cycled. When the patients don't have spontaneous ventilation, PCV does not offer any advantage while compared with VCV. In particular, VCV provides deceleration flow, while PCV can provide lower breathing work, which increases patient comfort if the respiratory demand increased and varied.

2. The nurse called 14 hr after admitted in ICU, the patient has a new onset of atrial fibrillation with RVR (rapid ventricle response), HR 135, MAP

85 mmHg, what would be the cause? Will you treat it? What if his MAP is 55 mmHg? When you will cardioverter him?

Keypoint: With the population aging and the increased morbidity of heart failure, the incidence of atrial fibrillation is rising. Initial assessment of new onset atrial fibrillation should include investigation of reversible causes and evaluation of potential cardiac function. The key points of new AF management include reducing the risk of systemic thromboembolism, controlling ventricular rate and rhythm control. If the patient is still symptomatic after the stroke risk and heart rate are under control, the next therapeutic goal is maintaining the sinus rhythm, antiarrhythmic drugs or ablation.

3. Jaundice is worse than preoperative, the surgeon question would it be caused by anesthetic reaction, your response?

Keypoint: Try to answer with the start of postoperatively jaundice differential diagnosis: postoperative jaundice is defined as increased bilirubin after operation. There are many possible causes, which can be divided into prehepatic, intrahepatic and posthepatic causes. The prehepatic cause is due to excessive bilirubin, which can be derived from hemolysis or absorption of hematomas, hemolysis after transfusion or erythrocyte destruction after cardiopulmonary bypass. The intrahepatic cause is damage to hepatocytes or bile duct epithelial cells, including total parenteral nutrition, hypoxia, ischemia, drugs, newly acquired viral hepatitis and septicemia. Patients with liver diseases may be more prone to jaundice and more serious. Extrahepatic biliary obstruction, including residual stones, stenosis and direct damage by abdominal surgery, may cause postoperative jaundice.

Halogenated inhalation anesthetics, including halothane, enflurane, isoflurane and desflurane, can cause metabolic hepatocyte damage. During the metabolism of these anesthetics, acetylated proteins may form new antigens and trigger antibody mediated immune responses. The possibility of postoperative immune hepatitis depends on the metabolic amount of anesthetics, and it is rare in enflurane, isoflurane and desflurane, while compared with halothane. Sevoflurane is unlikely to cause immune hepatitis, becauseit doesn't metabolize to trifluoroacetyl compounds.

4. Ulnar nerve injury: on postoperative day 4 at the surgical floor, the patient complains of left 5th finger numbness, how would you start the work up? The surgeon told the patient, this was caused by anesthesia, how would you differentiate a preexisting and a newly occurred nerve injury? If it indeed is new, should the anesthesiologist be legally responsible?

Keypoint: The causative factors of ulnar nerve injury include male, BMI >38 and prolonged bed rest after operation. In addition, many patients have contralateral nerve dysfunction after postoperative ulnar neuropathy, suggesting they may be prone to nerve injury. Interestingly, studies have shown that there is no ulnar nerve injury in the first two days after operation. For the general nerve injury, if it is sensory, the patient is certain to improve in 5 days usually; if motor function is abnormal, immediate neurological consultation is necessary.

## > 术 后 管 理 <

1. 在手术结束时，患者不能拔管。带管送至 ICU 后，ICU 护士问你如何设置呼吸机？容量控制和压力控制有什么区别？对该患者的通气有什么影响？你会选择哪种模式？

要点：必须知道基本知识：容量控制通气（VCV）和压力控制通气（PCV）是不同的通气模式，但不同的控制变量反映在模式。最佳通气模式的争论仍在继续，最优控制变量的辩论亦然。VCV 提供了一个预先设定的潮气量和每分钟通气量以保证安全性，需要临床医师正确的设置吸气流量、流量波形和吸气时间。VCV 应用中，当顺应性降低、气道阻力增加或主动呼气时，气道的压力会增加，因而可能增加呼吸机所致肺损伤的风险。PCV,则是通过设置限制传递到肺的最大气道压力,但可能导致潮气量和每分钟通气量的改变。在 PCV,临床医师应调节吸气压力达至合适的潮气量,但吸气流速和流量波形是由呼吸机确定的。VCV 和 PCV 的有益特性可以组合在所谓的双重控制模式,亦即容量定标(volume targeted)、压力限制(pressure limited)和时间循环(time cycled)。在患者没有自主呼吸时,PCV 与 VCV 相比并不提供任何优势。尤其是 VCV 提供减速流,PCV 可以提供较低的呼吸功,对呼吸需求提高和可变的患者,可增加患者的舒适度。

2. 在 ICU14 个小时后,护士报告患者有新发的心房颤动伴有快速心室率,HR 135 次/min,MAP 85 mmHg,你考虑什么原因? 如何处理? 如果他的 MAP 是 55 mmHg呢,如何处理? 何时考虑电复律?

要点:随着人口老龄化和心力衰竭的患病率增加,房颤发病率呈上升趋势。新发房颤患者的初始评估应包括可逆性原因的调查和对患者潜在心功能的评估。新发房颤处理的关键点包括降低全身血栓栓塞的风险,控制心室率和节律控制。对卒中风险和心跳速率得到控制后仍有症状的患者,维持窦性节律与抗心律失常药物或消融是下一步的治疗目标。

3. 黄疸比术前加重,外科医师问是否与麻醉作用有关,你的回答?

要点:回答从术后黄疸鉴别诊断开始。术后黄疸定义为术后出现胆红素升高,有许多可能的原因,可分为几类:肝前、肝内和肝后。肝前性的原因是由于过量的胆红素,可来自血肿溶血或吸收,输血反应的溶血或体外循环术后红细胞破坏。肝内原因包括肝细胞或胆管上皮细胞损伤,包括全肠外营养、缺氧、缺血、药物、新近获得的病毒性肝炎和败血症。有肝脏疾病的患者可能更容易出现这些情况,并更加严重。肝外胆道梗阻,包括残留结石、狭窄和腹部手术直接损伤,可能导致术后黄疸。

卤代吸入麻醉药氟烷、恩氟烷、异氟醚和地氟醚可产生代谢性肝细胞损伤。这些麻醉剂的代谢过程中,乙酰化修饰的蛋白质可能构成新抗原,并有可能触发抗体介导的免疫应答。术后免疫性肝炎的可能性取决于麻醉的代谢量,与氟烷相比,安氟醚、异氟醚和地氟醚引起术后免疫性肝炎很少见。七氟醚不大可能引起免疫性肝炎，因为代谢不产生三氟乙酰基化合物。

4.尺神经损伤：术后第 4 天在外科病房里，患者诉左手第五指麻木，你如何处理？外科医师告诉患者这是麻醉的原因。你如何区分术前存在的和新近发生的神经损伤？如果这确实是新发的，麻醉师应当负责吗？

要点：尺神经病变的诱发因素包括：男性、BMI>38 和术后卧床休息过长等。此外，许多患者出现术后尺神经病变，伴有对侧的神经功能障碍，提示这些患者可能易有神经损伤。有趣的是，有研究表明，术后前 2 天没有尺神经损伤的发生。对于一般的神经损伤，如果是感觉性的，患者在 5 天内几乎可以肯定会好转；如果运动功能异常，需要立即进行神经科会诊。

Jianzhong Sun

孙健中

# 3 Anesthesia management for total thyroidectomy

## 普外科手术病例——甲状腺手术麻醉

> **Basic information** <

A 35 years old female with Graves' disease for 3 years, she has been having difficult with medical management in control of her symptoms, but did not want to have the radiation treatment. She has been scheduled for a total thyroidectomy and the surgeon requests the anesthesia to do the preoperative preparation to get her ready for the surgery.

She complains easily agitated, anxious, and sweating, weight loss. She got tired easily with light activity. Lost 10 kg in last year. Noticed some voice change in last month or so but could not be any specific.

PE: BP 112/74, HR 110, RR 18, SpO$_2$ 99% RA; weight 68 kg.

Medications: methimazole 10 mg bid, propranolol 30 mg bid, VITs.

Lab: WBC 12.5, Hgb 11.2, Plat 150; TSH 0.23, free T3 201 and T4 2.8 were in normal range.

ECG: sinus tachycardia 108, non-specific ST–T changes.

## > 基 本 信 息 <

一位 35 岁的女性患弥漫性甲状腺肿 3 年,药物治疗很难控制她的临床症状,但她却不想接受放射治疗。她将接受择期全甲状腺切除术,外科医师要求麻醉医师做术前准备,以达到手术的安全。

主诉有容易烦躁、焦虑、出汗及体重减轻,轻微活动后就容易疲倦,去年体重轻了 10 kg。大约在上个月发现发音有些变化,但不知道具体原因。

体检:BP 112/74 mmHg,HR 110 次/min,RR 18 次/min,$SpO_2$ 99%(空气);体重 68 kg。

药物治疗:甲巯咪唑 10 mg,每天 2 次;普萘洛尔 30 mg,每天 2 次;维生素。

实验室检查:WBC $12.5\times 10^9$/L,Hgb 112 g/L,血小板 $150\times 10^9$/L;促甲状腺激素(TSH)0.23、游离 T3 201 和 T4 2.8,均在正常范围。

心电图:窦性心动过速 108 次/min,非特异性 ST - T 改变。

## > Preoperative management <

1. Grave disease:What is Grave disease, what is the etiology?

The surgeon asks you do the preparation for surgery, agree or refuse, why/why not? When would you consider the patient is ready for surgery? Specific on lab tests and clinical presentations?

Keypoint:this is an open question to test the knowledge of Graves disease and the implications for anesthesia management; specific knowledge of readiness for surgery during preoperative assessment; familiar with lab test and known the limitations.

2. Cardiac assessment:Would you get additional cardiac exam, such as echocardiograph, why/why not? Is it common that Grave disease could cause

cardiac problem?

Keypoint: it is not uncommon that either Graves disease presented with dysrhythmia or congestive heart failure, till further work up found out the underline cause of hyperthyroidism; this is more common in female and geriatric population; long term cardiac dysfunction deserves a thorough cardiac work up.

3. Preparation for hyperthyroidism: When would you consider the patient was in eudthyroid condition, normal free T3 (75~200 ng/dL) and T4 (0.8~2.8 ng/dL), TSH (0.5~6 UU/mL)? The surgeon tells that there is a gap between the normal lab values vs the clinical symptoms, the latter is more important, how do you respond? If so how do you explain her persistent tachycardia?

Keypoint: this is specifically test for knowledge of lab test, and to test whether the candidate truly understanding the results and their relation to clinical presentation.

4. Additional test: Do you have a concern of her recent voice changes? ENT consult? CT scan of her neck? If the patient was found to have one side vocal cord paralysis and the tracheal deviation towards to the left, how it would affect your anesthesia plan?

Keypoint: this is specifically related to anesthesia clinical practice, all thyroid surgery patients should be carefully assessed for his or her airway anatomy, so that a specific plan could be formed accordingly, remember this is an elective surgery!

5. Ophthalmopathy: The patient asked you in the PAC (preoperative anesthesia clinic), would the surgery cure or stop her eyes protrusion and improve visual problem?

Keypoint: this is a question for the knowledge beyond routine anesthesia practice but closely related, be able to answer the question certainly will put the anesthesia provider in a higher position; on the other hand, if frequently having the conversation with the surgeon, the question should not be difficult to answer.

6. Time for hormone replacement: the patient wants to know when the replacement therapy should be started, in OR or after the surgery? Any side effect (associated symptoms and signs) should she know and pay attention to, your response?

Keypoint: this is another seems non-anesthesia directly related question, but very practical about the patient after the surgery.

## > 术 前 管 理 <

1. 弥漫性甲状腺肿：什么是弥漫性甲状腺肿，其病因是什么？

外科医师要求你做手术准备，同意还是拒绝，为什么？ 你认为患者什么时候可以做手术？ 具体的实验室检查和临床表现是什么？

要点：这是一个开放性的问题，测试弥漫性甲状腺肿及其麻醉管理的相关知识；术前评估确定可以手术的具体知识；熟悉实验室检查并了解这些结果的局限性。

2. 心脏评估：你会做一些额外的心脏检查，如超声心动图吗，为什么？ 弥漫性甲状腺肿会造成心脏的问题吗？

要点：弥漫性甲状腺肿并发心律失常或充血性心力衰竭并不少见，有些患者先以心脏疾病的表现为主，直到进一步检查发现是甲状腺功能亢进而造成的。合并心脏问题更常见于女性和老年人群；长期的慢性心功能不全需要全面的心脏检查。

3. 甲亢的术前准备：什么样的情况下你认为甲状腺亢进的患者甲状腺功能是正常了？游离的 T3(75~200 ng/dL) 和 T4(0.8~2.8 ng/dL)，TSH(0.5~6 UU/mL) 达到正常值吗？外科医师认为，实验室正常值与临床症状之间有差距，后者更重要，你如何应答？如果是这样，你怎么解释她的持续性心动过速？

要点：这是专门测试实验室检查的相关知识，测试考生是否真正了解结果及其与临床表现的关系。

4. 其他检查：你是否担忧她最近的声音变化？需要五官科会诊吗？是否需要颈部的 CT 扫描？如果发现患者一侧声带麻痹，气管偏向左侧，它会如何影响你的麻醉计划？

要点：这是专门针对麻醉临床实施的问题，所有甲状腺手术患者均应仔细评估其气道解剖，这样才能形成一个相应的针对性的呼吸道管理的方案，记住这是一个择期手术。

5. 甲状腺眼病：患者在麻醉术前门诊问你，手术是否可以治愈或阻止她的眼睛前突并改善视力的问题？

要点：这个问题超出了临床麻醉的常规知识然而又密切相关，能够确切的回答问题可以使麻醉实施者提升到更高的水平。另一方面，如果经常与外科医师对话，这一问题应该不难回答。

6. 激素替代的时机：患者想知道什么时候应该开始甲状腺素替代治疗，是在手术室内或手术后？有没有她应该知道并注意的不良反应(相关的症状和体征)，你如何回答？

要点：这是另一个看似与麻醉非直接相关的问题，但对患者术后非常实用。

## > **Intraoperative management** <

1. Airway management：explain your plan for the airway management.

What if the CT shows a 3.5 cm tracheal left deviation? Let say you start with Glidescope and are not able to see the epiglottis and the cords, what would be your next step? Assume you would perform an awake fiberoptic intubation, describe your technique of airway nerve blocks, how do you test the block are adequate?

Keypoint: after the careful and thorough preoperative assessment, the candidate should be able to forma plan for the airway management, including plan A and B, even C. The candidate should be able to describe the steps for a complicated airway management.

2. Monitoring: will you place an arterial line, before or after induction? Explain why the arterial line would be superior to a cuff to monitor her blood pressure during surgery? The surgeon requests to place a NIM–ETT (with EMG electrodes), was it a reasonable request? How do you place it correctly? How it would help to prevent the injury to laryngeal nerve? Would it affect your anesthesia management, if so, how?

Keypoint: knows when to apply an invasive monitor, and the advantage and disadvantage of having an arterial line; knows the specific application for EMG-coupled ETT, and the special needed anesthetic technique (remifentanil infusion).

3. Threatening of thyroid storm: 90 min into the surgery, you noticed the HR 105 to 135, BP 110/65 to 145/93, concerned, why/why not? Your thought process for differentiate diagnosis, light anesthesia, thyroid storm, or malignant hyperthermia? And your management options. Assume this is a thyroid storm, what would you do? Would you ask the surgeon stop the surgery? Would a stat lab test for serum T3 level help the diagnosis? What would be your priority in controlling the storm? Supportive and symptoms control, then consider anti-hyperthyroidism, such as ventilation, hydration, cooling,

propranolol, treat dysthymia, steroid, iv PTU and/or iv iodine component (contrast or logol solution by NG prevent peripheral T4 to T3), and antibody be help?

Keypoint: several issues to test the candidate's clinical competency, 1) the ability to recognize and foresee such a crisis associated with this type surgery; 2) the ability to be able to differentiate the probable causes; 3) fast responses and actions; 4) be able to prioritize a resuscitation plan, etc.

Five "Bs": **B**lock synthesis (i.e. antithyroid drugs); **B**lock release (i.e. iodine); **B**lock T4 into T3 conversion (i.e. high-dose propylthiouracil[PTU], propranolol, corticosteroid and, rarely, amiodarone); **B**eta-blocker; and **B**lock enterohepatic circulation (i.e. cholestyramine), it has been report that the total thyroidectomy would be the last solution to control the storm).

4. Post sternal mass: Assume there was not even of the storm, but the enlarged thyroid gland extended behind the sternal, 3.5 hrs. into the surgery, the surgeon is still struggling to direct it free, could you do anything to help him? Another 30 min past, no progress rather there is another 500 mL blood lose. Would you advise him to call a CT surgeon? The surgeon told you that he suspected an injury to the left subclavian artery, what would you do at this point? And the total EBL (estimated blood lose) is about 1,800 mL.

Keypoint: the is a practical question directly related to the surgery, again a good sense of surgical complication, be able to prepare in advance, good communication skill with surgeon.

5. Coagulation disorder and transfusion: Now you noticed there is a significant oozing on the surgical field? What type test would help you to find out the cause of coagulopathy? What would be your transfusion threshold?

Keypoint: be able to recognize this acquired coagulation disorder and the properly and correct lab test; have a clear goal and threshold of transfusion.

6. Emergence and extubation：Finally the thyroid is totally removed and the surgeon started to close，explain your preparation for the emergence? Would you extubate the patient in the OR，why/why not? What is tracheal malacia，could it happen in this patient? How would you know in advance?

Keypoint：the standards for extubation，alteration when surgery is around the airway，be able to recognize the potential specific airway complications，and to have a backup plan.

> 术 中 管 理 <

1. 气道管理：说出你的气道管理计划。如果 CT 显示气管左偏 3.5 cm 呢？你一开始用可视喉镜（Glidescope），但看不到会厌和声带，那么你下一步怎么办？假设你将进行清醒纤维支气管镜插管，描述你的气道的神经阻滞技术，你如何测试阻滞是否完善？

要点：经过仔细彻底的术前气道评估，考生应该能够制订气道管理计划，包括计划 A 和 B，甚至 C。考生应该能够描述管理复杂气道的步骤。

2. 监测：你会放置有创动脉导管吗，是在诱导之前还是之后？解释为什么在术中行有创动脉优于袖带监测血压？外科医师要求放置 NIM‑ETT（带 EMG 电极的气管导管），这个要求合理吗？你如何正确放置？它如何有助于预防喉神经损伤？它会影响你的麻醉管理吗，如果会，是怎样影响的？

要点：知道何时使用有创监测，有创动脉的优缺点，知道 EMG 复合 ETT 及所需特殊麻醉技术（输注瑞芬太尼而不能用肌松药）的具体应用。

3. 甲状腺危象的威胁：手术开始 90 min 后，你注意到心 HR 从 105 到 135 次/min，BP 从 110/65 变为 145/93 mmHg，你担心吗，为什么？你如何进行鉴别诊断？是浅麻醉、甲状腺危象，还是恶性高热？你如何处理？假设这是甲状腺危象，你会怎么做？你会让外科医师停止手术吗？急查血清 T3 水平是否有助于诊断？什么是你控制危象的首选？支持治疗并控制症状，然后再考虑抗甲状腺功能亢进症，如机械通气、补液、降温、普萘洛尔、治疗心律失常、类固醇、静脉推注 PTU 和/或碘剂(经胃管给造影剂或卢氏液防止外周 T4 向 T3 转换)，抗甲状腺素球蛋白？

要点：测试考生的临床能力的几个方面：① 能够识别和预见到这种类型手术相关的危机的能力；② 能够区分可能的原因和鉴别诊断；③ 快速反应和处理的能力；④ 能否制订一个优先顺序复苏计划。

五"Bs"：阻止合成(即抗甲状腺药物)；阻断释放(即碘)；阻断 T4 向 T3 转化〔即大剂量丙硫氧嘧啶(PTU)，普萘洛尔，皮质类固醇，少见使用胺碘酮〕；β 受体阻滞剂；阻断肠肝循环(即考来烯胺)。已有报道，甲状腺全切除术是控制危象的最后手段。

4. 胸骨后肿块：假设没有甲状腺危象，但甲状腺肿大扩展至胸骨后。手术 3.5 个小时后，外科医师仍在努力完全切除，你能做些什么来帮助他吗？又过了 30 min，手术没有进展而患者又失血 500 mL。你会建议他请给心胸外科医师会诊吗？外科医师告诉你，他怀疑伤到左锁骨下动脉，对于这点你会做什么？总的估计失血量已经约 1 800 mL。

要点：这是一个直接关系到手术的实际问题，对于手术并发症敏锐的意识，能提前准备，并具备与外科医师良好的沟通技巧。

5. 凝血功能障碍和输血：现在你注意到在手术区域有一个明显的渗血，哪种检查会帮助你发现凝血功能障碍的原因？你的输血阈值是多少？

要点：能够识别这种获得性凝血障碍及恰当和正确的实验室检查；明确输血目标和阈值。

6. 麻醉苏醒和拔管：最后甲状腺完全切除了，外科医师开始关创面，解释你麻醉苏醒的准备？你会在手术室拔管吗，为什么/为什么不？什么是气管软化，在这个患者可能会发生吗？你怎么能事先知道？

关键点：拔管的标准，当手术部位于气道周围时的改变，能够识别可能的气道并发症，并有后备的计划。

---------------------------- > **Postoperative management** < ----------------------------

1. Hypocalcemia and laryngeal spasm: The patient was doing well and extubated in OR and transferred to PACU, 3 hrs later, you are called by the nurse to help the airway, the patient was in severe respiratory distress, a significant neck and chest muscle retraction are noticed, stridor could be easily heard, $SpO_2$ 84% to FS (facial shield $O_2$ 100%), what would be the likely cause? Any lab test might help? Your management options? Could this be prevented? Would a bilateral recurrent laryngeal nerves'（RLN）injury cause the same airway problem?

Keypoint: be able to recognize the severe laryngospasm, likely caused by accident remove of parathyroid glands during the surgery, a quick confirmation by serum calcium level, so as administered calcium intravenously, be able to handle emergency airway. In addition, be able to differentiate with the vocal cord injury associated with clinical presentations which mostly is resulted from RLN injury.

2. Neck hematoma: The patient was doing well and discharged to the floor, on postoperative day 3, her husband rushed to the nurse station for help, the patient had a sudden onset of severe difficult breathing and phonating, after talked to the surgeon, an emergency neck exploration has been posted. Explain your plan for anesthesia, induction and intubation? What if this was happening in anesthesia holding（preparation）room and you saw the patient was being cyanotic, what would do?

Keypoint: to test the candidate's sense and able to recognize this type airway emergency, the ability to communicate, and quick forming management plan; also a specific plan indeed a need to carry out a general anesthesia with endotracheal intubation.

3. Superior laryngeal nerve injury: The patient is a member of local church and actively involved in the choir. However, three months after she was still not able to sing, the examination revealed the left side vocal cord paralysis. She is very upset and sued the surgeon and hospital. Which nerve was mostly likely damaged? The surgeon told the hospital administrators "this was a team work, you, the anesthesiologist should bear some liability too", do you agree and how to defend?

Keypoint: know the anatomy and symptom associated with specific nerve injury; professionalism, always be able to defend your action, last good communication skills.

## > 术 后 管 理 <

1. 低钙血症和喉痉挛：患者手术做得很好，在手术室拔管后转入PACU，3个小时后，护士呼叫你来帮助处理患者的呼吸困难。这个患者发生了严重的呼吸窘迫，可以看到颈部和胸部肌肉收缩明显，听到明显的喘鸣音，FS(面罩吸100%氧气)时血氧饱和度84%，可能的原因是什么？哪种实验室检查可能会有所帮助？你的处理方法是什么？可以预防吗？假如这是双侧喉返神经损伤(RLN)的话，会造成相同的呼吸道问题吗？

关键点：能够认识到严重喉痉挛，可能是由于手术中意外切除甲状旁腺，快速确定血清钙水平，并静脉注射给予钙，能够处理急救气道。此外，能够与喉返神经损伤造成声带损伤的相关临床表现鉴别诊断。

2. 颈部血肿：患者手术顺利送回病房。术后第3天，她丈夫奔到护士站寻求帮助，患者突然出现严重呼吸和发声困难，与外科医师交流后，要行急诊颈部探查术。解释你的麻醉、诱导和插管计划？如果这种情况是发生在麻醉准备室，你这时看到患者发生青紫，你会怎么做？

要点：测试考生识别这类紧急气道的意识和能力，沟通及快速制订治疗计划的能力；还有需要进行气管插管全身麻醉时的具体计划。

3. 喉上神经损伤：患者是当地教会的一名成员，并积极参与唱诗班的表演。然而，术后3个月后她仍然不能够唱歌，检查时发现左侧声带麻痹。她很不高兴，起诉外科医师和医院。最有可能损伤了哪些神经？外科医师告诉医院管理者："这是一个手术团队工作，麻醉师也应该承担一定的责任"，你同意吗，并如何辩护？

要点：了解与特定神经损伤有关的解剖和症状；专业能力永远能够保护你的行为；最后是良好的沟通能力。

**Acknowledgement**

Dr. Huimin Huang, MD，PhD from Shanghai 9th People's Hospital translated the text to Chinese.

感谢上海交通大学附属第九人民医院黄慧敏医师的翻译。

Chuanyao Tong

童传耀

# 4 Ambulatory endoscopic surgery-ureteroscopic stone manipulation

## 日间内窥镜手术病例——输尿管镜碎石术

-------------------> **Basic information** <-------------------

A 55 years old female known for recurrent kidney stone with left flank pain, and nausea and vomiting for 3 days. She is scheduled for a transurethral laser stone lithotripsy in outpatient surgery center.

Other medical issues: DM2 (diabetes millets type 2), HTN (hypertension), CAD (coronary artery disease) and MI (past myocardial infarction), DES (drug eluting stent) ×3 3 years ago, COPD (chronic obstructive pulmonary disease), fibromyalgia, GERD (gastroesophageal reflex disorder), peripheral neuropathy in both low extremities.

Medications: metoprolol 50 mg bid, Cardizem 120 mg qd, lassie 40 mg qd, ASA 81 mg, Plavix 75 mg qd, metformin 500 mg bid, gabapentin 300 mg bid, Motrin 800 mg bid, Lisinopril 20 mg qd, albuterol prn, protonix, Nexium.

PE: BP 145 – 126/91 – 82, HR 88, RR 22, $SaO_2$ 92% RA, Weight 110 kg (BMI 41).

Lab: WBC 7.5, Hgb 10.5, Plat 120 k; Na 132, K 4.9, Cl 96, $HCO_3$ 28, BUN 27, Cr 1.9, Glucose 165. Hb1Ac 7.2.

ECG: atrial fibrillation, ventricular rate 108, nonspecific ST – T changes.

## 基 本 信 息

55 岁女性,肾结石复发伴左侧肋腹痛、恶心呕吐 3 天。拟于门诊手术中心行经尿道激光碎石术。

既往病史:2 型糖尿病、高血压、冠心病和陈旧性心肌梗死,3 年前放置 3 根冠脉药物洗脱支架,以及慢性阻塞性肺疾病、纤维肌痛、胃食管反流病和双侧下肢周围神经病变。

药物史:美托洛尔 50 mg,每天 2 次;地尔硫䓬 120 mg,每天 1 次;呋塞米 40 mg,每天 1 次;阿司匹林 81 mg,每天 1 次;波立维 75 mg,每天 1 次;二甲双胍 500 mg,每天 2 次;加巴喷丁 300 mg,每天 2 次;布洛芬 800 mg,每天 2 次;赖诺普利 20 mg,每天 1 次;沙丁胺醇按需使用;以及泮托拉唑和埃索美拉唑。

查体:血压 126~145/82~91 mmHg,心率 88 次/min,呼吸频率 22 次/min,吸空气时氧饱和度 92%,体重 110 kg(体重指数 41)。

实验室检查:白细胞 $7.5 \times 10^9$/L,血红蛋白 105 g/L,血小板 $120 \times 10^9$/L,钠 132 mmol/L,钾 4.9 mmol/L,氯 96 mmol/L,$HCO_3^-$ 28 mmol/L,尿素氮 9.61 mmol/L(尿素 4.81 mmol/L),血肌酐 167.96 $\mu$mmol/L,血糖 9.17 mmol/L,糖化血红蛋白 7.2%。

心电图:房颤,心室率 108 次/min,非特异性 ST - T 改变。

## Preoperative management

1. Is this patient ready for surgery?

This is an opportunity to evaluate patient, start with medical history and physical exam, and clearly address your concerns.

Suggested answer: I would first take a more detailed history and evaluate her medical conditions. In particular, I would like to ask the questions such as how does her physical activity changes recently, does her $SaO_2$ in room air always stay around 92%, etc. I will start the case, assuming she does not have any worsening symptoms recently.

2. Any additional tests needed, if so, what are they? How would the new information help your anesthesia planning?

Order tests for this patient only for acute exacerbation of symptom. In other word, you don't need new test if your management does not change.

Suggest answer: patient has a severe COPD, room air saturation is 92%, a quick room air arterial blood gas analysis would be very reasonable to assess the severity. The result may lead to optimize with supplemental $O_2$, and may using regional anesthesia to avoid intruding lungs, modify ventilation setting if general anesthesia is needed.

Keypoint: This is open question. You should assume the patient better (healthier) condition first.

3. What is her CHADS score (C-congestive heart failure, H-hypertension, A-age, D-diabetes mellitus, S-previous stroke)?

Specific knowledge question, state your understanding. You may politely ask examiner to restate this question if you does not understand the meaning of CHADS.

Suggested answers: CHADS score describe a new risk stratification schema (using point system) to assess perioperative stroke risk in patient with atrial fibrillation.

Keypoint: Review the content of CHADS.

4. The implication of her perioperative risk for stroke? And her risk for heart and lung?

It is time for you review this patient again, it is specifically for assessing the risk factors.

Suggested answers: This specific risk for CHADS is high in this patient. It is due to her pre-existed medical condition such as HTN, DM as well as the history of atrial fibrillation.

5. What is the highest risk factor for CHADS?

This is more specific question; you need to give very honest answer.

Suggested answer: The highest risk factor (points) should be the history of previous stroke.

Keypoint: It is question for medicine. Review the CHADS.

6. Since the risk factors for CHADS are all high, how do you manage this stroke risk?

Suggested answer: it is true the pre-existent risks are high, and current infection and possible sepsis, as well as surgical stress may even increase the risk of stroke. After a full discussion with the surgeon, I will start heparin therapy to reduce the risk.

Keypoint: In oral boards, it takes 3 steps to achieve the satisfactory score: 1. Know the challenge (risk), 2. Take the challenge (risk), 3. Manage the challenge (risk).

7. She has not taken her meds today, will you restart her all meds in the preoperative room?

Quite complicated medication list, you need to assess what are those medications for.

Suggest answers: I would stratify what is the purpose of medication and supplement the necessary medication if needed. Her Med include control DM, blood pressure and heart pill, reduce the chronic pain, improve the COPD, anti-coagulant for DES, and anti-reflex.

8. Does the Metoprolol considered to be necessary before surgery, why/why not? ASA? Albuterol? Metformin?

The broad range question is narrowing down to individual medication, you need know the recommendation for each medication.

Suggest answer: Assuming patient is asymptomatic at this time, the likelihood I will have the metoprolol (Beta-blocker) to start before surgery, and closely follow the patient to ensure she restart her other medication after surgery.

Keypoint:

1) COPD, albuterol is on PRN order, she don't needed if asymptomatic.

2) For GERD, Protonix, Nexium, don't needed since never be proven beneficial, just one dose.

3) For DM2, I would rely on IV insulin (slide scale) to control sugar level, oral hypoglycemic medication not only risk patient hypoglycemic medication (long duration), but also cause harm such as lactate acidosis, like metformin.

4) For anti-coagulant, ASA and Plavix are due to DES, or A-fib. The history is 3 years, and I prefer to discuss with her cardiologists before the surgery for the risk of stop those medications and "bridge solution". If the time not allow, I would not give the patient long-term anti-coagulant. I do understand the risk of thrombosis and give patient heparin SQ 5,000 unit before the surgery.

5) For chronic pain. Gabapentin, Motrin, it is chronic issue, rarely have any complication for a procedure, would resuming the medication after the surgery.

6) For blood pressure, Lisinopril, it has controversial benefit. Refractory hypotension if give before the surgery, rebounding hypertension if missed. My plan is to monitor the BP closely and treat the pressure accordingly during operation, and her blood pressure is stable at this time.

7) One dose of "Beta-blocker" right before the procedure to achieve

"myocardium protection" is unfounded. However, in a patient with significant cardiac history, and chronically on beta-blocker, it is quite beneficial to continue on, even it is right before the surgery.

9. The surgeon is complaining you are being "slow", stated that this is a relative urgent surgery should proceed right way, agree?

It is anesthesiologist's obligation to ensure the safety of this patient (reduce the mortality and morbidity).

Suggest answer: Agree it is urgent case, I do need time to know the patient and understanding the nature of her other underline co-morbidities. This time spent would lead to better management and reduced mortality and morbidity of this procedure.

Keypoint: you and the surgeon share the same responsibility for the patient's safety.

10. The surgeon state this is "emergency case"? Patient may develop Uro-sepsis if not treated right way, do you agree?

Communication with surgical colleague is very important. You and surgeon should share the same concerns about patient's safety.

Suggest answer: This procedure considers being urgent rather than emergent case. I do agree this case do have the URGENCE because the risk of sepsis. I would start the case after investigation of history and optimizing those risks and proceed as soon as I can.

Keypoint: Definition of the Emergency: Patient current vital sign is not stable, and vital sign drift toward worse direction despite adequate resuscitation. It is different from Urgent case.

11. Her glucose is 250 mg/dL, would you treat it, why/why not?

Hyperglycemia is common topic in oral boards. Review the guideline before the exam.

Suggest answer: I generally agree for treatment if the level is at or above 200 mg/dL, and it may trend up during the procedure due to surgical stress.

Keypoint: make decision and defend it.


12. Why do you select glucose level at or above 200 mg/dL for treatment? Not 150 mg/dL? Not 250 mg/dL?

It is very debatable the "true" good level of glucose to maintain during a procedure.

Suggest answer: A general consensus is to maintain the glucose level at 150~200 mg/dL. Higher would have worsening effect in wound infection and other complicaitons; if lower would have the risk of hypoglycemia.

Keypoint: The principal of management of glucose level during the surgery: avoid hypoglycemia. Titrating insulin to keep the blood glucose level below 200 mg/dL, (avoid diuresis induced by glucose). You need to be aware the risk of "ketoacidosis", electrolyte abnormality.


## > 术 前 管 理 <

1. 目前患者适合手术吗？

这是评估患者的时机，从病史和体格检查开始，并且要明确提出你的关注要点。

参考答案：首先进一步询问病史，评估病情。然后了解她最近体力活动水平有无改变，吸空气情况下氧饱和度能否维持在92%左右等。假如她最近症状没有任何加重，可以开始着手麻醉。


2. 需要做进一步检查吗？如果需要，应安排哪些检查？这些新的检查结果对你制定麻醉方案有何帮助？

对这个患者而言,除非病情突然加重才需要安排新的检查项目。换言之,如果你的麻醉方案没有变化,不需要给她安排新的检查。

参考答案:患者有重度慢性阻塞性肺疾病,吸空气下氧饱和度92%,动脉血气有助于评估其严重程度。这些结果可以指导优化氧疗方案,选择区域麻醉可以避免干扰肺功能;如果需要全身麻醉,应调整通气参数。

要点:这是一个开放式考题。你可以先假设患者目前状况较好。

3. 她的 CHADS 评分是多少(C-充血性心力衰竭,H-高血压,A-年龄,D-糖尿病,S-卒中史)?

知识细节考题,阐述你的见解。如果你不知道 CHADS 的含义,可以请考官重述一遍。

参考答案:CHADS 评分是一个新的风险分级系统(采用积分法),用于评估房颤患者的围术期脑卒中风险。

要点:复习 CHADS 评分系统。

4. 患者围术期脑卒中风险的影响因素? 发生心脏或肺梗死的风险?

这需要你重新回顾患者病情,尤其是要指出相关危险因素。

参考答案:这个患者的 CHADS 风险很高。这是由于她有相关的既往病史,比如高血压、糖尿病以及房颤病史。

5. CHADS 最高的危险因素是什么?

这是更深入的细节题,你需要非常坦率地回答问题。

参考答案:这个患者最高的危险因素(评分)是她的脑卒中病史。

要点:这是内科学考题。复习 CHADS。

6. 既然患者 CHADS 的危险因素评分都很高,你如何应对脑卒中风险。

参考答案:患者既往病史的危险因素确实很高,当前合并感染和潜在脓毒症,以及手术应激都会增加脑卒中风险。与外科医师充分讨论后,我会给予肝素治疗以降低风险。

要点：在口试过程中，三段式答案会获得较高的评分：首先知晓挑战（风险），其次接受挑战（风险），最后处理挑战（风险）。

7. 她今天还没有服药，你会在术前准备室内给她服用所有的药物吗？

她服用多种药物，你需要知道这些药物的治疗目的。

参考答案：我会梳理她服用药物的治疗目的，并且补充其他必要的药物。她服用的药物包括控制血糖、降血压、心血管药物、镇痛、改善慢性阻塞性肺疾病、冠脉支架术后抗凝和抗胃食管反流药物。

8. 术前必须给予美托洛尔吗，为什么/为什么不？阿司匹林、沙丁胺醇和二甲双胍呢？

提问试题从考察全面性转为针对单个药物，你需要知道每个药物的适应证。

参考答案：假如患者现在无症状，我可能会在术前给予美托洛尔（β受体阻滞剂），然后密切随访患者，并确保她术后开始服用其他药物。

要点：

1）对于慢性阻塞性肺疾病，沙丁胺醇是按需使用，如果她没有症状就不需要给。

2）对于胃食管反流症，不需要服用泮托拉唑或埃索美拉唑，因为没有证据表明术前单次剂量可改善患者结局。

3）对于 2 型糖尿病，我会选用静脉注射胰岛素（滑动胰岛素注射法）控制血糖，口服降糖药不仅会增加患者低血糖风险（作用时间长），还会引起乳酸代谢性酸中毒（二甲双胍）。

4）对于抗凝药物，阿司匹林和波立维是针对冠脉支架或房颤。已服药 3 年，我倾向于术前先跟她的心脏科医师讨论一下停药的风险和"桥接方案"。如果时间不允许，我不会给予患者长效抗凝药物。我知道患者有血栓形成风险，因此术前给予患者皮下注射肝素 5 000 U。

5）对于慢性疼痛，加巴喷丁、布洛芬，这是慢性疾病，对手术操作几乎没有任何影响，术后继续服用即可。

6）对于高血压，赖诺普利的作用有争议。如果术前服用可引起顽固性低血压,如果停药会引起反跳性高血压。我的计划是密切监测血压,术中针对性处理,目前她的血压是稳定的。

7)术前单次剂量β受体阻滞剂未发现有保护心肌作用。但是患者明确的心脏病史且长期服用β受体阻滞剂,因此继续服用对患者有利,即使是临近手术开始。

9.外科医师抱怨你"耽误时间",说这是相对紧急手术,应该立刻开始麻醉,你赞同吗?

麻醉医师的责任是保证患者的安全(降低死亡率和并发症率)。

参考答案:赞同,这是紧急手术病例,我花时间评估患者和疾病的性质。这些时间有助于提高麻醉管理质量,降低手术死亡率和并发症率。

要点:你和外科医师对患者安全负同等责任。

10.外科医师认为这是急诊手术病例,如果不立即手术,患者可能会继发尿脓毒症,你是否赞同?

与外科同事交流非常重要,你和外科医师对患者安全的关注是一致的。

参考答案:这个手术应该是紧急而不是急诊手术,我赞同这例手术符合紧急手术因为有脓毒症的风险。我会在调查病史后开始麻醉,并且尽最大努力规避这些风险,优化麻醉管理。

要点:急诊手术的定义:患者当前生命体征不稳定,尽管经过足够的复苏治疗,生命体征仍在恶化。这与紧急手术不同。

11.她的血糖是 13.89 mmol/L,你会处理吗,为什么?

高血糖是口试中常见的考点。考试前要复习指南。

参考答案:如果血糖高于 11.11 mmol/L,我一般会进行处理,患者血糖在术中可能会因手术应激而进一步增高。

要点:做出决定并给出你的理由。

12.你为什么会在血糖高于 11.11 mmol/L 时开始处理,为什么不是8.33 mmol/L或者 13.89 mmol/L?

术中血糖维持的最佳水平有很大争议。

参考答案：普遍共识是维持血糖水平在 11.11～13.89 mmol/L,过高可影响伤口愈合,低于 11.11 mmol/L 有发生低血糖的危险。

要点：术中处理血糖水平的原则是：避免低血糖；调节胰岛素用量维持血糖低于 13.89 mmol/L(避免高糖引起的利尿)；了解酮症酸中毒和电解质异常的风险。

## > **Intraoperative management** <

1. Are you going to give a general anesthesia for this case?

This is an expected question; it should be prepared for every case.

Suggest answer：I would do general anesthesia with endotracheal intubation. I select the GA not only because the complex of medical history but also the laser lithotripsy need to control the diaphragmatic move so the laser focus of the stone in kidney could relative easy.

Keypoint：You need make firm choice and defend on that choice. If you were challenged "why not", you need be ready for specific concerns.

MAC：patient may move；

LMA：patient may aspirate and breathing irregularly；

Spinal：hemodynamic swing and On Plavix.

2. Will you place an arterial line，why/why not?

Another decision to make，you make choice and defend your choice.

Suggest answer：In addition to ASA standard monitors，I like to have arterial line. I need it because of closely hemodynamic monitoring and multiple sampling to assess the ventilation status. It is quite challenge to ventilate the patient with COPD.

Keypoint：There are four good indications for arterial-line in general，but the patient very "sick" is not one of them.

1）Large hemodynamic swing in surgery is expected in this procedure.

2）Small hemodynamic swing is detrimental to patient.

3）Unable to monitor the patient blood pressure with regular blood pressure cuff（on By-pass）.

4）Multiple blood samples are needed to assess the patient's condition （ABG）.

3. Assume you decided for GA with endotracheal tube，how are you going to intubating this patient?

Routine question for anesthesia，your management should be ready.

Suggest answer：Assuming the airway examination is unremarkable. I would place select rapid sequence induction with close monitor hemodynamic. My plan is give lidocaine，propofol，and followed by succinylcholine.

Keypoint：State your plan short and precise.

4. Why don't you use "etomidate" for induction?

Defending your choice is better idea than not answer this question.

Suggest answer："Adrenal suppression"，even with just one dose of induction. I prefer to use propofol.

Keypoint：Etomidate is another induction agent with the profile of stable hemodynamics，especial suitable for patient with concurrent hypotensive and significant volume depletion（trauma or vital sign unstable）.

5. Would you consider giving a "Stress dose" steroid to the patient before the surgery?

This question is common but has new updated guideline.

Suggest answer：if patient is on Prednisone 10 mg every other day，it is small amount steroid，and this surgery consider to low stress surgery，I would continue her Prednisone and not supplement extra stress dose of steroid.

Keypoint: The concept "stress dose of steroid" changed. The regular 100 mg every 8 hours for any surgery is "overdose". New guideline prefers to tail the amount of steroid based on type of surgery. You can supplement the "stress dose" if the patient demonstrate "adrenal insufficient" sign during the procedure.

6. Thirty-five min into the surgery, the surgeon found the stone and fired the laser, shortly after you noticed the patient suddenly became more tachycardia HR 115, hypotensive 98/54, $SaO_2$ from 99% to 92% on $FiO_2$ 50%, what would be the likely causes?

This is a "what do you think" question, pay attention to vital sign changes while surgeon is doing something (hint).

Suggest answer: I believe the cause is bacteremia base on the nature of sudden onset during laser lithotripsy (stone contain bacteria). Other possibility include: heart ischemia and failure, pulmonary emboli, pneumothorax, pulmonary edema and possible injured or raptured kidney or ureter, etc.

Keypoint: good differential diagnosis (usually 4 or 5) is essential for oral board's exam.

7. Would you consider asking the surgeon to stop the surgery, why/why not?

Your response to must include notifying the surgeon, check the airway, and ventilation, there will not be treatment "options" until the etiology is identified.

Suggest answer: I would temporarily stop the procedure and ask surgeon to verify whether there is any injury to the kidney while I will focus on ventilation status. The treatment depends on what is the cause, and I will treat accordingly.

Keypoint: "Look, Listen, and Feel of the lung's compliance" are common three steps towards finding the cause of desaturation. Don't forget to talk to surgeon, it may cause by surgery.

8. Would this be caused by acute sepsis, why/why not?

This is "what do you think". Clearly state you're thinking process.

Suggest answer: Unless likely, but possible, because sepsis is a "process" which take time to development. In the nature of "sudden onset", I believe is bacteremia. (It is possible of septic shock as long as there is a decrease in blood pressure)

Keypoint: common are common.

9. Would you give beta blocker to decrease the heart rate (reduce the oxygen consumption) at this moment, why/why not?

Make sure what you are treated, defend your choice with reasons.

Suggest answer: assuming the patient's EKG shown no sign of ischemia and the tachycardia and hypotension is physiological response to "stress" or "hypovolemia". I would not initiate another dose of beta blocker at this time.

Keypoint: know what you treating.

10. Would you start vasopressor at this point, why/why not?

Make decision first and it is important to explain "why" or state the benefit of your new treatment.

Suggest answer: I would apply small dose of Neo-Synepherine to temporize blood pressure, and slow down the heart rate at same time.

Keypoint: Buy your time in order to find differential diagnosis.

11. The surgeon cannot detect "anything wrong" with the patient, do you still think it could be acute bacteremia?

When the examiner gives a hint, you are likely to follow up on that hint.

Suggest answer: Certainly, urinary stone may colonize bacterial growth. After the laser breaks the stone, bacteria may enter the blood circulation.

Keypoint: The hint in oral exam is very important clue for you to answer the correct question.

12. Assuming this is sepsis, what is your choice of vasopressor for the hypotension?

When the question starts with "assuming", it is what the patient has. You should very happy you have the diagnosis now.

Suggest answer: If the sepsis is agreed up the team, and patient blood pressure does not respond well to fluid resuscitation, cardiac output is higher than normal due to severe vessel dilation (septic hypotension), my next choice of vasopressor is phenylephrine drip (strong alpha effect).

Keypoint: flexibility and knowledge.

13. You have an ABG, pH 7.21, $PaO_2$ 145 mmHg, $PaCO_2$ 32 mmHg, $HCO_2^-$ 17, $SaO_2$ 100% on $FiO_2$ 50%, explain? Would you treat it, how? Fluid vs. vasopressor, why?

The correct interpretation of arterial blood gas is essential for anesthesia oral board.

Suggest answer: the respiratory status is acceptable, but patient has a metabolic acidosis. I would further investigate the cause of acidosis.

I will check the lactate level, and the base excess, calculate the "ion gap" to find out the cause. I would first found the cause and then treated accordingly.

Keypoint: There are several ways to identifying the cause of metabolic acidosis. Routinely, you start from respiratory status, then the metabolic status, then the possible mix respiratory and metabolic together.

14. Do you think patients may develope cardiogenic shock?

Pre-existent condition always the carry this risk of intraoperative worsening.

Suggest answer: Based on the severity of metabolic acidosis and previous heart condition, the cardiogenic shock is very high possibility.

Keypoint: It is better answer if your medical judgement also include this patient previous history.

15. If there is sign of cardiogenic shock seconday to the sepsis, what would be you additional management plan?

Make firm choice if medical condition is clearly defined.

Suggest answer: I would consider adding inotropic support if hypotension refractory to Nor-epinephrine drip (strong alpha and beta support).

Keypoint: Pharmacodynamics is another key in oral boards.

16. Patient is on insulin drip but the glucose on the ABG reach 350 mg/dL? Why?

The questions changed direction, you should quickly focused on new question.

Suggest answer: Surgical stress and possible sepsis all lead to increase "circulating catecholamine" and resisting the insulin, it may be the reason sugar high.

Keypoint: the stress induces hyperglycemia by counteract insulin effect.

17. Would you give insulin bolus because the glucose 350 mg/dL?

Make choice and defending your answer.

Suggest answer: Hyperglycemia could lead to diuresis, severe hypovolemia and hypo-perfusion (lactate acidosis); hyperglycemia may also indicate inadequate insulin which may lead to metabolic disorder such as ketoacidosis. I would increase the rate of insulin infusion to bring the glucose level slowly.

Keypoint：do not forget the possibility of "keto-acidosis".

18. Assuming "Keto" is negative，insulin infusion or bolus? Why infusion not bolus?

Make choice and defend it.

Suggest answer：I would increase the rate of insulin drip to put the glucose level under 200 mg/dL. I do not like the bolus option because it may lead to hypoglycemia（overdose）. Low the glucose level instantly（large amount insulin bolus）may lead to a significant osmolality swing（brain and pulmonary edema）and electrolyte imbalance（potassium shift intracellular）.

Keypoint：There are several ways to control the glucose level：drip，subcutaneous，or bolus，etc. The board examiner like to know what is your selection and why.

> 术 中 管 理 <

1. 你会选择给患者全身麻醉吗？

这是必考题，每个病例都要准备。

参考答案：我会选择气管插管全身麻醉。我选择全身麻醉不仅是因为患者病史的复杂性，而且激光碎石术需要控制膈肌运动，以便于激光聚焦肾结石。

要点：你需要给出确定的选择和支持理由。如果你被反问"为什么不是其他选择"，你需要准备好针对性的回答。

监测下麻醉管理：患者可能会动。

喉罩：患者可能会误吸和呼吸不规则。

脊髓麻醉：血流动力学波动，患者服用波立维。

2. 你会放置动脉导管吗，为什么？

需要你再次做决策，做出选择并给出理由。

参考答案：除了 ASA 标准监测外，我需要有动脉置管。因为我需要密切监测血流动力学，多次测血气以评估呼吸功能。慢性阻塞性肺疾病患者的呼吸管理很有挑战。

要点：放置动脉导管的常见 4 个适应证如下，患者"病情重"不是其中之一：

1）术中可能会出现大的血压波动。

2）患者不能耐受轻微血压波动。

3）常规血压计袖带法无法检测患者血压（体外循环）。

4）需多次采血监测病情（动脉血气）。

3. 假如你决定行气管插管全身麻醉，你如何给这个患者插管？

麻醉常规考题，明确归纳出你的方案。

参考答案：假设气道检查没有异常。我会选择在密切监测血流动力学情况下快速诱导麻醉。我的计划是给利多卡因和丙泊酚，然后琥珀胆碱。

要点：简洁而准确地给出你的方案。

4. 麻醉诱导为什么不选依托咪酯？

为你自己辩护比不回答问题更合适。

参考答案：即使是单次诱导剂量的依托咪酯也会有"肾上腺功能抑制"。我倾向于使用丙泊酚。

要点：依托咪酯是另一种麻醉诱导药物，具有血流动力学稳定的特点，尤其适合用于伴有低血压和明显血容量耗竭（创伤或生命体征不稳定）的患者。

5. 你会在术前给予患者应激剂量的类固醇吗？

这个考题很常见，但是指南有更新。

参考答案：患者隔天服用泼尼松 10 mg，属于小剂量类固醇治疗，这个手术被认为是低应激手术，我会维持她的泼尼松用量，但不会补充额外的应激剂量类固醇。

要点："应激剂量类固醇"的概念有变化。任何手术常规给予 100 mg，每 8 个小时 1 次的用量已经超量了。新指南倾向于根据手术类型给予不同剂量的类固醇。如果术中患者有肾上腺功能不足的症状，你可以在术中补充应激剂量的类固醇。

6. 手术开始后 35 min，外科医师找到结石并用激光碎石，你发现患者突然心动过速 HR 115 次/min，低血压 98/54 mmHg，氧饱和度从 99% 降至 92%（$FiO_2$ 50%），你认为是什么原因？

这是"你认为"类型的考题，在外科医师操作时（提示），应注意生命体征改变。

参考答案：我认为原因是菌血症，因为这是在激光碎石过程中突然出现的（结石内含有细菌）。其他可能的原因有心肌缺血和功能衰竭、肺栓塞、气胸、肺水肿，或者是肾脏、输尿管的损伤或破裂。

要点：在口试中一定要给出好的鉴别诊断（通常 4～5 个），但要有重点。

7. 你会考虑停止手术吗？为什么？

你的回答必须包括提醒外科医师，检查气道和通气。明确病因后才能提出处理方案。

参考答案：我会暂时中止操作，让外科医师检查肾脏有无损伤，同时我会关注患者呼吸状态。处理方案取决于具体病因，我会做出相应处理。

要点："检查管路、听呼吸音、感受肺顺应性"是诊断氧饱和度下降原因的常规三部曲。别忘了告知外科医师，因为有可能是手术操作引起的。

8. 这可能是急性脓毒症吗？为什么？

这是"你认为"类型的考题。明确给出你的诊断思路。

参考答案：不太像，但有可能，因为脓毒症是一个疾病过程，它需要时间来演化。基于"突然发作"的事实，我认为这是菌血症（有可能，只要发生血压下降）。

要点：优先考虑常见并发症。

9. 这个时候可以给予 β 受体阻滞剂降低心率吗（降低氧耗），为什么？

明确你要治疗什么，给出理由。

参考答案：如果患者的心电图没有任何缺血表现，这个心动过速和低血压是对"应激"和"低血容量"的生理反应。这时候我不会给予 β 受体阻滞剂。

要点：明确你在治疗什么。

**10.** 这时候你会给予缩血管药物吗，为什么？

首先作决定，重点是解释"为什么"或说出给予新治疗措施的益处。

参考答案：我会给予小剂量的去氧肾上腺素暂时提升血压，并且降低心率。

要点：给自己找出鉴别诊断争取时间。

**11.** 外科医师没有发现患者有"任何问题"，你是否还认为是急性菌血症？

当考官给出提示时，你最好能根据他的提示作答。

参考答案：当然还是这么认为，尿路结石可伴有细菌生长。激光使结石破碎后，细菌可能会进入血循环。

要点：在口试中，"考官提示"是你正确回答问题的重要线索。

**12.** 假设这是脓毒症，你选择什么血管收缩药治疗低血压？

当题目是以"假设"打头，这就是患者的真实状况。你应该为知道诊断结果而高兴。

参考答案：如果团队倾向于脓毒症诊断，液体复苏对患者血压没有明显作用，由于血管扩张，心排量高于正常（感染性休克），我接下来会选择去甲肾上腺素滴注（强烈的 α 受体效应）。

要点：灵活应对和知识储备。

**13.** 你有一个动脉血气结果：pH 7.21，$PaO_2$ 145 mmHg，$PaCO_2$ 32 mmHg，$HCO_3^-$ 17 mmol/L，$SaO_2$ 100% on $FiO_2$ 50%，如何解释？你会处理吗，如何处理？选择液体还是缩血管药物，为什么？

正确分析动脉血气结果是麻醉口试中的必考题。

参考答案：就患者动脉血气结果而言，呼吸功能尚可，但是患者有酸血症（代谢性）。我会找出酸血症的原因。

我会查看乳酸水平，碱剩余，计算"离子间隙"以找出原因。我会首先找出原因，再给予相应的治疗。

要点：有多种方式可以确定代谢性酸中毒的病因。一般而言，你可以先从呼吸功能着手，然后考虑代谢状态，再综合考虑呼吸和代谢因素。

14. 你认为患者可能会出现心源性休克吗？

术前合并疾病总是伴有术中恶化的可能。

参考答案：根据代谢性酸中毒的严重性和术前心脏病史，心源性休克的可能性很高。

要点：如果你在病情判断中加入患者的病史，这会更全面。

15. 如果出现继发于脓毒症的心源性休克症状，你如何进一步处理？

如果病情明确，就做出明确选择。

参考答案：如果去甲肾上腺素（强烈的 α 受体和 β 受体作用）滴注效果欠佳，我会考虑开始强心治疗。

要点：药代动力学是口试中的另一个重点。

16. 患者正在滴注胰岛素但是动脉血气中的葡萄糖高达 19.44 mmol/L，为什么？

考题变换了方向，你的注意力应快速集中到新问题上。

参考答案：手术应激和可能的脓毒症都可以引起"体循环内儿茶酚胺"增加和胰岛素抵抗，这可能是血糖增高的原因。

要点：应激引起的高血糖可以抵消胰岛素药效。

17. 在血糖 19.44 mmol/L 时，你会不改胰岛素负荷剂量吗？

做出选择并给出理由。

参考答案：高血糖可引起渗透性利尿、严重低血容量和低灌注（乳酸性酸中毒），高血糖也提示胰岛素用量不足，这会引起代谢性疾病如酮症酸中毒。我会增加胰岛素输注速度，以缓慢降低血糖。

要点：不要忘记酮症酸中毒的可能性。

18. 如果血酮体没有增高，选择胰岛素输注还是快速推注？为什么是输注而不是快速推注？

做出选择并给出理由。

参考答案：我会增加胰岛素滴注速度,使血糖水平降至 11.11 mmol/L。我不喜欢推注胰岛素,因为这可能会引起低血糖(过量)。迅速降低血糖(大剂量胰岛素推注)可能会导致显著的渗透压变化(脑和肺水肿)和电解质失衡(钾离子向细胞内转移)

要点：控制血糖有多种方式：滴注、皮下注射或静脉快速推注等。考官想知道你的选择和理由。

## > Postoperative management <

1. You and the surgeon decided that this patient would be admitted to ICU, her MAP(mean arterial pressure)is 73 mmHg and HR is 115 bpm while on norepinephrine 10 mcg/min and phenylephrine 100 mcg/min, would you extubate the patient, why/why not?

Patient need be awake, alert, and vital sign stable. Her vital signs are not considered stable while still on inotropic support.

Suggested answer：I would keep the patient intubated. I would admit the patient to ICU. This patient is likely to need a central line for vasopressor and inotropic infusion if she is remaining in sepsis. She needs continuous critical care support until her sepsis under control (when she is off inotropic drip).

Keypoint：Respiratory status is not the only criteria for extubation.

2. What if the patient was waking up, took good tidal volume and maintained adequate oxygenation? And is tiring. What if the patient was trying to pull her ETT?

It is a debatable question, controlled ventilation maybe needed for ICU care.

Suggested answer：I would prefer keeping this patient's airway protected as along as she still need inotropic support. She will be sedated by starting propofol infusion.

Keypoint: It is medical judgement. Patient could still be in septic shock at this time.

3. The patient had to be placed in PACU but there is no bed in ICU, what would be your next work up?

The examiner dictates the course of exam. In many situations, his questions do not follow your management direction. You probably did nothing wrong, but focus on new question.

Suggest answer: Patient needs blood culture, continue monitoring, volume resuscitation, broad-spectrum antibiotic, inotropic support, central lines and ICU care. Even though this patient is extubated for PACU, but the steps for sepsis management are the same.

Keypoint: focus on new question immediately.

4. How do you differentiate sepsis vs. septic shock?

Different stages of disease process. Definition for shock: there are evidences that the cardiac output does not meet the body's consumption need.

Suggest answer: Patient in sepsis will have symptom such as fever, increased heart rate and cardiac output, and hypotension due to severe vessel dilatation, etc. in shock stage, the patient's cardiac output does not meet the body need, which may reflect on patient's mental status.

Keypoint: Septic shock can lead to pulmonary edema, heart failure, cerebral stroke, multi-organ failure, and even death.

5. Would you consider cardioverter this patient because of unstable blood pressure while in a-fib (atrial fibrillation), why/why not?

Cardioversion is not treatment of hypotension in sepsis. Volume and inotrope are the treatment option.

Suggest answer: No, volume resuscitation, inotropic and vessel constriction support would be major measure to support the blood pressure.

Keypoint: Always treat the underlie causes.

6. Patient now is in ICU, blood pressure continue to be low despite volume resuscitation, norepinephrine and phenylephrine, any suggestion for the low pressure treatment?

This question tests the common pathophysiology of septic shock.

Suggest answer: Assuming patient CO (cardiac output) is still higher than normal, the likelihood of hypotension is due to nitric oxide mediated vessel dilation, a common pathophysiology of septic shock. I would recommend vasopressin drip (0.01~0.05 units/min).

Keypoint: persistent or refractory hypotension, we are focused on those 3 differentials:

Preload: hypovolemia.

Contractility: cardiac output (cardiogenic shock), heart rate, rhythm.

Afterload: vessel dilatation, viscosity (anemia) etc.

7. 3 hours later, assume the patient was extubated and off vasopressor in PACU, will you insist to be admitted to ICU?

It is your judgement, make the decision and explain why you made that decision.

Suggest answers: Patient returns to normal vital sign in such short duration may indicate transient bacteremia rather than "true" sepsis or septic shock. I prefer the patient admitted to ICU for overnight observation and continue on IV antibiotic.

Keypoint: It is your judgment. Patient off the drips may indicate volume resuscitation is "catching up, but the sepsis may still there."

8. 18 hours later, the troponin was 0.02 $\mu$g/mL, would you consider this was NONSTEMI (none ST segment elevation myocardial infarction)?

Elevated troponin (troponin leaking) after procedure has multiple causes.

Suggested answer: Yes, it is possible patient developed NONSTEMI. The diagnosis of NONSTEMI is made when a patient has symptoms of unstable angina, has no ST-segment elevation on the ECG, and has an elevation in cardiac enzymes.

Keypoint: understand this subject: the differential diagnosis of elevated troponins after a surgical procedure.

9. Are you suggesting the patient had ACS (Spontaneous acute myocardial infarction)?

The diagnosis would be more convincing if patient has coronary disease and hypotension during the procedure.

Suggest answer: It is possible. She does have very significant cardiac history. However she also develops sepsis or septic shock, and significant hypotension and tachycardia. The troponins may derive from systemic inflammatory response syndrome, tachycardia (high oxygen demand), hypotension (low oxygen supply).

10. Well, what is your management, now knowing the troponin is elevated?

I would focus on differential diagnosis.

Suggest answer: I would first make sure patient vital sign is stable, and supplement oxygen. I would pay special attention to the blood pressure and control the heart rate. Find the reason why the troponin is increased.

Keypoint: Differential diagnosis: concurrent heart ischemia, inflammation response, pre-existent stent dysfunction etc.

11. Would you consider cardiologist consultation? Why yes/why not?

Initiating the cardiac consultation to verify the heart condition and provide further treatment option if her troponin remaining and likely caused by MI.

Suggest answer: Patient's elevated troponin is concern; it may from the dysfunction of the stents. The cardiologist help delineate the severity of her disease and implement further treatment plan had the troponin is due to cardiac ischemia or the stent dysfunction.

Keypoint:

1) The first step in treating NONSTEMI is to stabilize the heart muscle to prevent further damage.

2) The cardiologist will need to decide whether to continue with "conservative" therapy (that is, drug therapy alone) or "aggressive" treatment such as angioplasty and re-stenting.

12. Would you think this patient is susceptible to cerebral stroke and POCD (postoperative cognitive dysfunction)? Why yes/why not?

This is the question for specific knowledge about our current understanding of POCD.

Suggest answer: Elderly patients, history of atrial fibrillation, valvular disease, renal disease, or previous stroke. The mechanism of developing perioperative stroke is not complete understood at this time. It is believe to be "inflammation reaction induced by surgical stress", or the thrombotic "plaque" from the injured vessel.

Keypoint: what are the risk factors for POCD.

13. What would be most common clinical presentations of stroke?

The presentation of stroke includes many different aspects.

Suggest answer: Patient's post-operative mental status, memory, speech, gross motor function and awareness of surrounding are the common signs to identify perioperative stroke.

Keypoint: it is very important to recognize the disorder; sometimes the symptom can be very elusive, and not sure about.

14. Would you order a head CT in ICU if you suspect a stroke, why/ why not?

You need professional consultation to help to manage the patient's condition.

Suggest answer: I would consult the neurologist to make the decision. I do not have sufficient knowledge to judge whether the head CT will be sufficient to make the diagnosis of small "ischemia stroke".

Keypoint: Perioperative stroke and POCD was associated with delayed recognition, infrequent intervention. Professional consultation is important part of medicine practice.

15. During the joint M & M (morbidity and mortality) conference, the surgeon pointed out there was a delay in surgery by anesthesia team, which he believed the main cause for the ineffective treating her urosepsis and sepsis shock, would you agree with this surgeon's statement?

Complications of surgical procedure, many times, are derived from the pre-existent disease.

Suggest answer: I would not agree with his assessment for "anesthesia delay" is the cause of urosepsis and the complications. I believe confirmed risk factor is "pre-existent" condition. Renal stone may culture the bacteria and lead to sepsis; her previous heart condition pushed her into cardiac shock under the stress of hypotension and tachycardia.

Keypoint: The identifiable risk factor is from pre-existent medical condition. It is rare that anesthesia evaluation cause sepsis.

16. The same surgeon states that spinal anesthesia maybe the better choice for this procedure than general anesthesia, what is your response?

We have very minimal data to prove that "different outcome" from different mode of anesthesia care for any surgical procedure.

Suggest answer：regional vs. general anesthesia has benefits and risks. No evidence one form is "better" than another in most our anesthesia practice.

Keypoint：Defending your position with good knowledge and polite altitude. "Social" science is very important part of medicine. You are not "less MD" than any other MDs.

## > 术 后 管 理 <

1. 你和外科医师决定患者应该送入 ICU,患者平均动脉压 73 mmHg,心率 115 次/min,输注去甲肾上腺素 10 μg/min,去氧肾上腺 100 μg/min,你会给患者拔管吗,为什么?

提示:拟拔管患者应该是清醒、警觉的,并且生命体征平稳。患者仍需要正性肌力药物支持时,生命体征不能认为是平稳的。

参考答案:我会保留患者气管插管,并将患者转送至 ICU。如果患者有脓毒症,需要放置中心静脉以便于输注血管活性药和正性肌力药。患者需要持续重症支持治疗直到脓毒症得到控制(不再需要滴注正性肌力药物)。

要点:呼吸功能不是拔管的唯一标准。

2. 如果患者苏醒,潮气量正常且氧合充足呢? 患者烦躁,如果她要拔掉气管导管呢?

这是争议性考题,ICU 治疗中有时是需要控制性通气的。

参考答案:只要患者还需要正性肌力药物支持,我就会维持机械通气。我会考虑泵注异丙酚镇静。

要点:这是医学判断力的体现,患者此时可能还处于感染性休克状态。

3. 患者必须放在 PACU,但是 ICU 暂时没有病床,你的下一步计划是什么?

考官掌控考试过程。很多情况下,他不会按照你的处理思路提问题。你没有答错任何问题,注意力转移到新的考题上。

参考答案:患者需要进行血液培养、持续监护、容量复苏、广谱抗生素、正性肌力药物支持、中心静脉导管和重症监护治疗。即使这个患者在 PACU 拔管,治疗脓毒症的方案不变。

要点:注意力迅速转移到新的问题上。

4. 你如何区分脓毒症和感染性休克?

这是疾病发展不同阶段。休克的定义是:有心排量不能满足全身氧耗需求的证据。

参考答案:脓毒症患者会有发热、心率和心排量增加,严重血管扩张引起的低血压等等。在休克阶段,患者的心排量不能满足全身需要,患者可有意识状态改变。

要点:感染性休克可引起肺水肿、心力衰竭、脑卒中和多器官功能衰竭甚至死亡。

5. 如果患者血压不稳又是房颤,你会考虑给予患者电复律吗?为什么?

电复律不是处理脓毒症低血压的方法。容量复苏和正性肌力药才是正确选择。

参考答案:不,容量复苏、正性肌力药和缩血管药物支持是提升血压的主要手段。

要点:选择对因治疗方案。

6. 患者现在 ICU 内,虽然经过容量复苏,给予去甲肾上腺素和去氧肾上腺,但血压仍然偏低,有什么处理低血压的建议?

这个考题考查感染性休克的病理生理常识。

参考答案:如果患者心排量仍然高于正常水平,低血压可能是由于一氧化氮介导的血管扩张,这是感染性休克的病理生理常识。我建议滴注垂体后叶加压素(0.01~0.05 U/min)。

要点：持续性或顽固性低血压，我们通常考虑 3 个鉴别诊断：

前负荷：低血容量。

收缩性：心排血量（心源性休克）、心率、节律。

后负荷：血管扩张、血液黏滞度（贫血）等。

7. 3 个小时后，假设患者在 PACU 内已经拔管并停用缩血管药物，你会坚持将患者送至 ICU 吗？

这是你的判断，做出选择并解释选择理由。

参考答案：患者在如此短的时间内恢复正常生命体征，提示可能是短暂的菌血症而不是"真"的脓毒症或感染性休克。我倾向于让患者在 ICU 内过夜，便于观察和静脉抗生素治疗。

要点：这是你的判断。患者停用药物提示容量复苏已经足够，但是脓毒症可能还存在。

8. 18 个小时后，测肌钙蛋白 0.02 $\mu g/mL$，你认为这是非 ST 段抬高型心肌梗死吗？

手术后肌钙蛋白增高（肌钙蛋白渗漏）可能有多种原因。

参考答案：是的，患者可能出现非 ST 段抬高型心肌梗死。患者有非稳定性心绞痛症状，心电图无 ST 段抬高和心肌酶谱增高可诊断为非 ST 抬高型心肌梗死。

要点：理解考查点，手术后肌钙蛋白增高的鉴别诊断。

9. 你是认为患者有急性冠脉综合征吗（自发性急性心肌梗死）？

如果患者有冠脉疾病和术中低血压，诊断可能会更明确。

参考答案：这是有可能的。她的确有显著的心脏病史。但是她出现了脓毒症或感染性休克，以及显著低血压和心动过速。肌钙蛋白增高可能是由于全身炎症反应综合征、心动过速（高氧耗）和低血压（低氧供）。

10. 你现在知道肌钙蛋白增高，你的处理是什么？

我会关注鉴别诊断。

参考答案：我首先要确保患者的生命体征平稳，并给予氧疗。我会更关注血压，并控制心率。找出肌钙蛋白增高的原因。

要点：鉴别诊断：伴发心肌缺血、炎症反应和既往冠脉支架功能障碍。

11. 你需要心脏专科医师会诊吗？为什么？

请心脏专科医师会诊可以确定心脏病情，提供进一步治疗意见，如果肌钙蛋白仍然很高则很可能由于心肌梗死引起的。

参考答案：肌钙蛋白升高值得关注，可能是由于冠脉支架的失效。心脏专科医师可以协助确定患者病情严重程度，如果确认肌钙蛋白增高是由于心肌缺血或冠脉支架失效，还可拟定下一步治疗计划。

要点：

1）第一步是处理非 ST 抬高型心肌梗死以稳定心肌，防止进一步损伤。

2）心脏专科医师需要决定是否继续保守治疗（药物治疗）或手术治疗比如血管成形术或冠脉支架置入术。

12. 你认为这个患者是发生脑卒中和术后认知功能障碍的高风险人群吗，为什么/为什么不？

这是考查术后认知功能障碍相关知识的细节题。

参考答案：老年患者，有房颤病史、瓣膜疾病、肾脏疾病或脑卒中病史。围术期脑卒中的发病机制还不是很清楚。目前认为可能是由于手术应激引起的炎症反应，或者受损血管的血栓斑块脱落。

要点：哪些是术后认知功能障碍的危险因素。

13. 脑卒中的常见临床表现是什么？

脑卒中的临床表现包括多个方面。

参考答案：患者术后的意识状态、记忆、言语、大体运动功能，以及对环境的认知是鉴别围术期脑卒中的常用指标。

要点：能识别这个并发症很重要，有时候患者的症状模棱两可，不太确定。

14. 如果你怀疑患者有脑卒中,你考虑在 ICU 内进行头颅 CT 检查吗,为什么?

你需要专科医师会诊来协助处理病情。

参考答案:我会咨询神经专科医师来决定。我缺乏足够的知识确定头颅 CT 是否足以诊断微小缺血性脑卒中。

要点:围术期脑卒中与未能及时诊断和积极干预有关。专科会诊是医疗过程中的重要部分。

15. 在死亡及并发症病例综合讨论中,外科医师指出该病例的麻醉工作存在拖延,并且认为这是尿脓毒症和感染性休克的主要原因,你同意这个外科医师的观点吗?

外科手术中的并发症,很多情况下是由于术前伴有疾病所致。

参考答案:我不同意外科医师认为"麻醉拖延"是尿脓毒症和并发症主要原因的观点。我认为确切的危险因素是患者的术前并发症。肾结石可能含有细菌并引起脓毒症,患者心脏病史以及低血压和心动过速,使病情加重至心源性休克。

要点:可确定的危险因素是术前伴有疾病。麻醉评估导致脓毒症是罕见的。

16. 该外科医师认为脊髓麻醉比全身麻醉更适合这个手术,你怎么作答?

关于不同麻醉方式造成某种手术结局不同的现有证据非常少。

参考答案:区域麻醉和全身麻醉各有利弊。在我们绝大部分麻醉实践中,没有证据表明某种方式优于另一种方式。

要点:用扎实知识和礼貌的态度维护你观点。谈话技巧是医学的重要部分。你不比其他的医学博士差。

**Reference**

[1] Angus DC, van der Poll T. Severe Sepsis and Septic Shock. N Engl J Med. 2013;369(9): 840 - 851.

[2] Vincent JL, De Backer D. Circulatory Shock. New Eng J Med. 2013;369(18): 1726 - 1734.

## Recommendations

Compare to your other exams in your professional career，the Oral board's exam is complete different exam. It is quite subjective due to pass or fail standard are based on board examiner judgment. It is paramount important for you to understand the process and read the books specifically prepare for oral boards.

Suggested reading list for US oral boards preparation：

1. Michael Ho：the essential oral boards review.

2. CJ. Gallagher et al.：Board Stiff Too.

3. Faust et al.：Anesthesiology Review.

4. Gupta et al.：Student Manuscript for Anesthesiology Oral Board Review.

5. DJ. Doyle：Hints for mastering the ABA Anesthesiology oral board Examination.

## 建议

与你职业生涯中的其他考试相比，口试是一种完全不同的考试。由于通过与否主要取决于考官的评判，口试相当的主观。了解考试过程和阅读口试备考书籍是非常重要的。

口试备考参考书目包括：

1. Michael Ho：口试实质评述。

2. CJ. Gallagher 等：口试真的很难。

3. Faust 等：麻醉学回顾。

4. Gupta 等：麻醉口试之学生手稿。

5. DJ. Doyle：掌握 ABA 麻醉口试建议。

Ming Xiong

熊铭

# 5 Anesthesia for total laryngectomy

## 耳鼻喉手术病例——全喉切除麻醉

> **Basic information** <

A 71 years old male with voice hoarseness for 3 months has been diagnosed with supraglottic mass (laryngeal cancer). He is scheduled for total laryngectomy, bilateral neck lymph nodes dissection, possible pectoralis flap transfer, and possible free flap transplant from the left forearm.

Other medical problems include 50 pack/year smoking history, chronic obstructive pulmonary disease (COPD) on home $O_2$ for 3 years, hypertension, hypothyroidism, and peripheral vascular disease (PVD).

Current medications: aspirin (ASA), simvastatin, gabapentin, albuterol inhaler, ipratropium inhaler, levothyroxine, lisinopril, and multi-vitamins.

Physical Exam: weight 77 kg, body mass index (BMI) 27, BP 140/92 mmHg, HR 74 bpm, RR 14/min, $SpO_2$ 91% on room air.

Electrocardiogram (EKG): Sinus rhythm at 65 bpm, with occasional premature ventricular contractions (PVCs). Possible left ventricular hypertrophy (LVH). Non-specific ST－T changes.

Pulmonary function test (PFT): forced vital capacity (FVC) 2.1 L, forced expiratory volume in the first second (FEV1) is 1.3 L and 65% predicted,

FEV1/FVC 60% predicted.

Arterial blood gas（ABG）at room air：pH 7.37，PaO$_2$ 76 mmHg，PaCO$_2$ 58 mmHg，HCO$_3^-$ 30 mEq/L，SaO$_2$ 92%.

Other lab results：complete blood count（CBC）and serum electrolytes are within normal limits.

## 基 本 信 息

病史：老年男性,71 岁,因声音嘶哑 3 个月诊断为声门上肿物(喉癌),现拟行全喉切除术、双侧颈部淋巴结清扫,备胸肌皮瓣转移,备左前臂游离皮瓣移植术。

其他病史包括：每年 50 包吸烟史、慢性阻塞性肺病(COPD)行家庭氧疗 3 年、高血压、甲状腺功能低下,以及外周血管病(PVD)。

现用药物：阿司匹林(ASA)、辛伐他汀、加巴喷丁、沙丁胺醇气雾剂、异丙托溴铵气雾剂、甲状腺素、赖诺普利和复合维生素。

体格检查：体重 77 kg,体重指数(BMI)27,血压 140/92 mmHg,心率 74 次/min,呼吸频率 14 次/min,吸入空气时外周血氧饱和度 91%。

心电图(EKG)：窦性心律 65 次/min,偶发室早。可疑左室肥厚。非特异性ST-T 段改变。

肺功能试验(PFT)：用力肺活量(FVC)2.1 L。第一秒用力呼吸容积(FEV1)1.3 L,为预计值 65%。FEV1/FVC 比例为预计值 60%。

吸入空气时动脉血气分析（ABG）：pH 7.37,PaO$_2$ 76 mmHg,PaCO$_2$ 58 mmHg,HCO$_3^-$ 30 mmol/L,SaO$_2$ 92%。

其他实验室检查结果：血常规和血清电解质检查结果正常。

## Preoperative management

1. Airway：How do you assess this patient's airway? Do you have any

specific concerns? Which of the following would provide the most important information regarding his airway situation: the patient's history and symptoms, physical exam findings, or computed tomography (CT) scan results?

Keyword: airway evaluation and difficult airway management are essential skills for anesthesia providers. This is especially crucial for airway diseases, because they may pose significant challenges for airway management.

A detailed history and meticulous physical exam are always good starting point. If the patient has developed dyspnea, this can be an indication of significant laryngeal stenosis. Furthermore, if the reclining position worsens the patient's dyspnea, this finding is particularly ominous for airway compromise — complete airway obstruction may ensue if general anesthesia is induced. In this scenario, awake fiberoptic intubation, or even awake tracheostomy, may be warranted instead.

Radiation therapy may be part of the regimen for some laryngeal cancer patients. This treatment modality may produce anatomical alterations in the upper and lower airways, and potentially make the tracheal intubation more difficult. Special attention should be given to assessing head/neck mobility, soft tissue edema and fibrosis, mouth opening, dentition, etc.

Imaging studies are another set of useful tools to evaluate the laryngeal tumor. They can be a great resource to identify the anatomical characteristics of the tumor, including its size, exact location, relationship with vocal cords and other airway structures, etc.

Many patients may have undergone indirect laryngoscopy by the surgeon in clinic prior to surgery. Surgeons may provide valuable information, such as the severity of laryngeal stenosis, the motility and bleeding potential of the tumor, etc. The importance of discussing the findings and plans with surgeons pre-operatively cannot be overemphasized.

2. Pulmonary: Please interpret the results of his ABG and PFT. Do you

have any concerns? Are there any additional tests or preparations needed that might be helpful to optimize his pulmonary condition?

Keyword: it is not uncommon for patients with COPD to demonstrate mild to moderate hypoxemia and respiratory acidosis, as indicated in this patient's ABG result.

The PFT result of this patient shows an FEV1/FVC ratio less than 70%, suggesting an obstructive pattern. Furthermore, his FEV1 is between 50% and 79% of the predicted value. This is consistent with his diagnosis of moderate COPD.

Perioperative pulmonary complications of non-cardiac surgeries are common, and they are associated with substantial morbidity and mortality. Major risk factors include: advanced age (over 65), functional status, type of surgery and length of surgical time, history of COPD, general anesthesia, history of cerebral vascular accidents, emergency surgery, long-term steroid use, obesity, history of smoking and alcohol use, etc. This patient has many of these risk factors. Therefore, he is much more likely to develop peri-operative pulmonary complications comparing to general population.

To decide if he needs any additional test or preparations to optimize his pulmonary status, we should again start from the basics: history and physical. Any recent deterioration in his functional status, increase in his oxygen requirement, COPD exacerbation or respiratory infection should prompt further investigation and treatment accordingly. As for physical exam, mild expiratory wheezing might be anticipated. In that case, it may be prudent to communicate with this patient's primary care physician to find out his baseline pulmonary function, and if any intervention is warranted.

In addition, the American Society of Anesthesiologists (ASA) advocates that all patients presenting for surgery should be questioned regarding smoking, and provided with an appropriate consult for smoking cessation. Abstinence starting 3~8 weeks before surgery will significantly reduce the incidence of smoking related complications.

3. Medications: How would you instruct the patient about his medications? Does he need to stop or continue his medication for the surgery, such as albuterol, ASA, statins, etc.? Why or why not?

Keyword: Albuterol and ipratropium are important COPD medications for this patient. He should be advised to continue his routine regiment for his COPD management.

As for statins, the ASA recommends that surgical patients should stay on cholesterol medications to reduce risk of death.

In general, patients should be advised to take their routine thyroid medication to maintain their euthyroidism.

Aspirin should be continued during the perioperative period when it is prescribed as the secondary prevention of cardiovascular diseases or stroke. On the other hand, interruption of aspirin in primary prevention does not increase the perioperative risk, except in patients with diabetes. Therefore, if this patient is taking aspirin for primary prevention, it could be stopped before surgery.

Lisinopril is an angiotensin-converting-enzyme (ACE) inhibitor. ACE inhibitors are associated with significantly higher incidence of perioperative hypotension. Although there is a lack of consensus among anesthesiologists, many institutes instruct patients to continue ACE inhibitors until the day before surgery, and not take them on the day of surgery. For this particular case, the use of vasopressors may be restricted. Therefore, it is reasonable to follow the above recommendation.

Gabapentin should be continued for better post-operative pain control.

Unless the patient has specific vitamin deficiency, multi-vitamins are usually not necessary before surgery. Anesthesiologists should also inquire about the use of herbs or other supplements, and make recommendations accordingly.

4. Cardiac risks: Does this patient need a cardiology consult prior to surgery? Why or why not? Please address your specific concerns. At the preoperative anesthesia clinic, the patient tells you that he suffered atrial fibrillation 3 years ago and it was resolved by cardiac ablation 1 year ago. What is your response?

Keyword: although this patient has no documented history of coronary or cerebrovascular diseases, he has multiple risk factors, including age, tobacco use, history of hypertension, and history of PVD. A detailed history and physical is warranted to assess his perioperative cardiac risk.

Assuming negative history and physical findings on this patient for previous history of cardiac infarction, severe valvular diseases, symptomatic arrhythmia, or uncompensated congestive heart failure, the combined surgical and patient characteristics will predict a risk of a major adverse cardiac event in the range of 1% ~ 5%. According to the 2014 ACC/AHA Guideline on Perioperative Cardiovascular Evaluation and Management of Patients Undergoing Noncardiac Surgery, the functional capacity of this patient should be carefully assessed to guide further cardiovascular testing. If the patient demonstrates moderate or greater functional capacity (≥4 Metabolic Equivalent of Tasks, METs), no further testing is required. For patients with poor or unknown functional capacity (<4 METs), anesthesiologists should discuss with surgeons and other health providers to determine whether further testing will impact patient decision making (e.g., decision to perform the original surgery without delay or willingness to undergo cardiac interventions prior to surgery). For this patient, it is very likely that delaying the surgery for cardiac interventions (if indicated) may post substantial risk for cancer to progress, and thus he may lose the best window for surgical treatment. In that case, further testing may not provide any benefit for this patient.

For patients with the history of atrial fibrillation, a baseline EKG is recommended. Previous cardiology notes, including workup, possible etiology, previous echocardiogram, and previous treatment, will provide valuable information. If the patient is now completely symptom free, and not taking any medication for rate control or anticoagulation, no further testing is needed other than baseline EKG.

5. Nutrition: How do you assess his nutrition status? Will it affect his postoperative recovery?

Keyword: poor preoperative nutrition status would bes associated with slower post-operative wound healing, more susceptible to infection, and higher chance of decubitus ulcers. Thus, it may increase perioperative morbidity and mortality, and causes longer hospital stay.

A thorough history and physical can provide good assessment for the patient's nutrition status. When taking history, poor oral intake, recent weight loss, deteriorating muscle strength/functional capacity, frequent mucosal sores or skin ulcers are all indicators of malnutrition. Physical findings for poor nutrition status include: loss of subcutaneous fat/muscle mass, skin ulcer/mucosal sores, peripheral edema, conjunctival pallor, etc.

Serum albumin and pre-albumin level may help to confirm the existence and evaluate the severity of malnutrition. However, these tests are generally not indicated except for serious conditions. If malnutrition is suspected, thorough discussion with surgeons and the patient may be indicated for interventions prior to the surgery.

6. Tracheal stoma: At the preoperative anesthesia clinic, the patient askes you what to expect to live with a tracheal stoma, any preparation and precautions he should take, your responses?

Keyword: after the surgery, the patient's feeling of his respiration will be very different, for example to inspire the air inspired through the nose and mouth becomes meaningless, rather to draw the air by chest; a lot secretions are expected from stoma and needs a special care. I will refer the patient to see the tracheal stoma care team and the surgeon for specific instructions.

> **术 前 管 理** <

1. 气道：你如何评估这位患者的气道？有什么需要特别注意之处吗？以下哪一点可能会为气道评估提供最重要的信息：患者的病史及症状、查体和 CT 扫描结果？

要点：气道评估以及困难气道处理是麻醉医师需要掌握的基本技能。这项技能对与气道疾病尤其重要，因为这些疾病可能会对气道管理构成严峻的挑战。

详细的病史采集以及细致的体格检查往往是通向成功的第一步。如果这位患者存在呼吸困难的症状，这可能提示他有严重的喉部（气道）狭窄。另外，如果前倾位导致呼吸困难症状加重，这尤其预示着气道危机的可能性——在全麻诱导后可能会面临气道完全堵塞的局面。在这种情况下，可能需要考虑行清醒纤支镜插管，甚至清醒气管切开术。

放疗可能是一些喉癌患者治疗方案的一部分。这种治疗措施可能会引起上呼吸道以及下呼吸道的解剖结构改变，从而可能导致困难气管插管。在气道评估过程中，尤其需要注意检查头颈部活动能力、是否存在软组织水肿或纤维化、张口大小以及牙齿状况。

影像学检查是评估喉部肿瘤的另一项重要手段。它们是确定肿瘤的解剖性状，包括其大小、具体位置，与声门及其他气道结构的解剖关系的重要信息来源。

很多患者在手术前会在外科门诊接受间接喉镜的检查。外科医师可能会就喉部狭窄程度、肿瘤活动性及出血倾向等提供非常有价值的信息。在手术前一定不可低估与外科医师讨论各项检查结果以及手术方案的重要性。

2. 呼吸系统：请分析该患者的动脉血气以及肺功能检查的结果。有什么需要特别关注之处吗？这位患者还需要为优化他的肺部功能而做更多其他检查或术前准备吗？

要点：患有 COPD 的患者常伴发轻到中度的低氧血症及呼吸性酸中毒，这位患者的 ABG 也证明了这点。

他的 PFT 结果显示 FEV1/FVC 比例低于预期值的 70%，提示其阻塞性疾病的特点。另外，他的 FEV1 介于预期值的 50%～79%。这个结果与他中度 COPD 的诊断是一致的。

非心脏手术的围术期呼吸系统并发症很常见，而且这些并发症往往增加围术期发病率和死亡率。导致围术期呼吸系统并发症的危险因素包括：高龄（65 岁以上）、体能状态、手术类型及时长、既往 COPD 史、全麻、既往脑血管意外史、急诊手术、长期使用类固醇激素、肥胖、吸烟及酗酒史等。这位患者有多项上述危险因素。因此，他罹患围术期呼吸系统并发症的可能性要高于普通人群。

要决定他是否需要做更多的术前检查或准备来优化他的肺部功能，我们需要从最基本的病史和查体着手。如果患者出现近期体能状态下降，或者日常吸氧需求量增加，或者 COPD 恶化，或者呼吸道感染，那么他需要接受进一步的检查及相应治疗。在这位患者的查体过程中有可能发现轻度呼气相喘鸣，这是意料之中的。在这种情况下，为保险起见，可以考虑与患者的家庭医师沟通，以了解该患者的基础肺功能状态，并决定是否存在进一步诊疗的必要。

另外，美国麻醉医师学会（ASA）倡议对所有术前患者都应当询问吸烟史，并为戒烟提供适当的宣教。在手术前 3～8 周戒烟能够显著降低吸烟相关的并发症。

3. 术前用药：你如何指导这位患者的用药？对于沙丁胺醇、阿司匹林和他汀类药物等他正在使用的药物，在手术前需要暂停还是继续服用？为什么？

要点：沙丁胺醇和异丙托溴铵气雾剂对这位患者是重要的 COPD 药物。他应该继续按照他的日常剂量来控制其 COPD 症状。

至于他汀类药物，ASA 建议手术患者应当继续其胆固醇药物，以降低围术期死亡率。

一般来说，手术患者需要继续其甲状腺药物以维持甲状腺的正常功能状态。

如果这位患者服用 ASA 是为降低心血管疾病或中风风险的二级预防用药，他应当在围术期继续服药。与此相反，如果 ASA 是作为初级预防的药物，除了糖尿病患者以外，中断它并不增加围术期风险。因此，如果这位患者是因为初级预防而服用 ASA,可以考虑手术前停药。

赖诺普利是一种血管紧张素转化酶(ACE)抑制剂。ACE 抑制剂与围术期低血压发生率显著性增加相关。虽然现在在麻醉界还没有达成共识,但是很多医疗机构都建议患者坚持服用 ACE 抑制剂直到手术前一天,然后在手术当天停药。对于这个病例而言,术中升压药的使用可能会受到限制。因此,上述建议是一个合理的选择。

坚持服用加巴喷丁有助于更好地缓解术后疼痛。

除非患者存在特异性某种维生素缺乏,一般不建议术前服用维生素。麻醉医师同时也应当询问患者是否服用草药或其他保健品,并给予相应的术前指导。

4. 心血管风险:这位患者是否需要术前心内科会诊? 为什么? 请解释你是否有特殊考虑。在术前麻醉门诊,患者告诉你,说他 3 年前曾患有房颤,并于 1 年前经心导管消融治愈。你这时候怎么想?

要点:虽然这位患者并没有明确心血管或脑血管病史,他却存在多项相关的危险因素,包括年龄、吸烟史、高血压史,以及外周血管疾病史。详尽的病史采集和体格检查有助于进一步评估他的围术期心血管风险。

假设该患者既往没有以下疾病的病史及查体表现:心肌梗死史、严重心瓣膜病史,伴明显症状的心率失常,以及失代偿的慢性心力衰竭史,综合考虑患者及手术因素,本患者发生围术期严重心血管并发症的概率大概在 1%~5% 范围内。根据 2014 年发表的美国心内科学院/美国心脏学会(ACC/AHA)关于非心脏手术患者围术期心血管风险评估及管理指南,需要对这位患者的体能状态予以仔细评估,以进一步指导是否需要更多的心血管检查。如果这位患者能够胜任中度及以上强度的体能活动(≥4 METs),则不需要进一步的检查。如果该患者体能状态较差或无法准确评估(<4 METs),麻醉医师有必要与外科医师以及其他专科医师协商讨论,进一步的检查是否会影响到患者对手术的决定(比如该手术需要立刻进行还是可以等到完成相关心血管诊疗后再做)。对于这位患者来说,如果因为相应的心血管诊疗(假设存在相关指征)而延误手术,很有可能致使癌症进一步发展恶化的风险大大增加,从而导致该患者错过有效手术治疗的窗口期。如果是这种情况,那么进一步检查可能并不能为患者带来任何益处。

对于有房颤病史的患者,建议予以术前基础 EKG 检查。既往心内科病历记录,包括各种检查、可能的病因、既往超声心动图,以及既往治疗记录,都能够提供有价值的信息。如果这位患者完全没有任何症状,也不再服用任何控制心率或抗凝药物,那么除了基础 EKG 以外,不需要其他更多检查。

5. 营养:你如何评估他的营养状态?这会影响他的术后康复吗?

要点:术前营养不良与以下多项围术期并发症都相关:术后伤口愈合缓慢、感染机会增加,以及褥疮机会增加。由此,它可能进一步增加围术期并发症率和死亡率,并延长住院时间。

详尽的病史和查体能够为患者的营养状况提供有效评估。如果病史中出现进食饮水障碍、近来体重下降、肌肉力量/体能状态恶化、频繁黏膜破溃或皮肤溃疡等,都提示营养不良的可能。体检中提示营养不良的表现包括皮下脂肪/肌肉容量流失、皮肤溃疡/黏膜破溃、外周水肿和睑结膜苍白等。

人血白蛋白及前白蛋白水平能够帮助确诊营养不良,并对其严重程度予以评估。但是除非是非常严重的营养不良,一般并不需要常规做这些检查。如果怀疑存在营养不良的状况,需要考虑与外科医师及患者做深入讨论,以决定是否需要在手术前给予相应治疗。

6. 气管造口:在术前麻醉门诊,患者问你,他今后生活可能都需要气管造口,需要如何准备以及注意什么。你如何回答?

要点:术后患者呼吸的感觉会不一样,比如通过鼻子和嘴巴吸气没有意义,而是应该通过胸部扩张吸气;造口有大量分泌物需要特殊护理。建议患者与气管造口护理团队以及外科医师商量,以获得专业指导。

> **Intraoperative management** <

1. Airway management: The attending surgeon walked in the operating room (OR), and told you and your team that he will perform an awake

tracheotomy first. What is your response? Will an awake fiberoptic intubation be a valid alternative to safely secure his airway? Would you provide sedation to assist surgeons for the awake tracheostomy? If yes, please explain your choice of medication, doses. How do you monitor and ensure the proper and adequate level of sedation?

Keyword: if the surgeon requested an awake tracheostomy for this patient, I would like to find out his rationale behind his decision. There are several scenarios that an awake tracheostomy is preferred.

The first scenario is with severe supraglottic or glottic mass/stenosis. Awake fiberoptic intubation could be challenging under these conditions. An awake tracheostomy may be a better choice for airway management.

The second scenario is with a significant bleeding potential from the laryngeal mass. Copious bleeding in the airway can be devastating. It not only obscures the view from the fiberoptic scope thus making intubation impossible, but it can also induce coughing, aspiration, and even asphyxiation. Awake tracheostomy with minimal disturbance in the upper airway can avert a potential disaster.

The third scenario is with a mobile supraglottic mass that could cause complete airway obstruction. Any manipulation in the upper airway should be minimized.

In anticipation of a highly challenging airway, minimal sedation is usually the best strategy to avoid any airway compromise. However, on the other hand, awake tracheostomy often sounds frightening to patients. Therefore, a thorough explanation of this procedure and a strong rapport from anesthesia providers are essential to relieve their anxiety. If after these efforts, the patient is still so nervous that he cannot stay still and being cooperative with the surgery, a sedative with minimal effects on respiration such as dexmedetomidine may be considered. The goal is for the patient to remain conscious (able to communicate with either voice or other means) and tolerate the procedure. Dexmedetomidine can be delivered with a bolus of $0.5 \sim 1$ mcg/kg in $10 \sim 20$ minutes, then followed by infusion of $0.2 \sim 0.6$ mcg/kg/hr, titrating to effect. Standard ASA monitors are mandated throughout the procedure. The patient should remain conscious or easily arousable until the airway is secured by tracheostomy.

2. Monitoring: How would you monitor the patient during the surgery? Would you consider to place an arterial line? If yes, please explain how the arterial line would help with your anesthesia management. What about the central venous pressure (CVP) monitoring or a pulmonary artery catheter (PAC)? Why or why not?

Keyword: standard ASA monitors, including EKG, blood pressure with minimal interval of every 5 mins, pulse-oximetry, oxygen concentration in the breathing system, end-tidal $CO_2$, and body temperature, are mandatory for this case.

If there is no contraindication, an arterial line should be considered. It can provide more information about intraoperative ventilation status and hemodynamic stability. This patient has a moderate COPD. Intraoperative end-tidal $CO_2$ may not accurately reflect his arterial $CO_2$ level. Furthermore, given this patient's pulmonary comorbidity, his baseline oxygen requirement, and the lengthy surgery, it is perceivable that he may need ventilation support after surgery. ABG monitoring can provide guidance for these clinical decisions. As previously discussed, although this patient has no significant history of coronary heart or cerebrovascular diseases, his multiple risk factors may pose him a higher chance for perioperative cardiac complications. With arterial line, more accurate and real-time hemodynamic monitoring could potentially reduce these complications. Before placing the arterial line, anesthesiologists should discuss with surgeons about the potential flap harvest site to avoid any injury.

If adequate peripheral venous accesses are obtained, a central line or the PAC is not indicated for this case. Although CVP may provide some information about intravascular volume, it is generally not a good indicator. Usually significant blood loss or large fluid shift is not anticipated in this kind of surgery. Close attention to surgical field, blood loss, urine output, vital signs, and respiratory variation in arterial pulse pressure can give acceptable estimate for the patient's intraoperative volume status. Based on the history and physical, assuming this patient does not have significant pulmonary hypertension, left or right heart dysfunction, PAC is not necessary. However, if previous tests (such as echocardiogram) indicate any of the above conditions, PAC should be considered.

3. Volume status: Assuming the patient had some difficulty with eating and drinking for the last 3 weeks, how do you assess his volume status? Are there any clinical exams and tests indicated? Would you consider a volume expansion with fluid bolus prior to the surgery? If yes, what is your choice of fluid, and how much volume? What is your end-point for this treatment?

Keyword: this patient is highly like to be dehydrated, malnutrition, and electrolytes abnormality. Detailed history and physical can help to reveal clues of dehydration. Weakness, dizziness, confusion, palpitation, low volume or dark color of urine is all symptoms that suggest dehydration. Hypotension (including orthostatic hypotension), tachycardia, dry skin/mucosa, decreased skin turgor are potential signs of dehydration.

If the patient has demonstrated symptoms and signs of moderate to severe dehydration, further investigation and intervention should be considered before the surgery.

If the patient just has mild dehydration without significant changes in vital signs, it is reasonable to proceed with the surgery without delay. Pre-treatment with 500~1 000 cc of Lactate Ringer (LR) before induction might help achieve hemodynamic stability. Close monitoring of perioperative fluid status is recommended (see the above section for details), and the goal is to maintain euvolemia.

4. Endotracheal tube (ETT) and ventilation: Following the tracheotomy and the creation of a tracheal stoma, a steel reinforced ETT was inserted. What is the indication of a reinforced ETT here? Could a regular ETT work instead? Is there any special consideration with the ventilator setup comparing to a regular trans-oral ETT?

Keyword: a reinforced ETT is specially designed to be resistant to kinking. They are particularly useful for some of the head and neck surgeries where the ETT has to be bent away from the surgical field for better exposure. Regular ETTs are susceptible to kinking with such maneuvers, and can subsequently cause ventilation difficult or ever impossible. If no reinforced ETTs are available, regular ETTs can be used. In that case, both anesthesiologists and surgeons have to pay close attention to the ETT, and avoid bending it in a sharp angle.

As for the ventilator set up, there is no special consideration for reinforced ETTs via tracheostomy or tracheal stoma or suggests to cut down the tidal volume because of decreased dead space (mouth to trach).

5. Nerve monitoring: The attending surgeon requests no paralysis during the surgery because of intraoperative electromyography (EMG)/nerve monitoring. Do you agree? Which nerves do you think he will monitor and how? How would you ensure the patient's immobility during the surgery?

Keyword: for neck dissection/exploration procedures, several nerves, including braches from the trigeminal nerve, facial nerve, spinal accessory nerve, vague nerve, hypoglossal nerve, phrenic nerve, and brachial plexus, could be potentially injuried. Intraoperative nerve monitoring can help surgeons to identify or confirm nerve branches with motor component, and thus minimize unintentional injury. The most commonly monitored nerves during these procedures are the facial nerve and the spinal accessory nerve. Muscle movements can be monitored via EMG activity or directly observed upon stimulation.

Intraoperative administration of neuromuscular blockade agents can interfere with such a nerve monitoring, and render it ineffective. Therefore, after the initial muscle paralysis for intubation, routine use of neuromuscular blockade medications should be discouraged.

To maintain intraoperative stability, balanced general anesthesia with continuous infusion of a potent opioid such as remifentanil is chosen by many anesthesia providers. Remifentanil infusion has strong analgesic effect, with relative less impact on cardiovascular system. Another unique characteristic of remifentanil is its fast offset, which allows a smoother and faster emergence after a lengthy procedure.

6. Field avoidance: After induction and ETT placement, the operating room (OR) table was turned 180 degree away. The patient's head was positioned on the other side of anesthesia machine. Under such condition, could you provide a list of precautions you should take from an anesthesiologist's perspective?

Keyword: turning the OR table 180 - degree away from the anesthesia providers will decrease airway accessibility. Therefore, close communication among anesthesia providers, surgeons and nurses are essential to protect the integrity of the airway.

Before the turn, extensions for the anesthesia circuit and the sample line should be either installed or immediately available. Fraction of inspiratory oxygen (FiO$_2$) of 100% is preferred before the turn to prepare for any interruption in ventilation. All the cables and lines on the patient should have enough length and be arranged in the way that turning will cause minimal disruption in patient caring. During the turn, anesthesia providers should stay at the head of the bed to guard the airway, and take the leading role in coordinating this process. After the turn, the position and connection of the ETT should be examined. A flexible connector could be inserted between the ETT and the anesthesia circuit to prevent disconnection.

During the whole procedure, anesthesia providers should stay vigilant for any potential disconnection or malposition of the ETT, notify surgeons immediately when it happens, and act accordingly.

7. New onset of intraoperative atrial fibrillation (AF): Three and half hours into the surgery, you noticed the patient's heart rate became irregular. How would you differentiate AF from other cardiac arrhythmia? Would you treat it? If yes, How? Would you tell surgeons to abort or wrap up the surgery as soon as possible? What do you think the underlining causes of his AF might be? Would you call the cardiologist for an emergent intraoperative consult? Would the new onset AF change this patient's perioperative outcome? If yes, what can be done to minimize the AF associated complications?

Keyword: Atrial fibrillation (AF) is one of the most common arrhythmias encountered in the OR. Characteristic features of AF include: absence of P waves, narrow QRS complexes, and irregular R – R intervals. Usually AF is easily recognized on anesthesia monitors. If there is any uncertainty, a 12 – lead EKG is recommended for definitive diagnosis.

Management of intraoperative AF depends on a few factors.

First, hemodynamic stability. For unstable AF, surgeons should be notified, and immediate cardioversion is warranted. If the unstable AF persists or recurs after cardioversion, intravenous bolus of amiodarone could be given before another attempt of cardioversion. Meanwhile, surgeons should be advised to either abort or speed up the surgery.

Second, ventricular rate. For stable AF, rate control should be achieved with the target ventricular rate under 100 bpm, ideally between 60 and 80 bpm.

Drugs of choice are beta blockers or calcium channel blockers, such as metoprolol or diltiazem.

For stable AF with a ventricular rate of $60 \sim 80$ bpm, no immediate treatment is required. However, possible underlying causes should be explored. The most common precipitating factors for AF are electrolyte abnormalities (especially hypokalemia or hypomagnesemia) and hypovolemia. Other potential causes include myocardial ischemia (this would have a high probability for this patient), pulmonary embolism, etc.

In general, cardiology consult is not necessary for intraoperative AF management. However, persistent or recurrent unstable AF may benefit from their input.

The loss of atrial kick secondary to AF may decrease the cardiac output by up to 30%, thus comprise the patient's cardiac function, and cause more perioperative complications. Vigilant monitoring and prompt treatment are key steps to minimize complications associated with intraoperative AF.

8. Fluids versus vasopressors: After 6 hours into the surgery, surgeons started working on the flap (with skin and muscle) for neck reconstruction. The patient's BP was trending down, and a fluid bolus of 1,000 mL LR was given. Hemoglobin level was checked with the result of 9.2 g/dL. You would like to administer phenylephrine. However, the attending surgeon strongly opposed this idea because he was concerned that the vasoconstrictive effect might cause ischemia to the flap. What is your response?

Keyword: the administration of vasopressors in microvascular free flap surgery is controversial. Many microvascular surgeons are still concerned about potential flap ischemia from intraoperative usage of vasopressors, despite recent studies that have shown no increase in flap failure or perioperative complications associated with pressors. On the other hand, too much intraoperative fluid administration (over 7 liters) is one of the contributing factors to free flap complications.

Intraoperative usage of pressors should be a joint decision between anesthesiologists and surgeons. If all the potential correctable causes of hypotension have been addressed, then a pressor should be considered to maintain hemodynamic stability, and this should be discussed with surgeons. Potential causes of intraoperative hypotension include intraoperative bleeding/hypovolemia, excessive anesthetic depth, cardiac ischemia/arrhythmia, abnormal electrolytes, allergic reaction, etc.

9. Emergence crisis: At the end of surgery, ETT tube was removed and the surgeons were maturing the stoma. Shortly after the patient's head was turned back to you, some pink foam secretion mixed with some fresh bright blood came out of the tracheal. Meanwhile, his $SpO_2$ was trending down to 80%. What are the most likely causes? How do you differentiate flash pulmonary edema vs. tracheal injury? What are your treatment options? Small facial mask with 100% $O_2$ had minimal effect. What is your next step?

Keyword: judging from the clinical presentation, two potential diagnoses should be considered: pink foam secretion suggests pulmonary edema, while fresh bright blood points to surgical bleeding. If symptoms are mild, vital signs and oxygen saturation level are relative stable, non-invasive intervention (such as gentle suction and supplemental oxygen via tracheal mask) can be attempted first. However, for this case, the patient's $SpO_2$ has dropped to a critical level of 80%, immediate tracheal suction followed by re-intubation via the stoma is probably the best choice to prevent further deterioration. After laryngectomy, mask ventilation or oral-tracheal intubation is not possible, and should never be attempted. Once the patient is stabilized, further examination and testing can be carried out for more definitive diagnosis and management.

Once the airway is secured, surgeons should carefully examine the stoma for any surgical site bleeding. Gentle suction and/or bronchoscopy may facilitate visualization of the bleeding site.

If pulmonary edema is suspected，cardiac dysfunction and fluid overload are the two most common underlying causes. A 12‑lead EKG, cardiac enzyme tests，chest X-ray，serum brain natriuretic peptide（BNP）level，and bedside echocardiogram may provide valuable information to guide the diagnosis and treatment. Diuresis may help alleviate the symptoms. Prolonged intubation and post-operative ventilation support may be indicated，depending on the patient's condition.

## > 术 中 管 理 <

1. 气道管理：主治外科医师走进手术室,告知你和你的团队,他将首先做清醒气管切开术。你会如何应对？纤维支气管镜引导下清醒气管插管将会是一个有效并安全的气道管理的替代措施吗？在协助外科医师行清醒气管切开术时,你会为患者提供镇静措施吗？ 如果会,请列举你将选择的药物及剂量。你将采用哪些监测手段来保障患者充分并安全的镇静程度？

要点：如果外科医师要求为这个患者做清醒气管切开术,我会和他探讨他做出这个决定的理由。以下几种情形,外科医师可能会选择清醒气切。

第一种情形是患者存在非常严重的声门上或声门狭窄。这种情形会对纤维支气管镜下清醒气管插管构成一定挑战。清醒气切或许是气道管理的更佳选择。

第二种情形是喉部肿瘤具有显著出血倾向。气道内大量出血可能诱发严重后果,它不仅可以使纤维支气管镜的视野模糊,从而导致无法进行气管插管,它还能诱发呛咳、误吸、甚至窒息。清醒气切可以最大程度地减少对声门上气道的扰动,从而避免可能的灾难。

第三种情形是活动性较强的声门上肿物,它可能造成气道的完全堵塞。在这种情况下需要尽量减少任何对声门上气道的扰动性操作。

当我们预期气道管理将会具有高度挑战性时,给予患者的镇静越少越好。这种策略有助于避免气道管理事故。然而另一方面,清醒气切往往会对患者造成很大心理压力。因此，麻醉医师向患者详细解释该手术操作，并提供强大的心理支持，有助于缓解患者的焦虑情绪。如果经过这些尝试后，患者仍然还是非常紧张，无法保持静止来配合手术，可以考虑使用一些呼吸抑制最小的镇静药物，如右美托咪定。镇静的目标是患者能够耐受手术的同时，仍然保持清醒的意识（能够通过语音或其他方式交流）。右美托咪定的给药方式是：$10\sim20$ min 内快速静脉注射 $0.5\sim1~\mu g/kg$，然后静脉维持 $0.2\sim0.6~\mu g/(kg\cdot h)$，根据患者的反应微调给药速度。整个手术过程都必须予以 ASA 标准监测。患者在术中应当保持清醒或轻易就能唤醒的意识状态，直到气管切开完成以确保气道安全。

2. 术中监测：手术中如何对这位患者进行监测？你会考虑放置动脉导管吗？如果会，请解释动脉导管如何能够协助术中麻醉管理。那么中心静脉压监测（CVP）以及肺动脉导管呢（PAC）？为什么？

要点：ASA 标准监测，包括心电图、至少每 5 min 一次的血压监测、血氧饱和度、呼吸系统内给氧浓度、呼末二氧化碳分压和体温等都是这个手术必须监测的指标。

如果没有相关禁忌证，可以考虑放置动脉导管。它能够为术中通气以及血流动力学提供更多信息。这位患者患有中度 COPD，术中呼末二氧化碳分压有可能不能准确地反映其动脉二氧化碳水平。另外，综合考虑这位患者的呼吸系统病史、基础吸氧需求，以及这个手术的时长，可以预见他很有可能术后需要机械通气支持。动脉血气分析有助于为这些临床决策提供指导数据。另外，如上文讨论，虽然该患者并没有明确心血管或脑血管病史，他存在多项危险因素，从而会增加他围术期心脏并发症的风险。动脉导管可以通过提供更加准确的实时血压监测，从而降低相关风险。在放置动脉导管之前，麻醉医师需要向外科医师询问皮瓣可能的采集部位，以免造成损伤。

如果能够建立足够的静脉通路，中心静脉或者肺动脉插管对于这个手术必要性不大。虽然 CVP 有可能为血管内容量评估提供一定信息，但是它往往不是一个好的评估指标。通常这类手术不会出现大量失血或体液转移。密切监测术野、失血量、尿量、生命体征，以及有创脉压呼吸变异度等，一般能够对患者的术中容量状态做出可以接受的评估。基于病史和查体，如果该患者不存在肺动脉高压，左心或右心功能不全，不需要放置 PAC。然而，如果既往检查（如超声心动图）提示有任何上述病变，可以考虑术中 PAC 监测。

3. 容量状态：假设该患者在过去 3 周内存在进食及饮水障碍，你如何评估他的体内容量状态？他需要做什么相关临床或化验检查吗？手术前你是否考虑给予补液扩容？如果是，你用哪种液体，给多少？这项治疗措施的终点是什么？

要点：该患者很可能出现脱水、营养不良和电解质异常。详细的病史和查体可以为脱水诊断提供线索。虚弱、眩晕、意识混乱、心悸、尿量减少或颜色加深等都是提示存在脱水的症状。低血压（尤其是体位性低血压）、心率加速、皮肤/黏膜干燥、皮肤弹性降低等都是脱水可能的体征。

如果该患者具有中度到重度的脱水症状和体征，有必要考虑术前的进一步检查和干预。

如果该患者的脱水表现轻微，不存在生命体征的改变，不要拖延直接手术是一个合理的选择。诱导前可以考虑给予 500～1 000 mL 的林格液（LR）预处理，这可能有助于维持其血流动力学稳定。围术期建议严密监测体液容量状态（具体措施参见上节），目标是维持其正常体液容量。

4. 气管内导管（ETT）和通气设置：在气管切开和气管造瘘后，气管内插入一个加强型 ETT。为什么要使用加强 ETT？能够用普通 ETT 来替代吗？与经口插管的普通 ETT 相比，在呼吸机的通气设置上有什么需要特殊考虑的吗？

要点：加强 ETTs 是一种特殊设计的气管内导管，具有抗打结扭折的特点。它们尤其常用于一些头颈手术，因为这些手术中有时会将 ETTs 从手术野处弯折，从而达到更好的暴露效果。这种操作很容易引起普通 ETTs 发生扭结，而导致通气困难，甚至无法通气。如果实在没有加强 ETTs 可以使用，可以尝试用普通 ETTs。这时需要麻醉医师和外科医师都注意术中 ETT 的位置，以免发生极度锐角弯曲的现象。

至于呼吸机的通气设置，对于经气管切开或气管瘘口插入的加强 ETT 不需要有什么特殊处理；或者是建议减少潮气量，因为无效腔量减少（由口到气管段的无效腔量）。

5. 神经监测：主治外科医师因为术中需要做肌电图（EMG）/神经监测而要求不要给肌肉松弛药物。你同意他的要求吗？他在术中会对哪些神经进行监测，如何监测？你如何能够保证患者在术中保持不动？

要点：在颈部清扫/探查术中，有些神经或其分支，包括三叉神经、面神经、副脊神经、迷走神经、舌下神经、膈神经和臂丛神经等，都有可能受到损伤。术中神经监测能够帮助外科医师定位并确认那些具有运动功能的神经（分支），从而减少意外损伤。在这些手术中，最常监测的神经是面神经和副脊神经。这些神经支配的肌肉运动可以通过刺激该神经后观测 EMG 或者直接观察肌肉收缩。

术中使用神经肌肉阻断药物可以干扰神经监测，而导致其失效。因此，在诱导时使用肌松药协助插管后，术中一般不建议常规使用神经肌肉阻断药物。

为维持术中稳定，很多麻醉医师选用均衡的全麻方案辅以静脉滴注强效阿片类药物，例如瑞芬太尼。瑞芬太尼滴注具有强效镇痛效果，而且它对心血管系统的作用相对较弱。瑞芬太尼的另外一个独特的性能是其药效时程非常短，这有助于患者在较长的手术后顺利迅速苏醒。

6. 远离术野：在麻醉诱导及气管插管完成后，手术台被旋转 180°。患者的头部位于麻醉机对面的位置。在这种情况下，从麻醉医师的角度看，你能列举出哪些需要注意的事项？

要点：手术台旋转 180°会造成麻醉医师无法有效接近气道区域。因此，术中麻醉医师、外科医师，以及手术护士间的密切交流对于保护气道的安全至关重要。

在转动手术台前，麻醉机呼吸回路以及采样管都需要有其相应的延伸管，要么已经安装好，要么可以立刻安装。吸入氧浓度（$FiO_2$）最好在转动手术台前设置为 100%，以便应对转动时造成的通气暂停。与患者直接连接的各条线路及管道都需要有足够的长度，而且最好排列有序，这样在转动时尽量减少对患者的影响。在转动时，麻醉医师需要随时保持在患者头部的位置，保护气道，领导并协调手术室团队完成患者的体位转换。转动完成后，气管插管的位置和连接需要重新检查。在 ETT 和麻醉机呼吸回路间可以放置一个可弯曲连接管，以防止意外脱开。

在整个手术过程中，麻醉医师需要对各种可能发生的 ETT 脱开或折断情况予以高度警惕。一旦发生上述情况,立即通知外科医师,并采取相应措施。

7. 术中新发房颤:手术进行 3.5 个小时后,你发现患者的心律变得不规则。你如何区分房颤和其他心律失常? 你会予以治疗吗? 如果会,如何治疗? 你会要求外科医师终止手术或尽快完成手术吗? 你认为发生房颤的内在原因是什么? 你会紧急传呼心血管内科做术中会诊吗? 这种术中新发的房颤会影响该患者的围术期预后吗? 如果会,你要怎样做才能减少房颤相关的并发症呢?

要点:房颤是手术室中最常遇到的心律失常之一。房颤的典型特征包括:P波消失、狭窄性 QRS 波型、不规则性 R－R 间隔等。通常房颤在麻醉监护仪上比较容易辨识。如果存在任何疑虑,建议做 12 导联心电图以便确诊。

术中房颤的处理措施取决于以下几点:

首先,血流动力学稳定性。对于不稳定型房颤,应当告知外科医师,并即刻行电转复。如果电转复后,不稳定型房颤仍然持续或再次发作,可以先给予静脉注射胺碘酮,然后再次尝试电转复。这时需要向外科医师建议要么终止,要么尽快完成手术。

其次,室性心率。对于稳定型房颤,室性心率应当控制在 100 次/min 以下,最好是在 60～80 次/min。可以选择的药物包括 β 受体拮抗剂和钙离子通道拮抗剂,例如美托乐尔和地尔硫䓬。

对于室性心率在 60～80 次/min 的稳定性房颤,不需要立刻采用任何治疗措施,但是有必要考虑调查其潜在的诱因。术中房颤最常见的诱因是电解质异常(尤其是低血钾或低血镁)和低血容量。其他可能的诱因包括心肌缺血(该患者最可能的原因)、肺栓塞等。

术中房颤通常不需要心内科会诊,但是如果出现顽固性或反复发作不稳定房颤,心血管内科的意见还是有重要价值的。

房颤可以造成心房丧失驱血功能,从而降低心输出量,降低程度可高达 30%。这些改变会进一步导致心脏功能受损,并增加围术期并发症。严密的监测和及时的治疗是降低围术期房颤相关并发症的关键步骤。

8. 补液还是升压药:手术进行 6 个小时后,外科医师为颈部重建开始着手皮瓣处理（包括皮肤和肌肉组织）。患者的血压缓慢下降，给予 1 000 mL LR 快速补液后，复查血红蛋白水平为 92 g/L。你计划使用去氧肾上腺素，但是外科医师表示强烈反对，因为他担心此药的血管收缩作用可能会导致皮瓣缺血。你如何应对？

要点：在显微血管游离皮瓣手术中使用血管升压药是存在争议的。虽然最新研究表明，术中使用血管升压药并不增加皮瓣移植失败率或围术期并发症，但是许多显微血管外科医师仍然坚信升压药可能会造成皮瓣缺血。另一方面，术中补液太多（超过 7 L）是引发游离皮瓣并发症的重要诱因之一。

术中是否使用升压药物需要由麻醉医师和外科医师协商共同决定。如果已经对可能造成术中低血压的各种可纠正诱因，都已经采取了相应措施，这时候应该考虑使用升压药来维持血流动力学稳定性。这一决定需要及时与外科医师沟通。可能造成术中低血压的诱因包括术中出血/低血容量、麻醉过深、心肌缺血/心律失常、电解质异常和过敏反应等。

9. 苏醒期危机：手术即将结束时，ETT 已拔除，外科医师正在做气管瘘口成型。当患者头部重新转过来后，一些粉红色泡沫状分泌物，夹杂着一些鲜红色新鲜血液从气管中流出。这时候，患者血氧饱和度下降至 80%。最有可能的诊断是什么？你如何鉴别是急性肺水肿还是气管损伤？你的救治方案是什么？如果面罩给100% 氧却收效甚微，你下一步会如何处理？

要点：根据上述临床表现，需要考虑以下两个主要的鉴别诊断：粉红色泡沫状分泌物提示肺水肿，而鲜红色新鲜血液则表明手术出血的可能。如果相关症状轻微，生命体征及血氧饱和度平稳，可以先尝试一些非创伤性治疗措施（比如轻柔吸引分泌物，以及通过面罩给氧）。然而，对于这个患者来说，他的血氧饱和度已经降至 80% 这一危险数值，为防止病情进一步恶化，立刻予以气管吸引，然后通过气管瘘口行气管插管可能是最佳处理方案。在全喉切除术后，面罩给氧或者经口气管插管都是不可行的，而且坚决不应当尝试。患者的病情稳定以后，可以做进一步的检查以便获取准确诊断，并指导治疗。

在确保气道安全以后，外科医师可以仔细检查气管瘘口，是否存在手术部位出血。轻柔吸引以及纤支镜可能有助于直接观察到潜在的出血点。

如果怀疑是肺水肿,那么心功能不全和补液过量是两个最常见的诱因。12 导联心电图、心肌酶谱检查、胸部 X 线片、血清脑利钠肽（BNP）水平,以及床旁心动超声都能够为指导诊断和治疗提供重要信息。利尿剂可以帮助缓解相关症状。取决于患者的病情,有可能需要术后延长气管插管以及机械通气支持。

---

> ### **Postoperative management** <

1. Pain management：How would you assess the patient's pain after surgery? What is your goal, and what is your plan for pain management?

Keyword：adequate pain control after surgery is not only crucial for patient's comfort and recovery, but it can also reduce risk of post-operative complications. Pain is highly subjective, and varies greatly among patients. Therefore, pain assessment should rely on each patient's own description, as well as some objective measurements.

When the patient is unconscious or unable to effectively communicate, vital signs, breathing pattern, facial expressions, and body movements could all be used for pain assessment. Common signs of pain include：tachycardia, hypertension, diaphoresis, tachypnea, breath holding or splinting, frowning or grimacing, moaning or crying, motor rigidity or restless, etc. If the patient is awake, self-report pain score is more reliable. The most commonly used pain assessment tools include：visual analogue pain scale, numerical rating pain scale, and Wong-Baker faces pain scale.

Multi-modal approach provides the safest and the most effective analgesia for post-operative patients. Acetaminophen and non-steroidal anti-inflammatory drugs（NSAIDs）are useful adjunctive analgesics for mild to moderate pain. Opioids are reserved for moderate to severe pain.

The goal of post-operative pain management is twofold：one is to relieve pain and provide comfort for each patient；the other is to minimize the medication associated side effects and complications. Frequent pain assessment is essential for post-operative pain management. At the same time, vigilant monitoring for over-sedation or respiratory depression should be implemented to prevent opioid overdose.

2. Pneumonia: On postoperative day (POD) 2, the patient remained on ventilator, chest X-ray (CXR) suggested bilateral infiltrates. The ICU physician wrote in progress note that this might be caused by improper intraoperative ventilation or ventilator induced lung injury (VILI). What is your response? Are there strategies to prevent this injury from happening?

Keyword: prolonged intubation is defined as the failure to extubate within 24 hours after the surgery. It is one of the serious post-operative pulmonary complications. The potential underlying causes should be investigated and treated accordingly. Based on the clinical picture described above, the following differential diagnoses should be considered: ventilator-associated pneumonia, aspiration pneumonia, congestive heart failure, atelectasis, COPD exacerbation, acute respiratory distress syndrome (ARDS), etc. Further testing, such as ABG, CBC, tracheal secretion culture, EKG, echocardiogram, serum BNP, serial chest X-ray, chest CT, may help with the diagnosis.

VILI is one of the known contributing factors to the development of ARDS, especially for patients with pulmonary comorbidities. However, there are no clinical symptoms, signs, changes in physiological variables, or bedside investigations that are specific to detect VILI. Therefore, it is easier to speculate than prove that improper intraoperative ventilation is the direct cause of post-operative respiratory failure.

Although the exact pathophysiological mechanism of VILI remains unclear, regional lung over-distention when ventilated at high volume, atelectrauma when ventilated at low volume, and biotrauma have all been suggested as the underlying causes of such injury. Multiple ventilation strategies have subsequently developed to reduce lung injury: lower tidal volume to limit lung over-distention; higher positive end-expiratory pressure (PEEP) to decrease atelactrauma, and recruitment maneuver to prevent atelectasis and minimize ventilation heterogeneity.

3. Emergency airway management: On POD 4, the surgeon posted an emergent neck exploration for flap hematoma and necrosis. What is your plan to secure the airway? What is your approach to avoid damaging the tracheal mucosa?

Keyword: as discussed above, mask ventilation or oral-tracheal intubation is not possible after laryngectomy. The only way to secure the airway under this condition is to intubate through the stoma.

The fresh created stoma is easy to be injured during ETT insertion, and the ETT could enter into a teared mucosal layer results in unable to ventilation. I would preforme this when the patient is awake and breathing spontaneously by instilling 2% lidocaine 2~4 mL into the stoma, then very gently advance the well lubricated ETT till and confirmed by etCO$_2$ waveform. Even, it is recommended to be guided by fiberoptic scope. Furthermore, low pressure, high volume ETTs has been proved to cause less ischemic mucosal damage. Manometer may be used to confirm the cuff pressure of the ETT.

4. Conversation with family members: After the surgery, the attending surgeon set up a meeting with the patient's family members. He explained the flap complication was due to tissue edema, which is partly caused by anesthesia fluids overload and vasopressor usage. What is your response?

Keyword: modern surgery is essentially a multidisciplinary team work. Effective communication among surgeons, anesthesiologists, nurses, surgical technologists, and other involving health providers can promote patient safety and decrease perioperative complications. Once an adverse event or complication occurs, a timely debriefing or huddle allows team members to review and analyze this event from different angles. Thus, it may provide insight into the potential causes, guide further treatment, and improve patient care.

As for the flap complication, a thorough and candid conversation should be initiated between surgeons and anesthesiologists, to explore all the probable causes based on current guidelines and evidence. If anesthesia is suspected as a potential contributing factor, the attending anesthesiologist should accompany the attending surgeon to the family meeting. We should present the truth to the patient and his family, express sympathy to them, and provide our expertise in explaining probable anesthesia related complications. It is our responsibility as a doctor to be honest, forthright, and always act in the patient's best interest.

## 〉 术 后 管 理 〈

1. 疼痛管理：你如何对患者的术后疼痛进行评估？你如何制定术后镇痛的目标，具体是怎样计划的？

要点：充分的术后镇痛不仅对于患者的康复和舒适至关重要，而且它还有助于减少术后并发症。疼痛具有高度的主观性，不同的患者对于疼痛的感受会有很大的差别。因此，疼痛评估不仅需要根据患者的主观描述来判断，而且也需要根据客观指标来衡量。

当患者意识不清，或者无法有效沟通时，生命体征、呼吸方式、面部表情、肢体运动等都可以用于疼痛评估。疼痛的常见表现包括心跳加速、高血压、大汗淋漓、呼吸加速、屏息式呼吸或保护型呼吸、皱眉或做鬼脸、呻吟或哭闹、运动僵硬或者烦躁不安等。如果患者足够清醒，自报疼痛分数是更加可信的疼痛评估手段。最常用的疼痛评估手段包括视觉模拟疼痛分级、数量化疼痛分级和 Wang-Baker 面部表情疼痛分级。

多模式方案能够为术后患者提供最安全最有效的镇痛管理。对乙酰氨基酚和非甾体抗炎药（NSAID）是治疗轻度到中度疼痛的非常有效的辅助镇痛药物。阿片类药物一般用于中度到重度疼痛的处理。

术后镇痛管理的目标需要从两个方面来考虑：一方面是缓解疼痛，使每一个患者尽量舒适；另一方面则是尽量减少与镇痛药物相关的不良反应和并发症。定时而频繁的疼痛评估对于术后疼痛管理具有重要意义。同时，也需要对可能发生的呼吸抑制或过度镇静制定严格的监测措施，以防止阿片类药物过量。

2. 肺炎：术后第 2 天，患者仍然需要机械辅助通气，胸部 X 线片提示双侧浸润性改变。重症监护医师在病程记录中写道：这有可能是术中不当通气或者呼吸机诱发的肺损伤（VILI）所致的结果。你如何反应？有什么方法可以避免这种损伤的发生吗？

要点：延长气管插管的定义是手术结束后 24 个小时以内无法拔除气管导管。它是一种严重的术后呼吸系统并发症。对于可能的潜在诱因，需要予以调查，并进行相应的治疗。根据上述的临床表现，需要考虑以下一些鉴别诊断：呼吸机相关的肺炎、吸入性肺炎、充血性心力衰竭、肺不张、COPD 恶化、急性呼吸窘迫综合征（ARDS）等。更多检查，例如 ABG、CBC、气管分泌物培养、EKG、超声心动、血清 BNP、系列胸片和胸部 CT 等都可能帮助明确诊断。

VILI 是导致 ARDS 的已知诱因之一，尤其是对于那些本身存在基础肺部病变的患者。然而，目前还没有任何一种临床症状，或体征，或生理指标的改变，或床旁检查，可以非常特异性地检测到 VILI 的存在。因此，术中不当通气直接导致术后呼吸衰竭的结论更可能是源于猜测，而不是直接的证据。

虽然 VILI 具体的病理生理机制目前尚不明确，但是潮气量过大导致的局部肺过张，潮气量不足导致的不张性肺损伤，以及生物损伤等，都认为是造成 VILI 的潜在诱因。由以上理论衍生发展出一系列通气策略，以降低可能的肺损伤：低潮气量可以限制肺过张，更高的呼气末正压（PEEP）可以减少不张性肺损伤，肺复张操作可以防止肺不张，并减少通气异质性。

3. 紧急气道管理：术后第 4 天，外科医师因皮瓣血肿坏死，拟行紧急颈部探查术。你计划如何确保气道安全？为避免气管黏膜损伤，你需要采取哪些措施？

要点：如上文讨论，在全喉切除术后，面罩给氧或者经口气管插管都是不可行的。在这种情况下，唯一可行的确保气道安全的方法是经气管瘘口行气管插管。

插入 ETT 时，很容易引起新造的气管瘘口损伤，ETT 可能进入撕裂的黏膜层导致无法通气。我会在患者清醒，保留自主通气的情况下，经瘘口滴入 2% 的利多卡因 2~4 mL，然后轻轻地置入充分润滑的 ETT，直到经 etCO$_2$ 波形证明导管在位。甚至是建议经纤维支气管镜引导下插管。另外，有证据显示，低压力高容量的 ETT 引起黏膜缺血性损伤的可能性较小。压力监测器可以用来核对 ETT 气囊压力。

4. 家属谈话：手术后，外科医师安排了一次家属会议。他解释说，皮瓣的并发症是组织水肿的结果，而组织水肿在一定程度上是因为术中麻醉补液过量和术中使用血管升压药。你如何应对？

要点：现代手术实际上是一个多科室的团队合作。外科医师、麻醉医师、护士、外科技术员，以及其他与手术相关的医务工作者之间的有效沟通，都有助于提高患者安全，减少围术期并发症。一旦发生了不良事件或并发症，及时的团队总结和汇报可以帮助团队成员，从各个不同的角度来回顾和分析这一事件。这样做有助于挖掘事件发生的潜在诱因，指导下一步的诊疗，从而改善患者的医疗质量。

对于皮瓣相关的并发症，麻醉医师有必要与外科医师进行详尽坦诚的对话，根据当前现有的证据和指南，探讨各种诱因的可能性。如果与麻醉相关的因素被认定为可能的诱因，主治麻醉医师应当与主治外科医师一起出席患者家属会议。我们需要向患者及其家属公布实情，向他们表达同情之心。如果存在可能与麻醉相关的并发症，向他们提供专业的说明和解释。作为一名医师，诚实且坦率，总是把患者利益放在首位是我们的天职。

Dongdong Yao

姚东东

# 6 Anesthesia management for left adrenalectomy of pheochromocytoma

## 嗜铬细胞瘤患者左肾上腺切除术的麻醉管理

> **Basic information** <

A 45 years old female with recurrent episodes of headache and tachycardia, diaphoresis, dizziness for 3 months and progressively getting worse. She has been diagnosed for pheochromocytoma of left adrenal gland and has been scheduled for laparoscopic left adrenalectomy.

Co-morbidities: hypertension (5 years), left thyroid tumor resected 5 years (unknown etiology), COPD (chronic obstructive pulmonary disease), IBS (irritable bowel syndrome), fibromyalgia.

PE: Wt 76 kg, BP 180/98, HR 89, RR 16, T 36.7, $SaO_2$ 97% on room air.

Medications: Diovan, HCTZ, albuterol, atrovent, lyric, Neurontin, albuterol inhaler as needed.

Lab tests: WBC 8.9, Hgb 11, Platelet 235; Na 138, K 3.3, Cl 99, $HCO_3^-$ 25, BUN 23, Cr. 1.5; 24 hr urine Vanillylmandelic acid (VMA) increased, serum eipnephrine 560 ng/mL, norepinephrine 25 ng/mL. Plasma and urine free metepinephrine were significantly elevated ($>$3.5 mg, normal$<$1.7 mg), urine 24 hrs VMA ($>$24 mg, normal$<$5 mg) and HVA (homovanillic acid$>$32 mg, normal$<$15 mg) were elevated as well.

ECG：SR 86，LVH，ST - T nonspecific changes.

PFT：TLV (total lung volume) 1,300 mL，FEV1 65% (predicted)，FEV1/FEV = 75%.

## 基 本 信 息

病史：45 岁女性患者，反复发作头痛、心动过速、出汗、头晕 3 个月，并逐渐恶化。诊断为左肾上腺嗜铬细胞瘤，拟行腹腔镜下左肾上腺切除术。

并发症：高血压 5 年、左甲状腺肿瘤切除术 5 年(病因不详)、慢性阻塞性肺病、肠易激综合征和纤维肌痛症。

查体：体重 76 kg，血压 180/98 mmHg，HR 89 次/min，RR 16 次/min，T 36.7 ℃，空气下 $SaO_2$ 97%。

用药：缬沙坦、氢氯噻嗪、沙丁胺醇、异丙托溴、lyric 和加巴喷丁，必要时使用沙丁胺醇吸入器。

实验室检查：白细胞 $8.9×10^9$/L，血红蛋白 110 g/L，血小板 $235×10^9$/L，钠 138 mmol/L，钾 3.3 mmol/L，氯 99 mmol/L，$HCO_3^-$ 25 mmol/L，尿素 4.09 mmol/L(尿素氮 8.19 mmol/L)，肌酐 132.6 $\mu$mol/L;24 小时尿香草扁桃酸 (VMA)升高，血清肾上腺素 560 ng/mL，去甲肾上腺素 25 ng/mL。血浆和尿游离钾肾上腺素显著升高(>3.5 mg，正常<1.7 mg)，尿 24 小时 VMA (>24 mg,正常<5 mg)和 HVA (高香草酸>32 mg，正常<15 mg)也升高。

ECG：窦性心律，86 次/min，左心室肥厚，ST - T 无特异性变化。

PFT：肺总容量 1 300 mL，FEV1 65%(预测)，FEV1/FEV = 75%。

## > Preoperative management <

1. Additional tests: any additional tests needed, such as echocardiography, arterial blood gas, etc.

Keypoint: open question format, the underline is to know whether the candidate consider this patient is ready for surgery? or any concern of perioperative complications.

2. What is pheochromocytoma, can you describe its clinical manifestations? Do this patient's symptoms and signs meet the profile? Would the surgery cure the disease? What would be the complications if left not treated?

Keypoint: knowledge about the disease and its associated pathophysiology and outcomes.

3. Pharmacological preparation: what is the typical pharmacological preparation, why? List the agent to be used, how long should the patient be on alpha-adrenergic blocker and how do you assess the preparation is therapeutically satisfied? Your colleague suggests adding beta blocker, do you agree?

Keypoint: adrenalectomy for pheochromocytoma is a classic case which requiring a through and careful planning and preparation, because of high perioperative morbidity and mortality. This question is to test the candidate's knowledge on the underline pathophysiology changes caused by excessive secretion of catecholamine resulted in intravascular volume depletion, the pharmacological preparation, the drugs, the duration, and the assess of the restoration of intravascular volume.

4. Why do not measure the plasma epinephrine directly, instead to measure the metepinephrine and 24 hr urine VMA?

Keypoint: underline the common lab tests and their implication of clinical diagnosis for the confirmation and severity.

5. Preoperative conversation: will you let your resident to obtain the anesthesia consent? Would it be different the preoperative conservation carried

by you versus your resident? How much would you discuss the possible intraoperative crisis, such as severe hypertension or hypotension, possible postoperative ventilation, etc. with the patient?

Keypoint: test the candidate's ability for an in-depth assessment for this special disease, knowledge of some details which may have impact on perioperative outcome, such as tachycardia, nutrition status, glucose control, etc.

6. The surgeon stated this is laparoscopic and is a minimal invasive surgery, why do you anesthesia make this such a big deal? Are you planning an A-line and/or central line? Why?

Keypoint: this is to test the potential view of complications from anesthesia and surgery, to know your professionalism, your ability to be able to defend your plan. Know how such an invasive monitoring would help/guide intraoperative management.

7. Do you concern about her lung? What would you do to avoid the possibility of postoperative ventilation?

Keypoint: to test your knowledge on COPD (chronic obstructive pulmonary disease), the diagnosis and treatment, and to be able to assess its severity, any additional test may want to sort or to improve her pulmonary function before the surgery.

## > 术前管理 <

1. 附加检查：任何额外的检查，如超声心动图、动脉血气等。

要点：开放性问题，目的是了解麻醉医师如何评价患者的术前准备，确定其适合接受手术？及对围术期并发症的关注。

2. 什么是嗜铬细胞瘤,你能描述它的临床表现吗? 这个患者的症状和体征是否符合? 手术会治愈这种疾病吗? 如果不治疗将会出现什么并发症?

要点: 关于疾病及其相关病理生理学和转归的知识。

3. 药理准备: 什么是经典的药理准备,为什么? 列出要使用的药物,患者应服用 α-肾上腺素能受体阻滞剂多长时间,以及如何评估术前准备达到满意的治疗? 你的同事建议添加 β 受体阻滞剂,你同意吗?

要点: 嗜铬细胞瘤行肾上腺切除术是一个经典的病例,需要周详和仔细的规划和术前准备,因为围术期的高并发症发病率和死亡率。这个问题是测试麻醉医师对下列病理生理变化的了解程度,包括过量分泌儿茶酚胺导致的血容量减少、药理准备、药物、持续时间和血容量恢复的评估。

4. 为什么不直接测量血浆肾上腺素,而是测量游离钾肾上腺素和 24 小时尿 3-甲氧基 4-羟基苦杏仁酸(vanil mandelic acid,VMA)?

要点: 明确常用的实验室检查及其对明确临床诊断和判断疾病严重性的意义。

5. 术前会话: 你会让住院医师去签署麻醉同意吗? 你与住院医师对患者的术前谈话是不同的吗? 你将如何与患者讨论机械术中潜在的危险,如严重高血压或低血压,术后可能的机械通气等?

要点: 测试麻醉医师对这种特殊疾病的深入评估的能力,可能影响围术期转归的一些细节知识,例如心动过速、营养状况和血糖控制等。

6. 外科医师说这是腹腔镜,一个微创手术,为什么麻醉医师看得这么严重? 你计划置入动脉导管和/或中心静脉导管吗? 为什么?

要点: 这是为了测试对麻醉和手术的潜在并发症的了解,了解你的专业性,执行麻醉计划的能力。知道各项侵入性监测将如何帮助/指导术中管理。

7. 你担心她的肺功能吗? 你会怎么做以避免术后机械通气?

要点：测试你对慢性阻塞性肺病诊断和治疗方面的知识,并能够评估其严重性,增加辅助检查或在手术前改善她的肺功能。

------------------------> **Intraoperative management** <------------------------

1. Monitoring: will you place an arterial line before induction or after induction, why or why not?

2. Would you consider place CVP (central venous line), PAC (pulmonary arterial catheter), or TEE (transesophageal echocardiography)? Explain how these invasive monitors would help/guide you for the anesthesia management?

Keypoint: the knowledge and skills for place such an invasive monitor and be able to interpret, and know the specific modality and clinical indication, be able to make proper clinical changes accordingly.

3. Choice of induction agents: your choice of induction agent, propofol or etomidate, why? Would ketamine be contraindicated, explain? At the time of intubation, MAP increased from 85 to 120 mmHg, treat? Anesthesia is too light? Choice of agent?

Keypoint: a common type question to test the knowledge on intravenous anesthetics, dose-response effect, and advantage and disadvantage when administered underline condition; your preparation and ability to handle the crisis, be prepared.

4. Maintenance of anesthesia: your choice of maintenance agent, propofol infusion vs. isoflurane, why? Choice of muscle relaxant, rocuronium vs. cisatracurium, why? Choice of narcotics, remifentanil infusion?

Keypoint: there is no absolutely right or wrong answer, just give your choice and defend the reason of your decision; same thing for choosing the muscle relaxant, be prepared to have the literatures to support your decision.

5. Intraoperative ventilation: how would you set up the ventilator? Would it be the same for the open surgery? How would you ventilate a patient with severe COPD?

Keypoint: test your knowledge on basics in mechanical ventilation and the choice of a proper mode for an indicated condition; test the concept for protective mechanical ventilation for COPD patient, and to prevent lung injury; also may test your response permissive hypercapnia and the evidence medicine.

6. Volume expansion: your goal of volume expansion? Would it be the same to the open laparotomy? How do you assess the patient's volume status intraoperatively?

Keypoint: despite of well preparation to expand the patient's intravascular volume, in the reality, the patient is still hypovolemic and requiring continue volume replacement during the surgery; test the candidate's knowledge on clinical modalities to measure/assess the intraoperative volume status, such as the fluctuation of blood pressure, respiratory variation of arterial line waveform; Flow-Trach measures cardiac output; the legs lifting test, etc.

7. Hypertensive crisis: all laparoscopic ports were inserted, the surgeon started dissection to explode the adrenal gland, there were several short episodes of hypertension, MAP from 85 to 110 mmHg, treat? Choice of agent? 30 min later, the MAP went to 160 mmHg and did not respond to NTG iv boluses, your response? Would start nitroprusside, bolus or infusion? What is the difference between these two nitro agents? Do you have a dose limit? Can you think of any other agent? How long could you let such a hypertension last? Would ask your surgeon to help, and how?

Keypoint: definition for hypertension crisis, how to make such a diagnosis while the patient is under general anesthesia? What would be the dangers if not treat promptly? Knowledge of pharmacology on the control of severe blood pressure elevation. Also, the candidate may be asked whether the hypertension crisis could cause acute cardiac ischemia, and the mechanism? The communication skill with the surgeon.

8. Persistent hypotension: 25 min later (after the adrenal gland was totally removed), MAP from 110 dived to 70 mmHg and continue falling, what was going? Treat with fluid, RBC, or vasopressors? Choice of vasopressors, why?

Keypoint: the candidate should be familiar with this type surgery and pay attention to the progress. In the matter of minutes, this is the time the patient would be from a over secreting catecholamine to lack of sufficient catecholamine to support the life once the tumor is removed, in which a life support plan should be activated, also this is to test the candidate's ability to differentiate from other common causes, such major bleeding, anaphylactic reaction, etc.

9. Your resident told you the patient has percutaneous emphysema in shoulders and neck, concerned, why/why not? Would you obtain a chest X-ray? To which extend, you might have a concern?

Keypoint: this is question of clinical judgement, the incidence is unique to laparoscopic surgery. Simple percutaneous emphysema is common and no other interventions are needed; however, it should warn for other potential complication, such as pneumothorax and/or pneumomediastinum; it is not an indicator of delayed emergence of $CO_2$ retention.

10. Explain your preparation for emergence, how would it be different from a non-COPD patient? The patient remained non-responsive, assume there was not residual anesthesia effect, explain the possible cause? $CO_2$ narcosis,

hypoglycemia? If the patient breathing adequate but still requiring epinephrine infusion，would you extubate the patient，why/why not? Where would be displacement for this patient?

Keypoint：test the basic knowledge and judgement on routine anesthesia emergence；ask the anesthesia recovery process in COPD patient，why it is slower? What are the specific considerations in this patient if a slower awakening occurs and the management plan.

## > 术 中 管 理 <

1. 监测：你会在诱导前或诱导后放置动脉导管吗，为什么或为什么不?

2. 你会考虑放置中心静脉导管，PAC 还是 TEE 吗? 解释这些创伤性监护如何帮助/指导你的麻醉管理?

要点：放置创伤性监测的知识和技能，知道并能够解释其特定模式和临床指征，能够根据监测结果临床进行相应的临床调整。

3. 诱导药物的选择：你选择的诱导药物，丙泊酚或依托咪酯，为什么? 氯胺酮是禁忌吗，为什么? 插管时 MAP 从 85 mmHg 增加到 120 mmHg，怎么处理? 麻醉太浅了? 选择何种药物?

要点：常见的问题，以测试对使用静脉麻醉药的掌握，其剂量-效应反应，以及在不同情况时的优劣；你预见和处理危机的能力，做好准备。

4. 麻醉维持：你会选择丙泊酚输注还是异氟烷吸入来维持麻醉，为什么? 选择罗库溴铵还是顺式阿曲库铵作为肌肉松弛剂，为什么? 选择瑞芬太尼输注吗?

要点：没有绝对正确或错误的答案，做出你的选择和给出你的理由；选择肌肉松弛剂也一样，用文献支持你的做法。

5. 术中通气:如何设置呼吸机?与开放手术是否一样?如何为重症 COPD 患者通气?

要点:测试你机械通气方面的基础知识以及在特定条件下选择适合的通气模式;测试您对 COPD 患者保护性机械通气的概念,预防肺损伤;也可以测试你对允许性高碳酸血症的反应和处理。

6. 补充血容量:你的目标是什么?与开放剖腹术相同吗?如何在术中评估患者的血容量状态?

要点:尽管术前已经充分扩容,实际上患者仍然血容量不足并且需要在手术期间持续补液;测试麻醉医师根据临床情况测量/评估患者术中血容量状态的能力,例如血压波动,动脉波形随呼吸变化;FlowTrach 无创测量心输出量;腿部举升试验等。

7. 高血压危象:所有腹腔镜口插入器械,外科医师开始操作暴露肾上腺,有几次短暂的高血压,MAP 从 85 mmHg 升至 110 mmHg,怎么处理?药物选择?30 min 后,MAP 达到 160 mmHg,并且硝酸甘油静推后无反应,怎么处理?开始使用硝普钠吗?推注还是泵注?两种硝基类药物有什么区别?有剂量限制吗?你能想到其他药物吗?你能让这样的高血压持续多久?会让外科医师帮助吗,如何帮助?

要点:高血压危象的定义,患者全身麻醉时如何做出诊断?如果不及时治疗会有什么危险?控制严重高血压的药理知识。此外,高血压危象是否会引起急性心肌缺血及其机制?与外科医师的沟通技巧。

8. 持续性低血压:当左侧的肾上腺完全切除 25 min 后,MAP 从 110 mmHg 降到 70 mmHg,并继续下降,什么原因?使用液体、RBC 或血管加压药治疗?选择哪种血管加压药,为什么?

要点:麻醉医师应熟悉这种类型的手术并关注进展。一旦肿瘤被去除,在几分钟内患者从过度分泌到缺乏足够支持生命的儿茶酚胺,此时应给予生命支持,麻醉医师需要排除其他常见原因,如大出血、过敏反应等。

9. 你的住院医师告诉你，患者肩膀和颈部有皮下气肿，是否担心，为什么/为什么不？你会做胸部 X 线检查吗？到什么程度你会担心？

要点：这是临床判断问题，腹腔镜手术特有的并发症。轻微的皮下气肿很常见，不需要其他干预；然而，它提示其他可能的并发症，例如气胸和/或纵隔气肿；它不是二氧化碳潴留延迟出现的指标。

10. 描述你的麻醉苏醒计划，它与非 COPD 患者有何不同？患者仍然没有醒来（有苏醒延迟），假设没有麻醉药残留，解释可能的原因？二氧化碳麻醉，低血糖怎么办？如果患者呼吸正常，但仍需要肾上腺素输注，你会为患者拔管吗，为什么/为什么不？这个患者术后去哪里？

要点：测试常规麻醉苏醒的基本知识和判断；考察 COPD 患者的麻醉恢复过程，为什么会延迟？该患者苏醒延迟的具体考虑和管理计划是什么？

## Postoperative management

1. The patient was remaining intubated and admitted to ICU, the respiratory therapist asked you for ventilator set up? Explain you goal for postop ventilation and transient for extubation? What is the difference between pressure support from SIMV, the best choice for COPD patient?

Keypoint: test the basic knowledge of mechanical ventilation for ICU patient and the goal for weaning; the ability to apply a specific mode to a special patient; be able to take COPD into consideration when set up the ventilation, what is it? How to assess your plan is correct/right?

2. Postoperative delirium: 24 hrs later, the patient was extubated, but she could not follow the command, did not know where she was, agitated, etc. The surgeon told the nurse and the patient's family members this was related to anesthesia, agree? Explain the causes of delirium and treatment options?

Keypoint: the definition of delirium, the diagnosis criteria, the underline causes, and the treatment options; also, to be able to defend your anesthesia plan, and the professionalism for the dispute from your surgeon colleague. May ask your knowledge on the recent scientific progress.

3. Pain management: will you place an epidural in advance before induction? If you decide to have an epidural placed before induction, will you consider startingthe epidural infusion intraoperatively

Keypoint: question for acute pain management; your judgement on the choice of epidural versus TAPB (transversus abdominis plane block) for postoperative analgesia and their specific indications, specific involved techniques for epidural and TAPB.

## > 术 后 管 理 <

1. 患者带气管导管进入 ICU,呼吸治疗师要求你设置呼吸机? 解释你的术后通气和快速拔管的目标? SIMV 和压力支持有什么区别,COPD 患者的最佳选择是什么?

要点:测试 ICU 患者机械通气的基本知识和脱管目标;特殊患者应用特定模式的能力;能够在设置通气时考虑到 COPD,如何设置? 如何评估你的设置是否正确。

2. 术后谵妄:24 个小时后,患者拔管,但她不能服从指令,不知道她在哪里,激动等。外科医师告诉护士和患者家属这与麻醉有关,你是否同意? 解释谵妄的原因和治疗选择?

要点:谵妄的定义、诊断标准、常见原因和治疗选择;能够与你的外科同事存在争议时为你的麻醉计划进行辩护的专业精神。可能询问你最近学科进展的知识。

3. 疼痛管理:你会在诱导前预先放置硬膜外导管吗? 如果你决定在诱导前放

置硬膜外置管,你是否会在术中开始硬膜外输注吗?

要点:急性疼痛管理问题;硬膜外与腹横肌平面阻滞(transversus abdominis plane block,TAPB)术后止痛的选择及其适应证,硬膜外和 TAPB 的具体技术。

## Reference

[ 1 ] Siperstein AE，Berber E，Engle KL，et al. Laparoscopic posterior adrenalectomy：technical considerations. Arch Surg. 2000；135(8)：967 - 971.

[ 2 ] Lenders JW，Pacak K，Walther MM，et al. Biochemical diagnosis of pheochromocytoma：which test is best? JAMA. 2002；287(11)：1427 - 1434.

[ 3 ] Kim AW，Quiros RM，Maxhimer JB，et al. Outcome of laparoscopic adrenalectomy for pheochromocytomas vs aldosteronomas. Arch Surg. 2004；139(5)：529 - 531.

[ 4 ] Asari R，Scheuba C，Kaczirek K，et al. Estimated risk of pheochromo-cytoma recurrence after adrenal-sparing surgery in patients with multiple endocrine neoplasia type 2A. Arch Surg. 2006；141(12)：1199 - 1205.

[ 5 ] Lee JA，Zarnegar R，Shen WT，et al. Adrenal incidentaloma，borderline elevations of urine or plasma metanephrine levels，and the "Subclinical" heochromocytoma. Arch Surg. 2007；142(9)：870 - 873.

[ 6 ] Berber E，Mitchell J，Milas M，et al. Robotic posterior retroperitoneal adrenalectomy：operative technique. Arch Surg. 2010；145(8)：781 - 784.

[ 7 ] Shen WT，Grogan R，Vriens M，et al. One hundred two patients with pheochromocytoma treated at a single institution since the introduction of laparoscopic adrenalectomy. Arch Surg. 2010；145(9)：893 - 897.

[ 8 ] Yeh MW. The changing face of pheochromocytoma：varied presentations，better outcomes. Arch Surg. 2010；145(9)：897 - 898.

[ 9 ] Pasternak JD，Seib CD，Seiser N，et al. Differences between bilateral adrenal incidentalomas and unilateral lesions. JAMA Surg. 2015；150(10)：974 - 978.

[10] Ramakrishna H. Pheochromocytoma resection：Current concepts in anesthetic management. J Anaesthesiol Clin Pharmacol. 2015；31(3)：317 - 323.

Yi Zhou，Renyu Liu

周一,刘仁玉

# 7 Anesthesia for hip surgery in elderly

## 老年患者髋关节手术的麻醉

-------------------------- > **Basic information** < --------------------------

A 77 - year-old female fell from her deck while raking leaves, resulting in a left humeral and femoral neck fracture 72 hours ago, and presented for ORIF of humeral fracture and hip hemiarthroplasty. She had been admitted into the internal medicine service for optimizing her medical conditions and pain control, and started anticoagulation prophylactically. She lived in her own house with her husband. Other significant medical problems included: diabetes, hypertension, CAD (coronary artery disease), hypothyroidism, osteoarthritis, and hyperlipidemia.

VITALS: BP 130/83 mmHg, HR 85, RR 18, Temp 37.3, Wt. 165 lb.

MEDS: Metformin, Glucotrol, Zocor (simvastatin, anti-cholesterol), Cozaar (ACEI), Atenolol, Lasix, Nifedipine, Synthroid, Heparin 5,000 U Q8 sc.

LAB: WBC 13.3, Hgb 10.4, Platelets 309, PT/INR normal; BMP normal; Glucose 194.

ECG: Sinus rate 83 with first degree A - V block, ST and T wave abnormality, consider lateral ischemia.

ECHO (2 years ago)：Dilated left atrium，the left ventricle chamber was normal sized；aortic valve area 0.90 cm²，peak gradient 41 mmHg，mean gradient 22 mmHg；mitral thickened，reduced excursion，regurgitation moderate；Estimated LVEF 50%．

X-rays：A complex comminuted left humeral head and neck fracture with displacement and left femoral neck fracture．

## 基 本 信 息

病史：77 岁老年女性，入院前 72 个小时在阳台修剪树枝时，不慎跌落致左肱骨、左股骨颈骨折，拟行左半髋置换术和左肱骨骨折切开复位内固定术。患者内科住院治疗，以优化她的术前条件，控制疼痛并开始预防性地抗凝治疗。患者和她的丈夫生活在一起，并住在自己的房子里。

既往史：糖尿病、高血压、冠心病、甲状腺功能减退、骨关节炎和高血脂。

生命体征：血压 130/83 mmHg，心率 85 次/min，呼吸频率 18 次/min，体温 37.3℃，体重 74.9 kg。

用药：二甲双胍、格列吡嗪、辛伐他汀（抗胆固醇）、科素亚（血管紧张素转化酶抑制剂）、阿替洛尔、呋塞米、硝苯地平、左甲状腺素钠、肝素 5 000 U 每 8 个小时皮下注射。

实验室检查：白细胞 13.3× 10⁹/L，血红蛋白 104 g/L，血小板 309× 10⁹/L，凝血酶原时间/国际标准化比值正常；电解质肝肾功能均正常；血糖 10.78 mmol/L。

心电图：窦性心律，83 次/min，Ⅰ度房室传导阻滞、ST－T 异常，考虑侧壁缺血。

心超（2 年前）：左房扩大，左室大小正常；主动脉瓣瓣口面积 0.90 cm²，最大压力梯度 41 mmHg，平均压力梯度 22 mmHg；二尖瓣增厚，移位减少，中度反流；LVEF 约为 50%。

X-rays：复杂粉碎性左肱骨头、肱骨颈部骨折伴移位，以及左股骨颈骨折。

## > **Preoperative management** <

The patient is scheduled for ORIF (open reduction and internal fixation) for the left humeral, and the hemiarthroplasty of her left hip. She has been brought to our Regional Nerve Block Service and received the left interscalene nerve and lumbar plexus blocks for postoperative analgesia. The patient was awake and stable, however it was noticed her $SaO_2$ was 92% on nasal cannula $O_2$ 3 L.

1. Do you want any additional tests before starting the anesthesia? Why/why not?

Keypoint: open question: optimization the patient's medication, risk prevention and preparation, etc.

2. How would you manage her medications, atenolol, synthroid, cozaar, etc.? How about her subcutaneous heparin? Should metformin be stopped, if so, what is your concern?

Keypoint: questions are for the knowledge of each drug-pharmacology, guideline on beta blocker, and side effects.

3. How is the preoperative assessment different in a geriatric patient from a normal adult (30~55 years old patient)?

Keypoint: question is on the knowledge of geriatric patient preoperative assessment, the difference in physiology, functional reserving, and the specific objective, even the response to anesthetics.

4. How would assess the patient with aortic stenosis and would it change your anesthesia plan? Why/why not?

Keypoint：the knowledge of aortic stenosis and anesthesia considerations and contraindication，recognize the potential crisis could happen during the surgery. Aortic stenosis is the word for crisis warning.

5. Your choice for the intraoperative monitoring，why?

Keypoint：knowledge of different invasive and noninvasive monitoring，know the limitations。

6. Would the preoperative regional nerve blocks help your anesthesia management，why/why not?

Keypoint：this is a complicated question，intraopeartive and postoperative comfort does not equal to a better outcome，there is not enough evidence yet to support the regional is better than GEA.

7. The patient complained of dyspnea after left interscalene nerve block. What are your differential diagnoses（DDX）? What would you do next?

8. 20 mins after interscalene nerve block，the patient developed the hoarseness and complained of difficulty talking on the way to OR. What is the most likely cause? How to proceed? Would you cancel the case，why/why not?

## ＞ 术 前 管 理 ＜

患者拟行左肱骨骨折切开复位内固定术（ORIF）＋左髋关节半髋置换术。患者在术前接受区域神经阻滞麻醉，包括左臂丛肌间沟神经阻滞和腰丛神经阻滞，用于术后镇痛。操作期间，患者清醒、平稳，但是在鼻吸氧 3 L 的情况下，其脉氧为 92%。

1. 在开始麻醉前,你需要做额外的检查么? 为什么/为什么不?

要点:开放性问题:如何优化患者的用药、预防风险及术前准备?

2. 你将如何处理她的用药,如阿替洛尔、科素亚、呋塞米等? 还有皮下肝素? 应该停用二甲双胍么? 如果停了,你需要关心什么?

要点:所有问题都跟每种药物的药理学知识、β受体阻滞剂的用药指南以及药物不良反应有关。

3. 老年患者的术前评估与正常成人(30～55 岁)有何不同?

要点:这是关于老年患者术前评估知识的问题,包括老年患者的生理学、功能储备,及老年患者特殊的检查甚至对麻醉药物反应的不同。

4. 如何评估患者主动脉瓣狭窄的程度? 它会改变你的麻醉计划么? 为什么/为什么不?

要点:主要考察主动脉瓣狭窄和麻醉禁忌证的知识,要认识到术中可能会发生的潜在风险。主动脉瓣狭窄是风险提示的关键词。

5. 你选择哪些术中监测手段? 为什么?

要点:了解创伤性和无创的监测手段,知道它们的局限性。

6. 术前的区域神经阻滞对于麻醉管理有帮助吗? 为什么/为什么不?

要点:这是一个复杂的问题,术中和术后的舒适不代表更好的预后,并没有足够的证据支持区域阻滞优于全麻复合硬膜外阻滞。

7. 左臂丛肌间沟神经阻滞后,患者主诉呼吸困难。你的鉴别诊断是什么? 你如何采取下一步行动?

8. 左臂丛肌间沟神经阻滞 20 min 后,在去手术室的路上,患者出现声音嘶哑,主诉讲话困难,最可能的原因是什么? 如何处理? 你会考虑取消这个手术吗?

## > **Intraoperative management** <

1. The patient is now in OR and ready for inducing general anesthesia. Your choice of induction agents and the doses, and explain?

Keypoint: a question of testing how the candidate understand the pharmacology and pathophysiology changes in this patient, based on her age, co-morbidities, recent injury especially significant blood lose from hip and humeral fracture, the choice of agent and dose do matter.

2. Would you place an arterial line? If so, would you place it before or after the induction? Why/why not?

Keypoint: to test whether the candidate could foresee the potential problem/crisis.

3. Any additional emergency medications that should be prepared? Why/why not?

Keypoint: how well the candidate has prepared mentally and medically.

Another IV was obtained (18G). A radial arterial line has been placed after induction. 25 mins later, the patient becomes hypotensive which did not respond to repeat boluses of ephedrine and phenylephrine. The continuing infusion of phenylephrine is not effective at all.

Meanwhile, the $SpO_2$ was low (80s%) and the $etCO_2$ waveform is ill appearing. The patient was immediately placed on 100% $FiO_2$ with manual ventilation.

4. What would be the likely cause of this life threatening condition?

Keypoint: this is asking for recognition of crisis, a quick diagnosis and rapid response to the presumed cause. Time is life-saving.

5. How would you confirm your diagnosis? What tests would be helpful?

Keypoint: additional test to assist quick diagnosis, and more to exclude other causes, such as TEE (transesophageal echocardiography) for this case.

6. How would you resuscitate this patient?

Keypoint: emphasize the concept of ACLS (advance cardiac life support), which is universal for any one with cardiopulmonary arrest.

7. Would the echo findings be helpful in assisting your original diagnosis?

Keypoint: again, ask the TEE to describe what might be the findings to either confirm or exclude a massive PE (pulmonary embolism) in this case.

8. Explain the hemodynamic changes caused by massive PE (pulmonary embolism).

Keypoint: ask the pathophysiological changes of a massive PE, including pulmonary and systemic circulations.

9. Can you describe the treatment/resuscitation strategy for a massive PE?

Keypoint: asking the knowledge of the principle treatment for a massive PE, besides aggressive resuscitation, specific towards the emboli including anticoagulation, thrombolysis, surgical embolectomy, endovascular retrieve emboli, or even ECMO (extracorporeal membrane oxygenation), and such a decision should be decided quick and unified with the entire care team.

Let us change to a different scenario. The induction is uneventful; the surgery has been started and all are going well. After placing the cement and the prosthesis into the femoral shaft, and the surgeon starts hammering.... At this time, the dramatic hemodynamics occurred (just as described above)?

10. What would be your differential diagnoses?

Keypoint：asking for possible other causes similar to PE，anaphylaxis，massive air or fat embolism，etc.，the candidate should be able to describe the differences among each underline cause.

11. Would TEE be helpful，if so，what would they find?（the same question asked in above）

12. Would the treatment/resuscitation plan be different from PE?

Keypoint：expect the candidate to stand his/her ground，ACLS comes the first to support the patient's life，then if time allowed to target each specific cause.

> 术 中 管 理 <

1. 患者现在手术室，并准备开始全麻诱导。你选择用什么药物诱导，以及诱导的剂量是多少，为什么?

要点：这是考察你对该患者药理学和病理生理学变化的了解程度，要结合患者的年龄、基本疾病和当前的损伤，尤其是因为髋关节和肱骨骨折导致的严重失血等情况一起考虑。所以诱导药物的选择和用量很重要。

2. 你打算行动脉穿刺置管吗? 如果是，你会在诱导前还是诱导后放置? 为什么/为什么不?

要点：考察你能否预见患者潜在的问题/危机。

3. 还需要准备哪些额外的抢救药物? 为什么/为什么不?

要点：考察你是否在精神上和医学知识上准备好了。

开放第二条静脉输液通道（18G）。麻醉诱导后，行桡动脉穿刺置管。25 min后，患者出现低血压，且重复静推麻黄碱、去氧肾上腺素无效，持续泵注去氧肾上腺素,仍无效。

同时,患者出现脉氧低(80%),etCO$_2$波形不良。立刻调高吸氧浓度致100%,并采取手动通气。

4. 这种危及生命的情况是什么导致的?

要点:考察对急症的快速识别、快速诊断和快速反应的能力。此时,时间就是生命。

5. 你如何验证你的诊断? 哪些检查于诊断有帮助?

要点:一些检查可以帮助快速诊断,更多的是帮助排除其他可能原因,如经食道超声心动可用于这种情况。

6. 如何复苏这位患者?

要点:强调高级心血管生命支持(advance cardiac life support,ACLS)的概念,这对任何一个心脏骤停的患者是通用的。

7. 超声检查结果有助于你的初步诊断吗?

要点:再次考察 TEE 的应用,在这个病例中,哪些发现可以证实或排除大面积肺栓塞的诊断?

8. 解释大面积肺栓塞引起血流动力学改变的原因。

要点:考察大面积肺栓塞,包括肺循环和体循环的病理生理改变。

9. 你能描述大面积肺栓塞的治疗和复苏策略吗?

要点:考察大面积肺栓塞的处理原则,除了快速复苏,还有针对栓塞的特殊治疗,包括抗凝、溶栓、手术切除栓子、血管内取栓,甚至体外膜肺。这些策略需要整个医疗团队的快速、统一决定。

让我们换个场景看一下:麻醉诱导平稳,手术开始一切顺利。在将骨水泥和假体置入股骨干后，外科医师开始锤击……在这个时候，出现了显著的血流动力学改变（如上所述）。

10. 你的鉴别诊断有哪些？

要点：考察类似肺栓塞的其他可能诊断，如过敏反应、大量的空气或脂肪栓塞等。需要你能够描述这些可能原因的不同点。

11. TEE 会有帮助吗？ 如果有，可能会发现什么？（上文中有同一个问题）

12. 这时的治疗和复苏策略于肺血栓栓塞有何不同？

要点：期望你可以站在自己的角度回答。ACLS 是支持患者生命的首要策略，而后，如果时间允许，再针对每一个具体原因采取措施。

## > Postoperative management <

This patient was treated in OR for an hour and half then transported to ICU for continuing resuscitation. Unfortunately，she passed away 12 hours later because the family decided to withdraw the life support. Next day，the medical care team sat down with her family members for debriefing. The patient's daughter who works in a malpractice law firm as paralegal，she has some questions for the care physicians.

1. The time of surgery："Knowing the risk of PE，if the surgery was performed earlier，could her PE be prevented?"

Keypoint：to test the candidate about the practice standard/guideline，the hospital policy on the timing surgery，and the number of incidence of PE despite the best practice nationwide.

2. Diagnostic tests for PE："There are many tests to help early detect the potential risks of PE；Did the anesthesia team order any of them? If they did，what are they? If not，why did not they order?"

Keypoint：a test whether the candidate has the ability to be able to defend his medical management plan，the knowledge of the limitation to be able to make the diagnosis of PE before the surgery，etc.

3. Skin test："If this was an anaphylactic reaction to the given antibiotics，should a skin test be performed prior to the administration?"

Keypoint：again，to test the knowledge and the ability to defend on the topic of anaphylaxis.

4. Anesthesia should be responsible? Finally，the surgeon said that the incident happened before the surgery started，so this had nothing to do with him，do you agree?

Keypoint：this is a question on professionalism，passion，and responsibility towards the patient and colleagues，it requires frequent thought and preparation so that the patient and family members would accept your explanation.

> **术 后 管 理** <

该患者在手术室抢救了 1.5 个小时之后被送至 ICU 继续复苏治疗。遗憾的是，因为家属决定停止生命支持，患者于 12 个小时后去世。第二天，整个医疗团队和患者的家属一起进行了病例讨论。患者的女儿是一位律师助理，就职于一家医疗事故律师事务所。她有一些问题要问医师：

1. 手术时机："假如知道有肺栓的风险，如果手术再早一点进行，那么是否可以防止发生肺栓塞？"

要点：考察你对操作准则/指南、医院对手术时机的政策，以及肺栓塞在全国范围内发生率的了解程度。

2. 肺栓塞诊断："有很多可以帮助早期诊断肺栓的检查，麻醉团队是否有实施其中任何一个？如果有，他们做了哪些？如果没有，为什么不做这些检查？"

要点：考察你对自己医疗处理方案的辩护能力，以及阐明术前能够做出肺栓诊断的局限性。

3. 皮肤实验："如果说这是抗生素引起的过敏反应，那么是否应该在给药前进行皮试？"

要点：再次考察你对过敏反应相关内容的了解情况和辩护能力。

4. 麻醉应该负责？最后，这位外科医师说这件事发生在手术开始之前，所以与他们无关，你同意吗？

要点：这是一个对患者和同事的关于职业精神、激情和责任的问题。需要你经常思考和准备，以便患者和其家属能够接受你的解释。

**Reference**

[1] Chatterjee S，Chakraborty A，Weinberg I，et al. Thrombolysis for pulmonary embolism and risk of all-cause mortality，major bleeding，and intracranial hemorrhage：a meta-analysis. JAMA. 2014；311(23)：2414 - 2421.

[2] Advanced Cardiac Life Support by American Hear Association.

[3] Tapson VF. Acute Pulmonary Embolish. N Engl J Med. 2008；358(10)：1037 - 1052.

[4] Liu HK，Chen WC. Fat Embolism Syndrome. N Engl J Med. 2011；364(18)：1761.

Chris C. Lee，Chuanyao Tong

李成付，童传耀

# 8 Anesthesia consideration for pneumonectomy

## 普胸手术病例——肺叶切除手术麻醉

································ > **Basic information** < ································

A 68 years old male patient has hemoptysis（cough with blood）for 2 months，CT and chest X-ray showed a left upper lobe mass with neck lymph nodes metastases. The subsequent biopsy confirmed this was a squamous cell cancer. He is scheduled for thoracotomy，left lobectomy and possible pneumonectomy. The patient weighs 120 kg and has lost 15 kg in last two months. Other medical problems are hypertension，chronic obstructive pulmonary disease，coronary artery disease with stable angina，chronic kidney disease with creatinine 2.1，GFR<25，type 1 diabetes，OSA（obstructive sleep apnea），and peripheral neuropathy.

PE：overweight but chronic illness appearing，full beard，BP 138/89，HR 89，RR 16，SaO$_2$ 91% on RA.

Meds：Lisinopril，HCTZ，ASA 81 mg，cardiazem，albutalol，atrovent，lasix，metformine，NTG. BiPAP 15 cmH$_2$O for 8 years.

LAB：WBC 8.9，Hgb 13.8，Hct 37，Platelet 213，Na 133，K 5.1，Cl 93，HCO$_3^-$ 32，BUN 32，Cr. 2.1，Glucose 179 mg/dL. BNP 560，HbA1c 7.2%.

ECG：SR 88 with RBBB，non-specific ST－T depression，question for old infarction in anterior and lateral regions.

## 基 本 信 息

病史：68 岁男性，咯血 2 个月，CT 和胸透显示左肺上叶及颈部淋巴结转移。活检确认为鳞状细胞癌。拟行开胸左肺叶切除全肺切除。患者体重 120 kg，近 2 个月内体重下降 15 kg。既往患有高血压、慢性阻塞性肺疾病、冠心病伴稳定型心绞痛、慢性肾病（肌酐 185.64 $\mu$mmol/L，GFR＜25 mL/min）、1 型糖尿病、阻塞性睡眠呼吸暂停及周围神经病变。

查体：超重，慢性病容，络腮胡，血压 138/89 mmHg，心率 89 次/min，呼吸 16 次/min，空气下血氧饱和度 91%。

药物：赖诺普利、氢氯噻嗪、肠溶阿司匹林 81 mg、硫氮草酮、沙丁胺醇、定喘乐、呋塞米、二甲双胍、硝酸甘油。使用 BiPAP 行无创正压通气 8 年（压力为15 $cmH_2O$）。

实验室检查：白细胞 $8.9×10^9$/L，血红蛋白 138 g/L，血细胞比容 37%，血小板 $213×10^9$/L，钠 133 mmol/L，钾 5.1 mmol/L，氯 93 mmol/L，$HCO_3^-$ 32 mmol/L，尿素氮 11.39 mmol/L（尿素 5.70 mmol/L），肌酐 185.64 $\mu$mol/L，血糖 10.0 mmol/L，B 型利钠肽 560 pg/mL，糖化血红蛋白 7.2%。

心电图：窦性心律 88 次/min，伴右束支传导阻滞，非特异性 ST－T 段降低，不排除前外侧区域陈旧性心肌梗死。

## Preoperative management

1. PFT（pulmonary function test）：would you like to have a PFT，why/why not? What would be a typical report of COPD patient? Explain how the report of PFT may help your anesthesia management?

Keyword：To understand pulmonary function test.

2. Does the patient need further cardiac work up? How about an echocardiography and stress test? What would you do if the stress test is positive, will you cancel the case, or the needs to have a cardiac catheterization?

Keyword: To understand cardiac function test.

3. Beta blocker: give the literature support beta blocker has a cardiac protective effect, would you start beta block on this patient, why/why not?

Keyword: To be familiar with the clinical application of preoperative use of beta blocker.

4. Do his medications need to be optimized, explain how?

Keyword: To understand how to optimize the patient pre-operative condition.

5. How would you assess this patient's perioperative risks and explain this to the patient and his family members? The patient asked you the likely chance of him being on ventilator postoperatively and how long?

Keyword: To understand how to talk to patient and family members.

6. How would you explain to this patient about his postoperative pain management? Your recommendation?

Keyword: To understand general rules of postoperative pain managements.

7. If patient has fever and cough, are you going to cancel the case?

Keyword: To understand how to diagnose the obstructive pneumonia.

> 术 前 管 理 <

1. 肺功能检查(PFT)：是否行 PFT，为什么？慢阻肺患者典型的 PFT 结果是什么？请分析 PFT 的结果如何有助于你的麻醉管理。

要点：掌握肺功能检查。

2. 是否需要进一步心功能评估？是否行超声心动图检查及负荷试验？若负荷试验阳性，是取消手术，还是需要行心导管置入？

要点：掌握心功能检查。

3. 有文献表明 β 受体阻滞剂具有心肌保护效应，是否对该患者开始 β 受体阻滞剂？为什么？

要点：熟悉术前 β 受体阻滞剂的应用。

4. 该患者用药是否需要优化？如何优化？

要点：掌握如何优化患者术前情况。

5. 你如何评估该患者围术期风险，以及如何向家属说明病情？患者咨询你术后呼吸机支持的概率及可能持续多长时间？

要点：掌握如何与患者及其家属进行术前谈话。

6. 如何向患者解释其术后疼痛管理？你的建议是什么？

要点：掌握术后疼痛管理常规。

7. 若患者出现发热、咳嗽，是否取消手术？

要点：掌握阻塞性肺炎的诊断。

## Intraoperative management

1. Monitoring, arterial line, before or after the induction, why/why not?

CVP，PAC，others?

Keyword：To understand the general rules of monitoring.

2. Will you place a DLT（double lumen endotracheal tube），why? Left or right，does it matter? Describe your steps to confirm the correction placement. What will you do if you are not able to place a DLT? Please explain other options.

Keyword：To understand how to do one lung ventilation.

3. OLV and hypoxemia：describe the OLV（one lung ventilation）set up，and when would you start OLV? Does it matter? 10 min after OLV，$SaO_2$ from 98% decreased to 90%，surprise? Explain the causes and what needs to be done to improve the patient's oxygenation?

Keyword：To understand the physiology of one lung ventilation induced hypoxia.

4. Robotic vs. open thoracotomy：if this was a wedge resection by robotic surgery technical，would your anesthesia management be different? Please explain?

Keyword：To understand the general rules of anesthesia care for robotic surgery.

5. Goal for hemodynamics：describe your goal to maintain BP and HR during surgery and why? 90 min into the surgery，MAP from 82 to 50 mmHg and HR from 85 to 125，treat with iv fluid or vasopressor? Why/why not? What might be the causes?

Keyword：To understand the general rules of hemodynamic managements.

6. Pain management：assume a thoracic epidural catheter is placed，will you

use it during the surgery，why/why not? Describe the process of placing an epidural catheter? If you are going to use the epidural，describe the choice of agent? Will it be different from postoperative analgesia?

Keyword：To understand epidural analgesia.

7. Emergence：describe your preparation for the emergence and extubation，would it be the same or different from a patient without COPD?

Keyword：To understand the general rules of extubation.

8. The patient suddenly develops hypotension，tachycardia and hypoxia. What can be the reasons? What is diagnosis and treatment?

Keyword：To understand what is the tension pneumothorax and what is the treatment.

> 术 中 管 理 <

1. 在诱导前或诱导后是否给予监护及连续动脉压检监测？原因是什么？是否应用中心静脉压、肺动脉导管及其他监测手段？

要点：掌握术中监护常规。

2. 是否置入双腔气管导管？为什么？选择左管或右管，这是否需要？请描述确定导管正确置入的步骤。如果未能正确置入双腔气管导管，你的下一步方案是什么？

要点：掌握单肺通气。

3. 单肺通气及低氧血症：请描述如何建立单肺通气？单肺通气的时机？选择时机重要吗？若单肺通气 10 min 后，血氧饱和度由 98% 降至 90%，是否奇怪？请解释分析造成患者低氧血症的原因及改善方法。

要点：掌握单肺通气所致低氧血症的生理。

4. 机器人手术对比开胸手术：若这是机器人辅助下肺楔形切除术，麻醉管理有何不同？为什么？

要点：掌握机器人手术麻醉管理常规。

5. 血流动力学管理目标：请描述你的术中血压和心率的理想水平，为什么？若手术进行 90 分钟后，平均动脉压由 82 mmHg 变为 50 mmHg、心率由 85 次/min 变为 125 次/min，是否需要静脉补液或使用血管升压药？为什么？可能的原因是什么？

要点：掌握术中血流动力学管理常规。

6. 疼痛管理：若已置入胸段硬膜外导管，术中是否应用？为什么？请描述放置硬膜外导管的过程。若术中通过硬膜外导管给药，应采用何种药物？与术后镇痛药物是否相同？

要点：掌握硬膜外镇痛技术。

7. 苏醒：对苏醒及拔管应做何种准备？对是否患有慢阻肺的患者是否有区别？

要点：掌握拔管适应证。

8. 若患者突然出现低血压、心动过速、低氧血症，原因为何？你的诊断和治疗方案是什么？

要点：掌握张力性气胸及其治疗。

-------------------- > **Postoperative management** < --------------------

1. Ventilator setting: despite the best trying, the patient seemed not ready

for extubation, he was admitted to ICU, would you consider changing his DLT to a regular ETT, why/why not? What if the intubation was a very difficult and DLT has to maintain? The ICU physician suggests to ventilate each lung separately, do you agree? Explain the pros and cons?

Keyword: To understand the general rule of airway management.

2. Hemothorax: in last 2 hours, the chest tube has put out 450 mL ($>$200 mL/hr), the patient has been given FFP $\times$4, RBC $\times$2, more FFP, factor VII. What is next step?

Keyword: To understand the general rules of blood transfusion and treatment of hemothorax.

3. New onset a-fib: 8 hrs after the surgery, the HR of the patient is 110 and irregular, MAP 90 mmHg, what is your response? 30 min later the MAP decrease to 70 mmHg, what you you do? What if his MAP is 50 mmHg, and your colleague suggested to perform cardioversion for him immediately, agree? Can you think why he had this new onset a-fib?

Keyword: To understand the treatment of A-fib.

4. Pain control: what would you do to his epidural if the blood pressure was not stable in ICU? 24 hour later, he is stable and the epidural is resumed, how will you keep the epidural running, 2 days or 3 days, why/why not? How do you convert to oral pain medication?

Keyword: To understand the general rules of postoperative pain managements.

5. Brachial nerve injury: 5 days later, the patient is transferred to the floor, he complains of his right hand being numbness, loss the grip strength and sensations, the surgeon tells him it is caused by anesthesia, agree? Will you request neurology consult? How do you differentiate a preexisting neuropathy

vs. new injury? If this is indeed caused by improper positioning, who should bear the primary responsibility?

Keyword：To understand the importance of positioning patients during the surgery.

6. Patient has confusion and inattention in ICU. What is the potential diagnosis and what is the treatment?

Keyword：To understand postoperative delirium.

## > 术 后 管 理 <

1. 呼吸机设置：多次尝试未能拔管，患者转入 ICU，是否考虑更换其将双腔气管导管更换为普通气管导管？为什么？若患者为困难气道而双腔管没有拔出，ICU 医师建议双肺分别通气，你是否同意？请解释其利弊。

要点：掌握气道管理常规。

2. 胸腔积血：近 2 个小时内，胸腔引流液达 450 mL（>200 mL/h），患者已输注 4 单位新鲜冰冻血浆、2 单位红细胞，血浆、凝血因子 VII。下一步治疗方案是什么？

要点：掌握输血适应证及胸腔积血的治疗。

3. 新发房颤：术后 8 个小时，护士呼叫患者心率达 110 次/min 且不规则，平均动脉压 90 mmHg，如何应对？若 30 min 后平均动脉压将为 70 mmHg，采取何种措施？若平均动脉压为 50 mmHg，同事建议立即除颤，是否同意？对此新发房颤如何解释？

要点：掌握房颤治疗。

4. 控制疼痛：若患者在 ICU 血压不稳定，如何处理硬膜外导管？24 个小时后,患者情况稳定,硬膜外导管恢复使用,你将如何应用? 是维持 2 天或 3 天? 为什么? 如何转变为口服止痛药?

　　要点:掌握术后疼痛管理常规。

　　5.臂丛神经损伤:5 天后,患者下地,诉右手麻木、丧失握力及感觉,手术医师告诉患者系由麻醉所致,是否同意? 是否需要神经科医师咨询? 如何鉴别早前存在的神经疾病及新的损伤? 若确实由于术中体位不当所致,谁应负主要责任?

　　要点:明确术中患者体位的重要性。

　　6.若患者在 ICU 中出现意识混乱及注意力涣散,可能诊断及其治疗是什么?

　　要点:掌握术后谵妄。

Zhongcong Xie

谢仲淙

# 9 Anesthesia management for pituitary tumor

## 脑外科手术病例——垂体瘤手术麻醉

-----------------------> **Basic information** <------------------------

A 58 years old male had persistent numbness of both hands and was evaluated for bilateral carpal tunnel release surgery. During the work-up, a pituitary tumor (0.9 cm × 0.9 cm) was found and the patient is now scheduled for trans-sphenoidal pituitary tumor resection.

Past medical history: HTN (hypertension), DM (diabetes millets type Ⅱ), OSA (obstructive sleep apnea), and hyperlipidemia.

Medications: Lisinopril, metformin, simvastatin and HCTZ.

Labs: WBC 6.7, Hgb 15.6, platelet 210; electrolytes are within normal range, glucose 146 mg/dL; using BiPAP (12 cmH$_2$O) for 5 years.

ECG: sinus heart rate 86, LVH, non-specific ST - T changes.

PE: weight 125 kg.

VS: BP 158/94 mmHg, HR 86, RR 16, SaO$_2$ 96% RA.

Airway: Mallampati Ⅲ with normal mouth opening but large tongue and mandible, prognathic chin.

## 基 本 信 息

病史：58 岁男性双手持续麻木,经诊断需要做双侧腕管松解手术。在治疗期间,发现一个垂体瘤(0.9 cm×0.9 cm),遂安排该患者进行经蝶骨垂体肿瘤切除术。

过去史：高血压、2 型糖尿病,睡眠呼吸暂停综合征和高脂血症。

药物：赖诺普利、二甲双胍、辛伐他汀和氢氯噻嗪。

化验：WBC 6.7 $\times 10^9$/L,Hgb 156 g/L,血小板 210 $\times 10^9$/L;电解质在正常范围内,葡萄糖 8.11 mmol/L;使用 BiPAP(12 $cmH_2O$)5 年。

心电图：窦性心率,86 次/min,左室肥厚,非特异性 ST-T 变化。

体格检查：体重 125 kg。

生命体征：BP 158/94 mmHg,HR 86 次/min,RR 16 次/min,空气下 $SaO_2$ 96%。

气道：Mallampati Ⅲ级,可正常张嘴,舌头、下颚肥大,下巴突出。

## Preoperative management

1. Systemic manifestations of secreting pituitary tumors: Do you think his previous carpal tunnel syndrome was related to his pituitary tumor? What are other symptoms and signs that might be also caused by a pituitary tumor?

Keypoint: The examinee should be able to recognize signs of acromegaly including soft tissue overgrowth and peripheral nerve compression. They should be able to describe incidentalomas, symptoms of optic chiasm compression, vs. secreting tumors acromegaly, Cushing's, infertility.

2. Pre-op assessment: Are any additional lab tests needed? How would these results help your anesthesia management?

Keypoint: The examinee should consider other endocrinopathies that can result from secreting pituitary tumors and could request BMP (basic metabolic profile), thyroid function studies, sleep study for OSA (obstructive sleep apnea), CBC(complete blood count) and type and screen in case of unexpected blood loss. They should perform a careful airway assessment given the elevated risk of difficult ventilation/intubation, and potentially request an endocrine consult for optimization prior to surgery.

3. Sleep apnea: What is sleep apnea? Are there different types? What risk factors are predictive of sleep apnea? How is it treated?

Keypoint: Describe obstructive and central types. Screening can be accomplished with STOP – BANG or similar tool, and definitive diagnosis is achieved with a sleep study and apnea hypopnea index (AHI). An AHI represents the number of apneic or hypopneic episodes in 1 hour. Normal<5, mild 5~14, moderate 15~29, severe ≥30. Treatment includes continuous positive airway pressure (CPAP) or bilevel positive airway pressure (BiPAP), surgical correction with uvulopalato-pharyngoplasty or diaphragmatic pacing.

4. Pituitary function: Review of the chart reveals elevated serum growth hormone concentrations, failure to suppress growth hormone concentrations after an oral glucose load and elevated IGF – I levels consistent with acromegaly. Describe the function of the anterior and posterior pituitary gland. What role do bromocriptine and octreotide play in the treatment of acromegaly?

Keypoint: Describe the secretion of ACTH, GH, prolactin, TSH, FSH, LH from the anterior pituitary and secretion of ADH and oxytocin from the posterior pituitary gland. Bromocriptine is a D2 agonist and suppresses GH release. Octreotide is an analogue of somatostatin and also inhibits GH release.

5. Hyperglycemia: What could explain his hyperglycemia? Would you treat it? Would you administer subcutaneous or IV insulin? What is your goal for his

blood glucose? Would tighter control (80～120 mg/dL) be better?

Keypoint：Growth hormone increases gluconeogenesis and lipolysis，and can also induce insulin resistance. Aggressive control of blood glucose may increase the risk of hypoglycemia and increased morbidity and mortality.

6. Hypertension：should his blood pressure be treated before the surgery，why/why not? What if it were 170/100 mmHg? What if it were 180/110 mmHg?

Keypoint：Discuss the perioperative complications of hypertension but also weigh the risk/benefit of surgery with the understanding that hypertension is unlikely to be resolved completely without curative surgery.

## > 术 前 管 理 <

1. 分泌性垂体肿瘤的系统表现：你认为他以前的腕管综合征与垂体瘤有关吗？其他哪些症状和体征也可能是由垂体瘤引起的？

要点：受试者应该能够识别肢端肥大症的体征，包括软组织过度生长和外周神经压迫。应该能够区分意外发现的肿瘤，视交叉压迫的症状与分泌性肿瘤肢端肥大症，库欣氏综合征和不育。

2. 术前评估：是否需要任何额外的实验室化验？这些结果将如何帮助你的麻醉管理？

要点：受试者应考虑可能由分泌性垂体肿瘤引起的其他内分泌病，并可能需要了解基础代谢检查（basic metabolic panel，BMP）、甲状腺功能、睡眠测试是否存在阻塞性呼吸停止；血常规、血型和筛选以防意外失血。考虑到较高的呼吸困难/气管插管的风险，应进行详细的气道评估；术前进行内分泌咨询以使患者情况尽量优化。

3. 睡眠呼吸暂停：什么是睡眠呼吸暂停？有不同的类型吗？什么风险因素预

示着睡眠呼吸暂停？如何治疗？

要点：描述阻塞性和中枢性类型。可以使用 STOP - BANG 或类似工具完成筛查，并通过睡眠测试和呼吸暂停低通气指数（AHI）进行明确诊断。AHI 代表 1 个小时呼吸暂停或呼吸不足的次数：正常＜5，轻微 5～14，中度 15～29，严重≥30。治疗包括持续气道正压通气（CPAP）或双相气道正压通气（BiPAP），手术矫正与悬雍垂腭咽成形术或膈肌起搏。

4. 垂体功能：化验结果显示血清生长激素浓度升高，口服葡萄糖也无法抑制生长激素浓度升高，IGF - 1 水平升高符合肢端肥大症。描述垂体前叶和后叶的功能。溴隐亭和奥曲肽在治疗肢端肥大症中有什么作用？

要点：垂体前叶分泌促肾上腺皮质激素、生长激素、催乳素、促甲状腺激素、卵泡刺激素和黄体生成素，垂体后叶分泌抗利尿激素和催产素。溴隐亭是 D2 兴奋剂并抑制生长激素释放。奥曲肽类是生长抑素，抑制生长激素释放。

5. 高血糖：如何解释他的高血糖？你会去治疗吗？你采用皮下注射还是静脉注射胰岛素？你的目标血糖是多少？严格的控制（4.44～6.67 mmol/L）会更好吗？

要点：生长激素增加糖异生和脂解，并且还可以诱导胰岛素抵抗。严格控制血糖可能增加低血糖的风险，并增加发病率和死亡率。

6. 高血压：他的血压手术前要治疗吗？为什么/为什么不？如果是 170/100 mmHg 呢？如果是 180/110 mmHg 呢？

要点：讨论高血压的围术期并发症，但也权衡手术的风险/益处，理解高血压在手术前不可能完全治愈。

## Intraoperative management

1. Difficult Airway：How will you secure his airway? What challenges can arise in the airway of acromegalic patients? The patient becomes apneic during

sedation or induction of anesthesia and mask ventilation is impossible. What would you do?

Keypoint：This question is open-ended but the examinee should be prepared for difficult mask ventilation and intubation with appropriate emergency equipment，video laryngoscope，FOI（fiberoptic intubation）etc. They should be able to describe a sedation plan and technique for an FOI if the airway exam indicates. They should be aware of the potential for difficult mask ventilation secondary to macroglossia，mandibular enlargement，and hypertrophy of laryngeal mucosa/cartilage.

2. Induction：Describe your anesthesia induction plan，choice of agents，doses，and explain why? Would you consider placing an arterial line? If yes，would you do this before or after induction? Why or why not? Are there risks to placing an arterial line?

Keypoint：Explain concern for airway and obstruction，and justify the decision to either maintain spontaneous ventilation or to give paralysis. What additional information would an arterial line provide? Would one be helpful to guide induction in the case of cardiac abnormalities，obtain arterial blood gases，or track hemodynamic instability?

3. Maintenance：Describe your plan to maintain anesthesia and your choice of agents. Do intravenous anesthetics and volatile anesthetics have the same effect on ICP? Explain? Would you use nitrous oxide，why/why not? What about ketamine?

Keypoint：Describe cerebral metabolic rate of oxygen （CMRO$_2$ ） and cerebral blood flow （CBF） effects of various anesthetics：

Nitrous oxide：CMRO$_2$ ↑ and CBF ↑

Ketamine：CMRO$_2$ ↑ and CBF ↑

IV anesthetics：CMRO$_2$ ↓ and CBF ↓

Volatile anesthetics: $CMRO_2 \uparrow$ and CBF $\downarrow$

4. Epinephrine: Sudden onset tachycardia (heart rate 120) and hypertension (180/110 mmHg) occur during local anesthetic infiltration. What is your differential? What would you do? Would you give more fentanyl, nitroglycerine, or others? Why?

Keypoint: The examinee should recognize intravascular injection or systemic effects of epinephrine that can result from local anesthetic infiltration. Other potential causes could be light anesthesia or arrhythmia.

5. Hyperventilation in neurosurgery: What ventilator settings would you use during surgery and does it matter? What is your goal of $PaCO_2$? Would hyperventilation to $etCO_2 < 25$ mmHg provide additional benefit? Harm?

Keypoint: Explain the effects of $CO_2$ on CBF reduction, as well as the potential for harm from extreme hypocapnea $< 25$ mmHg from vasoconstriction and ischemia.

6. Accidental extubation: The surgery is proceeding uneventfully when your ventilator leak alarm starts to sound. Your $etCO_2$ waveform is lower in amplitude but present. The $SaO_2$ is 97% but starts to fall. What would you do? What might be happening?

Keypoint: Recognize the potential for accidental extubation when sharing the airway or when the bed is turned. Troubleshooting should involve 100% $FiO_2$, manual ventilation, and recognizing mechanical malfunction such as disconnection or extubation vs decreased CO (cardiac output) or bronchospasm.

7. Bleeding vs. VAE (venous air embolism): 70 min into the surgery, the MAP suddenly decreases from 85 to 35 mmHg, and HR increases from 89 to 133. What are likely causes? How would you confirm your suspicion? How

would you manage his hypotension and tachycardia?

Keypoint：A differential diagnosis could include：bleeding，anaphylaxis，arrhythmia，venous air embolism，and pulmonary embolism. The examinee should pay attention to end-tidal $CO_2$ levels，initiate pressors，notify surgeon，and prepare for massive transfusion or supportive care of VAE.

8. Emergence and extubation：explain your plan for emergence，assuming that this was a difficult airway. The surgeon requests a deep extubation to minimize the bleeding，would you agree? How would you extubate the patient?

Keypoint：Weigh the risk of residual blood in the oropharynx or airway despite throat packing，and potential for aspiration and stage 2 of anesthesia，apnea，or laryngospasm if extubating deep against the benefit of avoiding coughing and bleeding with an awake extubation. The examinee could consider giving IV lidocaine to minimize coughing.

9. Disposition：Should the patient be admitted to Neuro ICU for postoperative care，why/why not?

Keypoint：The examinee should express post-operative monitoring concerns：hypoglycemia，polyuria，respiratory distress，bleeding，or OSA.

## > 术 中 管 理 <

1. 气道困难：你将如何保护他的气道？肢端肥大症患者的气道可能出现什么情况？如果在镇静或麻醉诱导期间，患者呼吸暂停，并且不能进行面罩通气，你会怎么做？

要点：这个问题是开放式的，但是受试者应该为可能发生的面罩通气困难和插管困难准备适当的应急设备，如视频喉镜和纤维支气管镜（fiberoptic intubation，FOI）。如果气道评估提示需要FOI，应能够陈述镇静的方法和技术。还应考虑到继发于巨舌、下颌骨增大和喉部黏膜/软骨肥大导致面罩通气呼吸困难的可能性。

2. 诱导:描述你的麻醉诱导计划,药剂的选择和剂量,并解释为什么? 你考虑监测有创动脉压吗? 如果是,你打算在诱导之前还是之后? 为什么或者为什么不? 放置动脉导管有风险吗?

要点:解释气道的情况和梗阻的风险,并阐明保持自主通气还是使用肌肉松弛剂的原因。有创动脉压提供什么附加信息? 在合并心脏异常、进行动脉血气分析,或监测血流动力不稳定的情况,动脉导管对于诱导会有帮助吗?

3. 维持:描述你如何维持麻醉和选择药物。静脉麻醉药和吸入麻醉药对颅内压的影响相同吗? 请解释为什么? 你会用氧化亚氮吗? 为什么/为什么不? 氯胺酮呢?

要点:描述脑氧代谢率($CMRO_2$)和脑血流量(CBF),以及各种麻醉药对其的影响:

氧化亚氮:$CMRO_2$ ↑ 和 CBF ↑

氯胺酮:$CMRO_2$ ↑ 和 CBF ↑

静脉麻醉药:$CMRO_2$ ↓ 和 CBF ↓

吸入麻醉药:$CMRO_2$ ↑ 的 CBF ↓

4. 肾上腺素:行局麻药浸润时突发心动过速(心率 120 次/min)和高血压(180/110 mmHg)。如何鉴别诊断? 如何处理? 你会追加芬太尼、硝酸甘油或其他吗? 为什么?

要点:受试者应该认识到可能是局麻药浸润时肾上腺素进入血管或其全身性作用,其他可能的原因包括麻醉偏浅或心律失常。

5. 神经外科手术中的过度通气:你在手术过程中如何设置呼吸机? 为什么? 你的 $PaCO_2$ 的目标是什么? 过度通气至 $etCO_2 < 25$ mmHg 能否提供额外的益处或危害?

要点:解释 $CO_2$ 对 CBF 减少的影响,以及由于极端低二氧化碳<25 mmHg 引起的血管收缩和缺血的潜在危害。

6. 意外拔管：手术正在顺利进行，呼吸机泄漏报警，etCO$_2$波形存在，但是幅度较低。SaO$_2$是97%，也开始下降。你会怎么做？可能发生什么？

要点：识别在共享气道或床转动时意外拔管的可能性，故障排除应包括100%的FiO$_2$、手动通气，识别机械故障，例如气道环路断开或拔管，以及心排出量降低或支气管痉挛。

7. 出血与VAE（静脉空气栓塞）：手术70 min，MAP突然从85 mmHg降至35 mmHg，HR从89次/min增加至133次/min，可能的原因是什么？你会如何确诊？你如何处理低血压和心动过速？

要点：鉴别诊断可包括出血、过敏反应、心律失常、静脉空气栓塞和肺栓塞。应注意监测呼吸末CO$_2$水平，给升压药、通知外科医师，并准备大量输血或VAE的支持性治疗。

8. 苏醒和拔管：假设这是一个困难的气道，陈述你的苏醒计划。如果外科医师要求深麻醉拔管以尽量减少出血，你同意吗？如何拔管？

要点：深麻醉拔管在避免咳嗽和出血方面优于清醒拔管。但是有咽喉填塞，以及口咽或气道残留血块、误吸可能、全麻二期、呼吸暂停或喉痉挛的风险。可以考虑静脉给予利多卡因以减轻咳嗽。

9. 术后安排：患者术后是否送神经外科ICU监护？为什么/为什么不？

要点：受试者应考虑到术后的并发症，如低血糖、多尿、呼吸抑制、出血和阻塞性睡眠呼吸暂停等。

## > **Postoperative management** <

1. Intracranial bleeding：He is extubated in the OR，and transported to PACU awake and responsive；30 min later，he complains of headache and left-sided visual loss. What are your response and management options?

Keypoint: Recognize focal neurologic deficits after pituitary surgery concerning for compression or bleeding. The examinee should immediately notify surgeon and prepare to return to the operating room.

2. Evacuation hematoma: an emergent head CT suggests a hematoma in the left cavernous sinus and the surgeon wanted to do an emergent exploration to stop the bleeding. How would you manage the airway if there were also a lot of blood clots in the posterior pharyngeal-larynx? Would you require any additional monitors or laboratory studies?

Keypoint: Be able to recognize emergent surgery and the need for immediate intubation in a difficult airway. Be prepared for massive blood loss and hemodynamic instability with large IV access and invasive monitoring.

3. NMR（muscle relaxant）: The patient's muscle relaxation had been reversed with IV glycopyrrolate and neostigmine at extubation, and now you choose to give succinylcholine for re-intubation. Should the dose be adjusted? Do you expect the duration of succinylcholine be changed?

Keypoint: Understand the unpredictable but usually prolonged duration of action of succinylcholine after administration of reversal agents.

4. Postoperative Nausea and Vomiting（PONV）: The patient is recovering well after the re-exploration. He however is experiencing severe nausea and vomiting in the ICU. You review the anesthetic record and discover that no anti-emetics were given. What are risk factors for postoperative nausea and vomiting? What are treatment options?

Keypoint: Risk factors include: Non-smoking status, opioid medications, female gender, history of PONV or motion sickness. The presence of 4 factors is associated with PONV rates of as high as 80%. Potential other factors include long duration of surgery, certain types of surgery, such as major abdominal and gynecologic surgery. Treatment options include ondansetron, droperidol, metoclopramide, scopolamine, dexamethasone, aprepitant.

5. DI/CSW/SIADH: On POD ♯1, the patient develops polyuria. How common is polyuria after a pituitary surgery? What might be happening? How would you differentiate diabetes insipidus from cerebral salt wasting syndrome or syndrome of inappropriate anti-diuretic hormone? If the patient appears hypovolemic with high serum sodium levels and low urine sodium levels, how would you treat?

Keypoint: Describe the workup of polyuria after pituitary surgery and describe a differential diagnosis. Workup would include urine output, serum and urine $Na^+$ levels, and assessment of volume status.

| | CSW | SIADH | DI |
|---|---|---|---|
| Volume Status | Hypovolemic | Euvolemic or hypervolemic | Hypovolemic |
| Serum $Na^+$ | Low | Low | High |
| Urine $Na^+$ | High | High | Low |
| Urine output | High | Low/Normal | High |
| Serum Osm | Low | High | High |
| Urine Osm | High | High | Low |
| Treatment | Na and fluid replacement | Volume restriction | Fluid replacement and DDAVP |

CSW: cerebral salt wasting; SIADH: syndrome of inappropriate anti-diuretic hormone; DI: diabetes insipidus.

6. The patient continues to demonstrate loud snoring and signs of obstruction with $SaO_2$ 84%. What would you do? Would you apply CPAP or NIPPV? Would you use an oral airway or nasopharyngeal airway? How does CPAP or BiPAP work in patients with OSA?

Keypoint: understand that non-invasive positive pressure ventilation

(NIPPV) is relatively contraindicated after pituitary surgery due to the risk of pneumocephalus. Additionally, nasopharyngeal airways may cause direct trauma near the surgical site. NIPPV assists with the maintenance of open alveoli, decreased V - Q mismatch and redistribution of lung water.

7. Adrenal insufficiency: On POD #2, the patient develops refractory hypotension and is nauseated and vomiting. His $Na^+$ is 126 and $K^+$ is 4.9. What might be going on? If adrenal insufficiency, is this likely primary or secondary adrenal insufficiency? How would you treat it?

Keypoint: recognize clinical signs of secondary adrenal insufficiency after pituitary surgery and treat appropriately with pressors and electrolytes as appropriate, in addition to steroid replacement.

8. Complication and communication: The surgeon explains the postoperative bleeding to the patient's family, and says: "The bleed occurred when his anesthesia got light and his blood pressure was higher". What is your response?

Keypoint: Open ended question, the examinee should demonstrate teamwork and professionalism with a focus on providing the best patient care. It is important not to shift blame to the surgeon.

> **术 后 管 理** <

1. 颅内出血:患者在 OR 中拔管,送至 PACU 后清醒并有反应:30 min 后,患者诉头痛和左侧视力丧失。你如何反应和处理?

要点:了解垂体手术后由于压迫或出血引起的局灶性神经功能缺陷,应立即通知外科医师并准备返回手术室。

2. 清除血肿:紧急头部 CT 表明左海绵窦血肿,外科医师打算急诊探查以止血。如果在咽喉后部有很多血块，你如何管理气道？需要额外的监测或化验吗？

要点：能够处理急诊手术以及困难气道时快速插管。准备好粗大的静脉通路和有创监测以防大量失血和血流动力学不稳定。

3. NMR（肌肉松弛剂）：患者拔管时静注格隆溴铵和新斯的明拮抗肌松药，现在你给予琥珀酰胆碱再次插管。是否调整剂量？你认为琥珀胆碱的作用时间会变化吗？

要点：应用拮抗剂后琥珀酰胆碱作用时间难以预测，通常延长。

4. 术后恶心呕吐（PONV）：患者开颅探查后恢复良好，然而在 ICU 严重恶心和呕吐。你检查麻醉记录发现没有给予止吐药。术后恶心呕吐的危险因素是什么？如何治疗？

要点：危险因素包括非吸烟状态、阿片类药物、女性、PONV 史或晕动病史。如果同时存在 4 个危险因素，则 PONV 发生率高达 80%。潜在的其他危险因素包括手术持续时间长，某些类型的手术如腹部和妇科大手术。治疗选择包括昂丹司琼、氟哌利多、甲氧氯普胺、东莨菪碱、地塞米松和阿瑞匹坦。

5. 尿崩症/脑性盐耗综合征/抗利尿激素异常分泌综合征：术后第 1 天，患者发展为多尿。垂体手术后多尿常见吗？可能发生什么情况？如何区分尿崩症与脑性盐耗综合征以及抗利尿激素异常分泌综合征？如果患者出现低血容量，伴高钠血症和低尿钠，你如何治疗？

要点：垂体手术后多尿时的检查项目和鉴别诊断；需检查项目包括尿量、血清和尿钠离子水平，以及容量状态。

| | CSW | SIADH | DI |
|---|---|---|---|
| 容量状态 | 减少 | 正常或减少 | 减少 |
| 血钠浓度 | 低 | 低 | 高 |
| 尿钠浓度 | 高 | 高 | 低 |

（续表）

| | CSW | SIADH | DI |
|---|---|---|---|
| 尿量 | 高 | 低/正常 | 高 |
| 血清渗透压 | 低 | 高 | 高 |
| 尿渗透压 | 高 | 高 | 低 |
| 治疗 | 补钠和补液 | 控制容量 | 补液和 DDAVP |

CSW：脑性盐耗；SIADH：抗利尿激素异常分泌综合征；DI：尿崩症。

6. 患者继续表现出大声打鼾和阻塞迹象，$SaO_2$ 84%。你怎么做？你应用 CPAP 还是 NIPPV？你用口咽通气道还是鼻咽通气道？CPAP 或 BiPAP 在 OSA 患者中如何起作用？

要点：由于气颅的风险，垂体手术后无创正压通气（NIPPV）是相对禁忌的。此外，鼻咽通气道则可能造成手术部位附近直接创伤。NIPPV 有助于维持肺泡开放、降低 V/Q 不匹配，以及肺水的再分配。

7. 肾上腺功能不全：术后第 2 天，患者出现顽固性低血压并恶心呕吐。他的 $Na^+$ 为 126 mmol/L，$K^+$ 为 4.9 mmol/L。可能发生了什么？如果是肾上腺功能不全，这是原发性的还是继发性的？你如何治疗？

要点：识别垂体手术后继发性肾上腺功能不全的临床症状，除了类固醇替代外，还可以适当地用升压药物和电解质进行治疗。

8. 并发症和沟通：患者术后出血，外科医师向家属解释说"出血是由于麻醉较浅导致的血压较高"。你的反应是什么？

要点：开放式问题，受试者应该展示团队精神和专业精神，重点是给患者提供最好处理，而不是将责任推给外科医师。

References

[ 1 ] Seidman PA, Kofke WA, Policare R, et al. Anaesthetic complications of acromegaly. Br J Anaesth. 2000；84(2)：179 - 182.

［2］Lugo G，Pena L，Cordido F. Clinical Manifestations and Diagnosis of Acromegaly. Int J of Endoc. 2012.

［3］Duncan AE. Hyperglycemia and perioperative glucose management. Curr Pharm Des，2012;18(38)：6195－6203.

［4］Anesthesia for Neurologic Surgery. Drummond JC. Miller's Anesthesia，7th Ed. 2010.

［5］Effects of Anesthetics on Cerebral Blood Flow and Cerebral Metabolic Rate. Patel PM. Miller's Anesthesia，7th Ed. 2010.

［6］Brian JE Jr. Carbon dioxide and the cerebral circulation. Anesthesiology. 1998；88(5)：1365－1386.

［7］Ausiello JC，Bruce JN，Freda PU. Postoperative assessment of the patient after transsphenoidal pituitary surgery.Pituitary. 2008;11(4)：391－401.

［8］Stoelting's Anesthesia and Co-Existing Disease，5th Ed. Hines RL. pp. 402－405. 2008.

［9］Oxygen Delivery Systems. Nicholau TK. Miller's Anesthesia，7th Ed. 2010.

［10］McCoy EP，Mirakhur RK. Comparison of the effects of neostigmine and edrophonium on the duration of action of suxamethonium.Acta Anaesthesiol Scand. 1995;39(6)：744－747.

［11］Kopelovich JC1，de la Garza GO，Greenlee JD，Graham SM，Udeh CI，O'Brien EK. Pneumocephalus with BiPAP use after transsphenoidal surgery.J Clin Anesth. 2012;24(5)：415－418.

［12］Postoperative Nausea and Vomiting. Apfel C. Miller's Anesthesia. 7th Ed. 2010.

Sunny Chiao，Zhiyi Zuo

左志义

# 10 Anesthesia management for left carotid artery stent placement

## 置入颈动脉内支架的麻醉管理

> **Basic information** <

The case: a 70 years old female with recurrent TIAs and scheduled for an urgent carotid stent placement.

A 70 - year-old 80 kg woman with recurrent TIAs is brought to the endovascular suite for an urgent left carotid stent placement under monitored anesthesia care. CTA (computer tomography angiogram) demonstrated severe LICA (left internal carotid artery) stenosis and an occluded right internal carotid artery.

The patient has a long-standing history of hypertension, myocardial infarction (MI) 1 year ago with congestive heart failure post MI requiring multiple hospitalizations.

Physical examination: BP 170/105 mmHg, P 68 R 20, T 37.5℃, $SpO_2$ = 88% RA.

MEDS (medications): Lisinopril 10 mg daily, Diltiazem CD 180 mg daily, furosemide 40 mg daily, NTG prn, clopidogrel 75 mg daily, aspirin 81 mg daily. Heparin infusion.

LABS: Hgb 12.5 gm/dL; Na 130 mEq/L; K 5.2 mEq/L.

## 基本信息

一个 70 岁女性反复短暂脑缺血发作,急诊行左颈动脉内支架手术。

病史:70 岁女性,体重 80 kg,反复性缺血性意识丧失,急诊入院后准备在监护麻醉下实施左颈动脉放置支架。CT 血管造影显示严重的左侧颈内动脉狭窄和右侧颈内动脉完全堵塞。

患者有长期高血压病史,1 年前由于心肌梗死后出现心力衰竭需要多次住院治疗。

体检:血压 170/105 mmHg,心率 68 次/min,呼吸 20 次/min,体温 37.5℃,空气下的氧饱和度 88%。

用药:赖诺普利每天 10 mg,地尔硫䓬每天 180 mg,呋塞米每天 40 mg。需要时服用硝酸甘油,氯吡格雷每天 75 mg,阿司匹林每天 81 mg。静脉滴注肝素。

实验室检查:血红蛋白 125 g/L,钠 130 mmol/L,钾 5.2 mmol/L。

## Preoperative management

1. How urgent is this procedure? Why?

Keyword:Question to test the medical judgment, risk and benefit about necessity of delayed procedure, whether the patient was optimized for the procedure.

2. How does the CTA result influence the urgency?

Keyword:Question is on the knowledge of TIA and carotid artery stenosis work up and value of CTA on carotid stenosis evaluation.

3. Preoperative use of ASA and clopidogrel influence urgency? Why?

Keyword:Question about knowledge on the impact of antiplatelet (anticoagulants) on carotid stent procedure, whether anticoagulants deem to delay the surgery?

4. Does the plan for monitored anesthesia care change after obtained the patient's CV (cardiovascular) status? Why or why not?

Keyword: Open-ended question: test knowledge whether the information on cardiac function is adequate? Whether patient was optimized with her cardiac status.

5. The patient has a history of 2 - pillow orthopnea but must lie flat on the angiogram table. How will you manage?

Keyword: Question to test candidates about their adaptability. Knowledge about cardiac status on the impact of carotid stent procedure.

6. Cardiac catheterization 8 months ago demonstrated EF of 25%. At that time, 3 drug-eluting stents were placed successfully. Need more information? What? Why?

Keyword: Question about knowledge of congestive heart failure on anesthetic choice. Knowledge on anesthetic consideration on drug eluting stent and dual antiplatelet therapy. Question about the risk of coronary artery stent thrombosis.

7. Current ECHO shows unchanged EF. Given this information, how will you manage orthopnea during MAC?

Keyword: Question about knowledge of anesthetic choice with compromised left ventricular systolic function. What is the advantage and disadvantage of general versus MAC anesthesia choices in regard of carotid artery stent placement? Whether there is any contraindication of different anesthetic modalities?

8. A colleague suggests 100 mg intravenous furosemide. Do you agree? Why or why not?

Keyword: Question on the knowledge of intraoperative management of congestive heart failure. Test the candidate knowledge on pharmacology and physiology effect of administration of furosemide.

9. Why is this patient hyponatremia? Differential diagnosis?

Keyword: Question the knowledge about differential diagnosis of hyponatremia; also test the candidate about clinical implication of hyponatremia.

10. Could CHF cause hyponatremia? How? Mechanism?

Keyword: Question about pathophysiological consequence of congestive heart failure, whether congestive heart failure itself or pharmacological agents lead to hyponatremia?

11. Why might the K be elevated in the face of furosemide? Mechanism and implications?

Keyword: Question the knowledge about pharmacological effect of furosemide, test candidate about hyperkalemia significance and treatment options.

12. INR drawn in pre-procedure area is 2.5. Why do you think INR is elevated?

Keyword: Question the basic knowledge about how INR being affected? Test the candidate about intrinsic and extrinsic coagulation pathway.

13. How is heparin therapeutic effect monitored?

Keyword: Question the knowledge about the pharmacological effect of heparin.

14. Could clopidogrel or aspirin account for the elevated INR? Why or why not?

Keyword：Question the knowledge about anticoagulants like clopidogrel and aspirin，test candidate about their anticoagulation pathway.

15. What is your differential for elevated INR? Does this result affect your anesthetic plan?

Keyword：Question the knowledge about which anticoagulation pathway will lead to elevation of INR? Also test candidate about how to adjust anesthetic plan when patient has coagulopathy for carotid stent placement，test the knowledge how to balance the anticoagulation to prevent coronary artery stent thrombosis versus concerns of intraoperative bleeding.

## 术 前 管 理

1. 这个手术有多么迫切？为什么？

要点：考核医疗判断，推迟手术的风险与益处，以及患者是否已经完善手术前的准备工作。

2. CT 血管造影的结果对于手术的紧迫性有无影响？

要点：考核 CT 血管造影的知识，颈动脉狭窄的成因，以及 CTA 对颈动脉狭窄的评估作用。

3. 术前服用阿司匹林和氯吡格雷是否对手术的紧迫性有影响？为什么？

要点：了解抗血小板药物(抗凝药)对颈动脉支架置入术的影响，服用抗凝药是否应推迟手术？

4. 你所获得的患者心血管功能信息对于你准备的监护麻醉方案有无影响？为

什么？

开放式问题：考核目前了解的患者的心功能是否已经足够？患者的心脏状态是否已优化？

5. 患者习惯用两个枕头防止睡眠呼吸困难，而此术式期间患者必须要求躺平，你如何处理？

要点：考核应试者的适应性。掌握心功能状态对颈动脉支架置入术的影响。

6. 8个月前心导管检查证实左室射血分数25%，当时成功的放置了3个药物洗脱支架。你需要更多信息吗？你还想知道什么？为什么？

要点：掌握充血性心力衰竭对麻醉选择的影响，采用药物洗脱支架和双抗治疗时麻醉应考虑的问题，冠状动脉支架血栓形成的风险。

7. 近期超声心动图显示左室射血分数无变化。根据这个情况，你在监护麻醉时如何处理端坐呼吸？

要点：考核左室收缩功能受损的麻醉选择，颈动脉支架置入术时全麻与监护下麻醉的优缺点，以及禁忌证。

8. 你的同事建议静脉推注100 mg呋塞米。你是否同意？为什么？

要点：掌握充血性心力衰的围术期处理，呋塞米的药理学和生理学。

9. 为什么患者有低钠血症？你的鉴别诊断是什么？

要点：掌握低钠血症的鉴别诊断和临床意义。

10. 患者的充血性心力衰竭是否可以造成低血钠？怎样？机制如何？

要点：掌握充血性心力衰竭的病理生理影响，了解充血性心力衰竭本身或者治疗用药是否会导致低钠血症。

11. 为什么在应用呋塞米后会出现血钾升高？机制和对患者的影响？

要点：掌握呋塞米的药理作用，高钾血症的影响和处理。

12. 术前检查 INR 结果是 2.5，你认为 INR 为什么会升高？
要点：掌握 INR 的基础知识，内源性和外源性凝血通路。

13. 如何监测肝素的抗凝效果？
要点：掌握肝素的药理作用。

14. 氯吡格雷或阿司匹林是否会导致 INR 升高？为什么？
要点：掌握抗凝药，如氯吡格雷和阿司匹林相关知识，包括作用机制。

15. 对于 INR 升高你的鉴别诊断是什么？该结果是否对你的麻醉方案有影响？
要点：考核何种抗凝通路会导致 INR 升高；行颈动脉支架置入术的患者伴有凝血功能异常时如何调整麻醉方案；如何合理的抗凝，即要防止冠状动脉支架血栓形成，又要防止术中出血。

> **Intraoperative management** <

1. Is there any special monitoring other than routine ASA standard needed? Why/why not?
Keyword：Question the knowledge about variable invasive and noninvasive monitoring，knowing their potential and limitation.

2. Is neurologic monitoring needed during stent placement? Why/why not?
Keyword：Test candidate what is prefer versus standard the neurological monitoring during carotid stent placement.

3. Monitored anesthesia care is planned for the procedure. Does this change your monitoring requirements? Why/why not?

Keyword: Question the knowledge about monitoring requirements for different type anesthetic techniques.

4. While placing monitor, the patient states she cannot breathe and asks to sit up. What will you do?

Keyword: Test candidate's adaptability when encountered any unexpected clinical scenario, also question the knowledge and management skill about respiratory distress.

5. Will you proceed with this case and if so, how? What factors go into your decision?

Keyword: Test candidate's medical judgment; determine the risk and benefit ratio and risk stratification.

6. After consulting with the surgeon, you decide to postpone case (if examinee wants to proceed under general, surgeon is uncomfortable and wants more medical optimization). As you go to inform the patient, she has developed a complete right hemiparesis and aphasia and is very agitated. BP has increased to 220/130. What will you do?

Keyword: Test candidate adaptability when face acute clinical condition changes. The quick differentiate diagnosis and prepare for back up plan?

7. Surgeon suspects acute carotid occlusion and requests general anesthesia for emergent endovascular procedure to restore cerebral circulation. You agree? Why/why not?

Keyword: This asking for recognition of acute deterioration of patient medical conditions, Ask candidate to form a quick comprehensive anesthetic plan and rapid response to situation, avoid delay and potential neurological complications.

8. How will you induce the anesthesia? Choice of agent? Why?

Keyword: Test the knowledge of anesthetic induction agent, how it will impact on hemodynamics during carotid artery stent placement?

9. Goals for BP during induction? Would you use succinylcholine for induction? Why/why not?

Keyword: Question the knowledge about cerebral auto regulation, also the relationship between cerebral perfusion pressure and intracranial pressure (ICP), determine how cerebral blood flow regulated by the blood pressure and ICP?

10. Is hyperkalemia a concern? Why/why not?

Keyword: Question the implication of hyperkalemia during the induction.

11. Why does hyperkalemia occur? What is mechanism for potassium increase with succinylcholine?

Keyword: Question the knowledge about causes of hyperkalemia and specific mechanism of succinylcholine-induced hyperkalemia.

12. Surgeon requests propofol administration for cerebral protection. How does propofol provide cerebral protection? Any other methods can be used for cerebral protection? Mechanisms?

Keyword: Question the knowledge about any methods and their mechanisms of cerebral protection. Whether there is cerebral protective effect of propofol?

13. Surgeon requests BP>200 systolic until artery is reopened? You agree?

Keyword: Question the knowledge about blood pressure management during severe carotid artery stenosis. How to maintain cerebral blood flow when one side carotid artery occluded?

14. With respect to the brain，the monitoring of systolic BP is more important BP? Why/why not?

Keyword：Test the knowledge of candidate what it is an important factor to determine cerebral blood flow? How systolic and diastolic blood pressures contribute cerebral perfusion pressure?

15. How would you accomplish that level of hypertension? Defend your choice?

Keyword：Question the candidate's knowledge how to use pharmacological agents to raise the blood pressure? Give the clinical reasoning to support your selection.

16. With BP 210/100，you notice a 2 mm ST segment depression in inferior leads. What would you do? Why?

Keyword：Clearly there is conflict interest here，question the knowledge how to balance cerebral protection and myocardial protection?

17. You inform surgeon，who says that if you lower BP，the patient will have a bad neurologic outcome. What would you do? Why?

Keyword：Again test the knowledge and management skills when there is a conflict interest to deal with vital organs protection，balance the priority without compounding the complications.

## > 术 中 管 理 <

1. 是否需要除了常规 ASA 以外的特殊监测？为什么？

要点：掌握不同有创和无创监测的相关知识及其作用和局限性。

2. 在放置支架时是否需要中枢神经功能监测？为什么？

要点：掌握颈动脉支架置入时神经功能监测方法。

3. 此术式计划采用监护麻醉，是否会改变你的监测需求？为什么？

要点：掌握不同麻醉方式对麻醉监测的要求。

4. 你在放置监测时，患者抱怨她不能呼吸要求坐起来。你如何应对？

要点：考核遇到临床突发事件的应变能力，对呼吸窘迫相关知识的了解和处理能力。

5. 你是否准备继续手术？如果是，如何实施？哪些因素会影响你的决定？

要点：考核考生的医学判断能力，平衡治疗的风险和利益之间的关系。

6. 和外科医师交流后，你决定延迟手术（如果考生想做全麻，外科医师心里不踏实，要求术前进一步完善）当你去告诉患者时，她出现了完全性的右侧偏瘫和无语，并且非常躁动，血压升高到220/130 mmHg，你如何应对？

要点：考生面对紧急的临床病情变化时的应变能力，能否迅速进行诊断和鉴别诊断，并准备应急备用方案。

7. 外科医师怀疑急性颈动脉闭塞，建议全麻下急诊放置支架术式恢复脑血流循环。你同意吗？为什么？

要点：考核对患者病情恶化的认知，能否尽快制订全面的麻醉方案。对实际情况做出快速反应，从而避免拖延和可能的神经系统并发症。

8. 你如何麻醉诱导？应用什么麻醉药诱导？为什么？

要点：考核对麻醉诱导药的了解，及其在颈动脉支架置入术中对血流动力学的影响。

9. 诱导期间血压控制的目标是什么？你诱导时是否应用琥珀酰胆碱？为

什么？

要点：掌握脑血流自动调节的知识，脑灌注压和颅内压的关系，以及血压和 ICP 如何调控脑血流。

10. 你顾及高血钾吗？为什么？

要点：掌握诱导时高血钾的影响。

11. 为什么会发生高血钾？应用琥珀酰胆碱造成高血钾的原因是什么？

要点：高血钾的原因，以及琥珀酰胆碱导致高血钾的具体原因。

12. 外科医师建议应用异丙酚保护大脑，异丙酚如何提供脑保护？有其他的脑保护措施吗？机制如何？

要点：掌握脑保护的方法及其机制；异丙酚脑保护的机制。

13. 外科医师要求在颈动脉开放以前，收缩压控制在 200 mmHg 以上，你是否同意这个决策？

要点：掌握严重颈动脉闭塞时术中的血压管理；一侧颈动脉闭塞时如何维持脑的血流灌注。

14. 对于大脑来说，收缩压的监测比血压重要吗？为什么？

要点：决定大脑血流的哪个因素最重要，收缩压和舒张压如何影响脑灌注压。

15. 你如何去达到想要的血压水平？为什么？如何为你的理论提供依据？

要点：考核如何应用药物升高血压。说出临床理由支持你的决定。

16. 当血压到 210/100 mmHg 时，你注意到了在下壁导联出现 2 mm 的 ST 段压低，你应如何应对？为什么？

要点：如何平衡脑保护和心肌保护。

17. 你告诉了外科医师,他回答说如果你降低血压,患者会有不良的中枢神经预后,你应该如何做? 为什么?

要点：掌握重要脏器保护的相关知识和方法,以及如何在实施中避免发生并发症。

## > Postoperative management <

1. Patient had uneventful left carotid artery stent placement，given the patient preoperative status，how would you determine whether patient is ready to be extubated?

Keyword：Question the knowledge about extubation criteria，differentiate and identify the pulmonary and cardiac components may contribute respiratory distress after the extubation. Question the knowledge about prolong intubation and neurological exam.

2. After arrived in PACU，patient continued to have hypertension BP 200/100 mmHg，what is your approach? Why?

Keyword：Question the knowledge about blood pressure management post carotid stent placement. Test the knowledge about pathophysiological consequence of cerebral blood vessels response post stent placement.

3. Also in the PACU, the nurse reported to you that patient had new onset LBBB comparing to baseline ECG，what types cardiac workup are necessary to this new finding?

Keyword：Question the knowledge about the potential cardiac effect after carotid stent placement. Also test the candidate what are the algorithms for cardiac work up when patient has new onset ECG findings?

## > 术 后 管 理 <

1. 成功的实施了左颈总动脉支架,根据患者术前状况,你如何决定患者术后是否可以拔管?

要点:掌握拔管的标准,呼吸或心脏的因素均可能引起拔管后呼吸抑制。了解延长插管和神经系统查体的知识。

2. 到达恢复室后,患者仍然有高血压 200/100 mmHg,你如何处理? 为什么?

要点:颈动脉内支架置入术后的血压管理,以及脑血管的反应和相关的病理生理影响。

3. 在恢复室,护士告诉你患者心电图出现新发生的左束支传导阻滞,根据新的发现,你认为需要哪些检查?

要点:颈动脉内支架置入术后对心脏可能的影响,以及对新发心律失常的处理流程。

## > Additional Topics <

### Substance Abuse

19 - year-old healthy male was scheduled to have an outpatient knee arthroscopy for probable MCL injury. During your preoperative questioning, he admits to regular use of cocaine — the last use being last night. Preoperative vital signs BP 110/60, Pulse 80, RR 15, SpO$_2$ 100% on room air.

1. Will you proceed with the anesthetic? Why or why not?

Keyword: Question about anesthetic implication when patient administers recreation drugs. Necessary evaluation process for safe anesthesia for patient undergo ambulatory surgery.

2. How does cocaine use affect anesthetic management? Mechanism?

Keyword: Test the specific knowledge about cocaine effect on central nervous and cardiovascular system.

3. If you agree to proceed would you admit the patient postoperatively? Why or why not?

Keyword: Question the knowledge of consequence effect on patient who consumes cocaine.

**Pain management**

An obese 23 - year-old woman complains of severe abdominal pain and is nearly hysterical 5 hours after open cholecystectomy under general anesthesia. She has a history of opiate addiction and was receiving suboxone (naltrexone) orally preoperatively.

1. What would you recommend? Why?

Keyword: Question the knowledge about pain management when patient has history of opioid addition.

2. Would an epidural be appropriate now? Why/why not?

Keyword: Question the knowledge about epidural efficacy on abdominal surgery, particularly for a rescue measure.

3. Where should the epidural be placed? Drugs? Why? Alternative approaches to management?

Keyword: Question the knowledge about epidural dermatomes coverage for abdominal surgery. Also how to use multimodal analgesia approach to control abdominal surgery?

## Seizure management

A 14 – year-old healthy child underwent an uneventful appendectomy for a ruptured appendix. Anesthetic agents used included sevoflurane, fentanyl and rocuronium. Ten minutes after arrival in the recovery room, the child has a grand mal tonic-clonic seizure (traditionally referred as grand mal seizure) and you are called to assess the patient.

1. Initial approach and management? What agent would you use to stop the seizure? Why?

Keyword: Question the knowledge about how to response acute event like seizure, what are most important steps such as airway, breathing and circulation ABC etc.

2. Would you re-intubate the patient? How decide? Seizure controlled and patient is post-ictal. What evaluation would you do? Why?

Keyword: Question the candidate how to make the judgment on airway management after patient had an episode of seizure? Also test the candidate knowledge about seizure differential diagnosis and management process.

3. Colleague suggests this could just be from fever (temp on arrival to RR was 38.5). Agree? Another colleague suggests CT scan and neurology consults. You respond?

Keyword: Question the knowledge abut seizure disorder. Any anesthetic agents can cause seizure episode? Whether neurology consultation necessary?

## Pulses oximetry reading differentials

An otherwise healthy 20 – year-old patient with no previous medical history presents for a laparoscopic appendectomy. Prior to induction, you notice the $SpO_2$ is reading 85%.

1. The patient is not cyanotic nor tachypneic. Your approach?

Keyword: Question about the knowledge how pulse oximeter works? The potential factors which may interfere to its reading?

2. Could this reading be inaccurate? Plethysmogram traces pulse reliably with pulsatility index$>3$. What will you do?

Keyword: Still question the knowledge how to differential pulse oximetry false reading versus true reflection of hypoxemia?

3. Colleague suggests getting a venous blood gas from the IV. Could this test help you? How?

Keyword: Question the knowledge what specific test can help to determine the potential causes of low pulse oximetry reading.

## End-tidal $CO_2$ and cardiac output

During a liver resection, the end-tidal $CO_2$ suddenly falls from 35 to 16, accompanied by hypotension. You suspect air embolism. Surgeon states air embolism is not possible and believes the patient has suffered a "cardiac event".

1. Could an intraoperative myocardial infarction present with a fall in end-tidal $CO_2$?

Keyword: Question the knowledge about the relationship between end-tidal $CO_2$ and cardiac function? Whether end-tidal $CO_2$ can be a surrogate for CO?

2. How — what is the mechanism?

Keyword: Question the knowledge about dead space, how it reflects cardiac function?

3. Could you differentiate between the two problems? How?

Keyword：Question the knowledge how to clinically differentiate air-embolism versus myocardial infarction? What other modality is useful other than end-tidal $CO_2$?

---

> **附 加 主 题** <

## 滥用毒品

19 岁健康男性在门诊手术室实施膝关节腔镜修补内交叉韧带损伤。在你术前评估时,患者承认常规应用可卡因,最后一次是昨天晚上。术前生命体征：血压 110/60 mmHg,心率 80 次/min,呼吸 15 次/min,空气下氧饱和度 100%。

1. 你是否决定继续麻醉？为什么？
要点：患者应用成瘾性药物时的麻醉要点；日间手术的麻醉为了保证麻醉安全需要做哪些必要的术前评估。

2. 可卡因是如何影响麻醉管理的？机制如何？
要点：掌握可卡因对中枢神经系统和心血管功能的影响。

3. 如果你同意继续手术麻醉,术后你是否会留患者住院？为什么？
要点：掌握滥用可卡因对患者麻醉后的影响。

## 疼痛管理

23 岁的肥胖女性,全麻下实施开放性胆囊切除术,5 个小时后抱怨严重的腹痛,近乎歇斯底里。她有阿片类药物依赖病史,术前口服丁丙诺啡。

1. 你有什么建议？为什么？

要点：阿片类药物成瘾患者的疼痛管理。

2. 现在放置硬膜外置管是否适合？为什么？

要点：硬膜外麻醉对腹部手术的作用，尤其是作为补救措施的时候。

3. 硬膜外应该什么水平置管？应用什么类药物？为什么？还有其他的处理办法吗？

要点：腹部手术时硬膜外麻醉的作用范围的知识，以及如何应用多模式镇痛。

## 癫痫的管理

14岁的健康儿童由于阑尾破裂顺利实施了阑尾切除术。术中应用七氟醚，芬太尼和罗库溴铵麻醉。术后到达恢复室10 min后，你被呼叫因为患者出现全身性阵发性痉挛和癫痫表现（俗称癫痫大发作）。

1. 你首先应当如何处理？用什么药控制癫痫的继续发作？为什么？

要点：遇到紧急情况，如癫痫发作时的处理，最重要的措施包括ABC，气道、呼吸和循环等。

2. 你是否需要给患者再插管？如何决定？癫痫控制住了但是患者出现癫痫后意识不清，你如何进行下一步评估？为什么？

要点：癫痫发作后的气道管理，以及癫痫的鉴别诊断和处理原则。

3. 你的同事建议患者的癫痫与发热有关（到达复苏室时体温为38.5℃）？你是否同意？另一个同事建议CT扫描并请神经内科会诊，你如何应对？

要点：掌握癫痫发作的知识。哪些麻醉药可能诱发癫痫发作。是否有必要请神经内科医师会诊。

## 氧饱和度读数的鉴别

20 岁健康没有明显病史的患者来做腔镜下阑尾切除术。诱导之前,你注意到患者的氧饱和度的读数只有 85%。

1. 患者没有发绀或呼吸困难,你应该如何应对?
要点:氧饱和度的工作原理,哪些因素可能影响其读数。

2. 这个读数是否不正确? 可是氧饱和度曲线的波动指数大于 3 而且曲线图像可靠,你如何做下一步处理?
要点:如何鉴别氧饱和度的伪读数和真正缺氧。

3. 你的同事建议查静脉血的血气,这个检查是否对你有帮助? 机制如何?
要点:掌握哪些检查有助于确定低氧饱和度的原因。

## 呼末二氧化碳和心输出量

在肝切除术中,呼末二氧化碳水平从 35 mmHg 突然降到 16 mmHg,同时出现低血压。你怀疑是气栓所致。而外科医师说气栓不可能,他认为患者出现了心脏的问题。

1. 术中患者发生心梗是否会出现呼末二氧化碳下降?
要点:呼末二氧化碳与心功能的关系;呼末二氧化碳能否代表心排血量?

2. 呼末二氧化碳水平如何反映心室功能?
要点:无效腔的相关知识以及如何反映心功能。

3. 呼末二氧化碳水平是否可以鉴别术中气栓还是心肌梗死? 如何区别两者的不同?
要点:临床工作中如何鉴别气体栓塞和心肌梗死? 除呼末二氧化碳,是否有其他可行的方式。

**Reference**

［1］Morgan & Mikhail's Clinical Anesthesiology.

［2］Frederick A Hensley Jr，Donald E Martin and Glenn P Gravlee：A practical approach to Cardiac Anesthesia.

［3］Yao & Arusio's Anesthesiology — problem-oriented patient management.

［4］李立环 & 彭勇刚,临床麻醉学热点,心血管问题剖析.

［5］Brian A. Hall & Robert C. Changtigian. Anesthesia：A comprehensive Review.

Yonggang Peng

彭勇刚

# 11 Anesthetic management for complex posterior spinal fusion and instrumentation

复杂后路脊柱融合术及脊柱矫形器械置入术的麻醉管理

······> **Basic information** <······

A 55 year-old woman，presents for complex posterior spinal fusion（PSF）reconstruction & instrumentation（$T_1$ to sacrum），due to kyphoscoliosis and neuropathic pain resulting from MVC（motor vehicle collision）and thoracic paraplegia. SSEP（somatosensory evoke potentials）monitoring has been requested by the surgeon.

Past medical history：1）Spinal Cord Injury（SCI），S/P（status post）MVC in 2000. No motor function and sensation from $T_4$ level and below. Associated neurogenic bowel and bladder disorders；2）Depression and 3）Osteoporosis.

PSH（past surgical history）：

1）Status post anterior and posterior thoracic spinal fusion，2000.

2）Hardware removal and Herrington rod insertion，2001 & 2002.

3）Intrathecal pump & catheter insertion and replacements，2004 and 2007.

4）Cervical spinal laminectomy，2007.

5) IVC (inferior vena cave) filter placement, August, 2010.

Medications: Allegra 60 mg BID, ASA 81 mg QD, Advil 600 mg PRN, Benadryl 50 mg QHS PRN, Bupropion SR 150 mg, 2 tabs QAM, Celebrex 200 mg BID, Ditropan XL 10 mg QD, Flexeril 20 mg TID, Lyrica 100 mg TID, Neurontin 300 mg, 3 caps TID, Hydrocodone-APAP 7.5/325 mg, 2 tabs TID, Pericolace 50/8.6 mg 2～4 tabs Qhs, PRN and Intrathecal Pump: Baclofen (519 mcg/d), Clonidine (78 mcg/d), and Fentanyl (259 mcg/d). Its battery checked preoperatively without problem. Pump to be refilled 3 months later after the procedure.

Allergy: Morphine-Hallucination and IV Dye.

Social History: Smoked 1ppd x 5yrs but quit 3 months PTA. Denies alcohol or drug abuse. Former RN (registered nurse), divorced and unemployed since 2000. Review of System (ROS): noncontributory.

Physical Exam: 162 cm, 84 kg; BP 125/84 mmHg, HR 100, and $SaO_2$ (RA) 96%. Mallampati (MP) I, edentulous, TM distance greater than 3FB, and full range of motion of neck (FROM). CV: $S_1 S_2$, RRR w/o m. Lungs: CTA (clear thoracic auscultation bilateral). Neurological: A + Ox3 (awake and oriented in place, time, date) in no acute distress. Paraplegia below the T4 level. Extremity: No edema.

Lab: H/H 12.3/37, BMP WNL (basic metabolic profile is within normal limit), $Ca^{++}$ 8.4 and Phos 3.4. PT 13.8, PTT 30, and INR 1.1.

EKG. NSR (normal sinus rhythm).

CXR: NAD (no acute disease).

PFT: restrictive lung disease (RLD, moderate).

Stress Echocardiography: Negative stress test for ischemic abnormality. LV (left ventricle) and RV (right ventricle) sizes and functions are normal. PAP (pulmonary artery pressure) 28 mmHg. Left ventricular ejection fraction (LVEF) 60%. No valvular diseases.

> **基 本 信 息** <

病史：患者，55 岁女性，因脊柱后侧突畸形，车祸（MVC）引起的神经病理性疼痛和胸段以下截瘫，拟行 T1 至尾骨复杂后路脊柱融合术（PSF）（重建）及脊柱矫形器械置入。外科要求监测体感诱发电位（SSEP）。

既往史：① 2000 年因车祸导致脊髓损伤（SCI）。T4 节段以下感觉及运动功能丧失，合并神经源性肠道及膀胱功能障碍；② 抑郁症；③ 骨质疏松症。

手术史：

1）2000 年行胸段脊柱前路及后路融合术。

2）2001 年和 2002 年行内固定取出术及哈灵顿棒（Herrington Rod）植入术。

3）2004 年和 2007 年行鞘内注射泵和导管置入及置换术。

4）2007 年行颈椎椎板切除术。

5）2010 年 8 月行下腔静脉滤器置入术。

目前用药：非索非那定 60 mg BID，阿司匹林每天 81 mg，雅维 600 mg PRN，苯海拉明 50 mg QHS PRN，安非他酮 SR 150 mg，2 tabs QAM，西乐葆 200 mg BID，奥昔布宁 XL 10 mg QD，环苯扎林（Flexeril）20 mg TID，普瑞巴林（Lyrica）100 mg TID，加巴喷丁 300 mg 3 caps TID，氢可酮-对乙酰氨基酚 7.5/325 mg 2tabs TID；鞘内注射泵：巴氯芬 519 $\mu g/d$，可乐定 78 $\mu g/d$，芬太尼 259 $\mu g/d$。手术前确保泵电池充足，术后 3 个月再次向泵内注药。

过敏史：吗啡—出现幻觉及静脉染料。

个人史：吸烟 5 年，1 包/天，戒烟 3 个月。无饮酒史及药物滥用史。曾为注册护士，2000 年车祸后失业，离异。系统回顾：无特殊。

体格检查：身高 163 cm，体重 84 kg，BP 125/84 mmHg，HR 100 次/分，氧饱和度 $SaO_2$（空气）96%。气道：Mallampati（MP）I，缺齿，甲颏距大于 3 指，颈部活动自如；心血管系统：$S_1S_2$，正常心率，律齐，无杂音；肺：呼吸听诊清晰；神经系统：神志清醒，定向力正常，T4 以下瘫痪；四肢：无水肿。

实验室检查：血红蛋白 122 g/L，血色素 37%。电解质肝肾功能正常，$Ca^{2+}$ 2.1 mmol/L，磷 1.1 mol/L。PT 13.8 S，PTT 30 S，IVR 1.1。

心电图：正常。

胸片：正常。

肺功能：限制性肺功能障碍(中度)。

应急超声心动检查：心肌缺血阴性，左右心室大小及功能正常。肺动脉压 28 mmHg，左心室喷血指数 60%，无瓣膜性疾病。

---

## > Preoperative management <

The patient presents for complex posterior spinal fusion (PSF) reconstruction & instrumentation, T1 to sacrum.

1. What preoperative tests and/or preparation should the patient have before starting the anesthesia for this incoming major spine surgery?

Keypoint: This patient does not need any additional test before this incoming major spine surgery, but she needs lots of preparations as follows.

This patient should be prepared psychologically and physiologically for major spine surgery and the postoperative course.

First, preoperative coaching of deep breathing, coughing and incentive spirometry should be emphasized. Patients with evidence of lung diseases, e.g., asthma, COPD (chronic obstruction lung disease) or parenchymal lung disease, should have bronchodilator therapy or aggressive pulmonary toilet preoperatively; as a result, reducing risk.

Second, the patient should be informed if an intraoperative wake-up test is planned and reassured that she will feel no pain or discomfort during the wake-up test. In addition, the patient should be reassured that the wake-up test will be brief and that anesthesia providers will be there to keep her safe and as comfortable as possible. The patient and her family members should understand the wake-up test is frequently requested by surgeon. It is also useful to rehearse the wake-up test during the preoperative visit and at home.

Third，the patient should be told that she will be asked to open eyes and move her extremities to follow verbal commands during the anesthesia emergence，including squeezing hands.

Finally，the patient should have adequate intravenous access (14~16 ga × 2，in addition to central venous line) and be type & cross-matched for four units PRBC prior to this major surgery.

2. What are major risks in patient with scoliosis or kyphoscoliosis?

Keypoint：

1) Restrictive lung disease：Respiratory impairment proportional to angle of lateral curvature (Cobb angle).

a) Decreased total lung capacity (TLC)，vital capacity (VC)，and functional residual capacity (FRC)，but FEV1/FVC usually is normal by calculation. If VC＜40% of predicted，postoperative mechanical ventilation probably necessary.

b) Increased A-a (alveoli and arterial) gradient and alveolar hypoventilation and hypoxemia.

2) Chronic hypoxemia leads to pulmonary hypertension (PH) and cor pulmonale.

3) Mitral valve prolapse (MVP) is seen in 20% of children/young adults affected with idiopathic scoliosis.

3. What are the pulmonary hypertension (PH) definition and its severity by echocardiography? How to manage patient with PH intraoperatively?

Keypoint：

1) PH is defined as a syndrome with elevated mean pulmonary artery pressure (mPAP) equal or greater than 25 mmHg at rest，or 30 mm Hg with exercise. PH can be either primary PH or secondary PH.

2）Severity of the PH by Echo：Doppler Echo can approximate systolic pulmonary artery pressure（sPAP）. Mean PAP can be approximated because mPAP ＝ 0.61×sPAP＋2. A systolic PAP of 40 mm Hg typically implies a mean PAP more than 25 mmHg ＝ PH.

a）Mild：25～40 mmHg.

b）Moderate：41～55 mmHg.

c）Severe：greater than 55 mmHg.

3）Intraoperative anesthesia management：

a）Avoid elevations in pulmonary vascular resistance（PVR）：prevent hypoxemia，acidosis，hypercarbia，hypothermia and pain. Provide supplemental oxygen at all times.

b）Maintain SVR：Decreased SVR dramatically reduces BP and CO due to "fixed" PVR.

c）Maintain preload.

d）Maintain sinus rhythm.

e）Avoid myocardial depressants and maintain myocardial contractility.


4. What aspects of the history and physical examination （H&P） are especially important before starting the anesthesia for this incoming major spine surgery?

Keypoint：

History：The patient should be specifically asked if she has history of difficulty airway（intubation）. Cardiopulmonary reserve should be assessed by questioning the patient about shortness of breath，dyspnea on exertion，exercise tolerance，and so on. As a rule，generally，the patients who can exercise normally will have good cardiopulmonary function reserve. Pulmonary symptoms such as episodes of wheezing or cough may indicate parenchymal lung disease and change perioperative management. Patients with muscular dystrophy，marfan syndrome and neurofibromatosis should be questioned about symptoms indicating abnormal cardiac conduction such as syncope or palpitation.

Physical examination (PE): should focus on airway, heart and lungs. Mallampati (MP), TM distance, and range of motion of neck (ROM) should be examed. Wheezing or rales suggest obstructive airway disease or parenchymal lung disease. On exam of the heart, it should include auscultation for murmurs, gallops, looking for signs of pulmonary hypertension, and right ventricular failure (engorged neck veins, an enlarged liver resulting from passive liver congestion and lower extremity edema), etc.

5. What should you consider in ordering pre-medications for the patient undergoing this incoming major spine surgery?

Keypoint: I would avoid the heavy premedication with benzodiazepines and opioids in patients with morbid obesity with obstructive sleep apnea (OSA), history of difficulty airway, neuromuscular disease, evidence of pulmonary hypertension, impaired gas exchanges, or markedly decreased pulmonary function. Use of an antisialagogue (Glycoppyrolate) may be helpful because many of these surgical procedures are performed in the prone position and copious secretions may wet tape securing the endotracheal tube and causing self extubate accidently during the surgery. Preoperative prophylaxis with high-dose corticosteroids may be considered for patients with a pre-existing neurologic deficit.

6. Why the preoperative neurologic assessment and documentation is important?

Keypoint: A preoperative neurologic assessment is very important because patients who have pre-existing neurologic deficits are at increased risk for developing spinal cord injury (SCI) during scoliosis or kyphoscoliosis corrective surgery. In addition, it is essential to document preoperative neurological function or focal neurological lesions in order to distinguish them from changes associated with the surgical correction & instrumentation，and avoid confusion about intraoperative or postoperative neurological complications.

## > 术 前 评 估 <

患者拟行 T1 至尾骨复杂后路脊柱融合术（PSF）重建及脊柱矫形器械置入。

1. 在开始麻醉前，患者需要做什么额外术前检查或准备么？

要点：患者不需要做额外的检查，可以接受复杂脊柱外科大手术，但患者需要做以下术前准备：

对于脊柱手术和术后病程，患者应在心理和生理方面做好准备。

首先，应强调指导患者深呼吸、咳嗽和刺激性肺活量测定法。有肺部疾病的患者，例如哮喘、慢性阻塞性肺疾病（COPD）或实质性肺病，术前应该支气管扩张剂治疗或进行侵入性肺部灌洗，预防风险。

其次，如果术中计划唤醒试验，应该告知患者，并向患者确保他们不会感觉到疼痛或不适。另外，应向患者说明唤醒试验非常简短，麻醉医师会在旁边保证安全并让患者尽可能舒适。患者和家人应该了解外科医师术中可能频繁进行唤醒试验，在术前访视期间以及在家里练习唤醒试验都很有用。

再次，患者应该知道，在手术结束时，需要按照医师的口头指令睁眼及移动所有的肢体包括握手等。

最后，患者应该有足够的静脉通道（除了中心静脉外，还需要建立 2 条 14～16 号静脉通道，并行血型和交叉配血检测，备血 4 个单位。

2. 脊柱侧弯或者脊柱后侧突畸形患者术前评的主要风险是什么？

要点：

1）限制性肺病：其严重程度与 Cobb 角的大小呈正相关：

a）肺总量（TLC）、肺活量（VC）和功能残气量（FRC）都下降，但 FEV1/FVC 基本正常。如果肺活量<预测值的 40%，则术后可能需要机械通气。

b）导致血氧分压差（肺泡和动脉）梯度增加，肺泡通气不足和低氧血症。

2）慢性低氧血症：导致肺动脉高压和肺心病。

3）二尖瓣脱垂：20%儿童及青少年脊柱侧弯中并有二尖瓣脱垂。

3. 肺动脉高压（PH）定义是什么？如何用超声心动图评估肺动脉高压严重程度？术中如何管理合并 PH 的患者？

要点：

1）肺动脉高压是休息时平均肺动脉压（mPAP）等于或者＞25 mmHg，或者运动时等于或者＞30 mmHg 的综合征。分原发及继发性肺动脉高压两种。

2）心脏超声可评估 PH 严重程度。多普勒超声可估测肺动脉收缩压（sPAP），而 mPAP 约＝0.61×sPAP＋2。sPAP 为 40 mmHg，意味着 mPAP＞25 mmHg，也就是存在肺动脉高压。

a）轻度：25～40 mmHg。

b）中度：41～55 mmHg。

c）重度：＞55 mmHg。

3）合并肺动脉高压患者的术中麻醉管理：

a）避免肺血管阻力增加：防止低氧血症、酸中毒、高碳酸血症、低温和疼痛。总是持续吸氧。

b）维持周围血管阻力（维持后负荷）：由于肺血管阻力"固定不变"，周围血管阻力减小将导致严重低血压及低心输出量。

c）维持前负荷。

d）维持窦性心律。

e）避免心肌抑制剂，维持心肌收缩力。

4. 对于此类大型脊柱手术麻醉前，病史和体格检查最重要的方面是什么？

要点：

病史：通过重点询问患者是否有困难气道病史。询问有无呼吸急促、运动时呼吸困难和运动耐力等来评估心肺功能储备。一般而言，能够正常运动的患者通常具有良好的心肺功能。存在发作性喘息或咳嗽等肺部症状可提示实质性肺病，应调整术中管理方案。对于肌营养不良、马方综合征和神经纤维瘤的患者,应该了解有关心脏传导异常的症状,如晕厥或心悸。

体检:应当重点检查气道、心肺、Mallampati 分级、甲颏距离和颈部活动度。喘息或啰音通常提示阻塞性气道疾病或实质性肺病。在心脏检查时,应该听诊心脏杂音和奔马律,寻找肺动脉高压和右心室衰竭的表现(充盈的颈静脉,肝淤血所致的肝脏肿大和下肢水肿)等。

5. 对于此类大型脊柱手术,术前用药时应该考虑什么?

要点:对于存在病理性肥胖合并梗阻性睡眠暂停综合征、神经肌肉疾病、困难气管插管史、肺动脉高压、气体交换障碍或肺功能明显下降的患者,尽可能避免使用大剂量强效的术前苯二氮䓬类镇静和阿片类药物。使用止涎剂(格隆溴铵)很有必要,因为许多这些外科手术是在俯卧位进行,而大量分泌物可能会浸透固定气管内导管的胶布而使导管脱出。对于某些已存在的脊髓神经损伤,可以考虑术前预防性应用大剂量激素。

6. 为什么术前神经系统评估和记录很重要?

要点:术前神经系统评估很重要,是因为在脊柱侧弯或脊柱后侧凸的手术中,已存在神经缺陷的患者发展为脊髓损伤(SCI)的风险增加。此外,有必要记录术前神经功能,以避免与术中或术后神经系统并发症混淆。

## Intraoperative management

The patient is now in OR and ready for inducing general anesthesia.

1. How do you monitor this patient? Any special monitors?

Keypoint:ASA standard monitors (BP, EKG, pulse oximetry, etCO$_2$, core temperature), Foley catheter for urine output (UOP), SSEP, invasive BP monitoring with artery line, CVP and BIS monitoring.

2. Is any invasive intra-operative monitoring really necessary?

Yes, it is necessary to place artery line and central line catheters.

Keypoint:

1) During invasive intra-operative arterial pressure monitoring in this patient, what level shall BP transducer be positioned and zeroed? Why? What is your MAP goal intraoperatively?

a) Arterial catheter is used for continuous blood pressure monitoring beat by beat. During invasive intra-operative arterial pressure monitoring in this patient, BP transducer is positioned and zeroed at her external ear to maintain accurate perfusion and oxygen delivery to the major organs such as brain, heart, kidney, spinal cord and eyes.

b) It will also be easy to obtain blood samples for arterial blood gas (ABG), electrolytes and hematocrit (Hct) measurements.

c) Maintain MAP > 60 mmHg in young healthy patients, and MAP > 85mmHg in older patients with/without co-existing diseases, for adequate spinal cord perfusion. Higher MAP is acceptable as soon as dissection is complete.

2) Why CVP line is necessary in this patient? How do you monitor CVP in the prone position?

a) In addition to central filling pressure monitoring and intravascular volume assessment, CVP line is indicated in this patient because large blood loss is expected in this major posterior spine reconstructive surgery, and the patient is at risk for hemodynamic instabilities secondary to massive blood loss, pneumothorax PE/VAE (pulmonary embolism/venous air embolism), MI (myocardial infarction) or CVA (cerebral vascular accident) which request norepinephrine or epinephrine administration, as well as postoperative access for TPN (total parenchymal nutrition) use.

b) In the prone position, CVP may be a misleading indicator of right and left ventricular end-diastolic volume. More importantly, it is more useful to monitor CVP trends, but not absolute numbers.

3) Is PA catheter indicated in this patient? Why/why not?

I would not place pulmonary artery (PA) catheter in this patient because there is mild pulmonary hypertension in this patient. In addition, wedge pressure is not accurate in the prone position.

a) A pulmonary artery (PA) catheter is rarely placed in routine scoliosis or kyphoscoliosis surgery, unless the patients have co-existing diseases such as cardiomyopathy from Duchenne muscular dystrophy, pulmonary hypertension (moderate or severe) or right ventricular failure in order to optimize volume replacement therapy.

b) Placing PA catheter is an invasive procedure associated serious complication such as rupture of pulmonary artery with a mortality rate of 50%, increased in patients with pulmonary hypertension. Risk and benefit ratio must be considered. TEE (transesophageal echocardiography) can be placed intraoperatively, as needed.

3. What options for spinal cord monitoring intraoperatively? What is the incidence of neurologic complications in scoliosis surgery? Which patient is at highest risk?

Keypoint:

1) They include: electroneurophysiologic monitoring: somatosensory evoked potential (SSEP), motor evoked potentials (MEP) such as transcranial stimulation (TeMEP), and electromyography (EMG), as well as wake-up test.

2) In the most recent incidence report of the Scoliosis Research Society (2006), the incidence of complete or partial paraplegia was 0.26%. Of note, the combined anteroposterior spinal fusion and instrumentation procedures had a significantly higher incidence of spinal cord injuries (1.12%) compared to anterior (0.0%) and posterior (0.21%) procedures alone.

3) Patients are at highest risk for developing paraplegia if they have a severe rigid deformity (greater than 120 degrees), kyphosis, neurofibromatosis, congenital

scoliosis, or pre-existing neurologic deficits and if they require more invasive instrumentation.

4. What's evoked potential (EP)? What's somatosensory evoked potentials (SSEP)?

Keypoint: EP monitoring noninvasively assesses neural function by measuring electrophysiological responses to sensory or motor stimulation such as SSEP, TcMEP, EMG, etc. SSEP tests the integrity of the peripheral nerve, the dorsal spinal cord, and the sensory cortex. It may be useful and is popular during the instrumentation of the spine.

5. What variables affect SSEP?

Keypoint: Five main variables, including:

1) Primary disease and neural damage.

2) Technical: inexperienced neurophysiological monitoring personnel, electrical interference (artifact or cautery), etc.

3) Physiologic: Triple H (Hypothermia, Hypoxemia and Hypotension), global or nerve ischemia, and anemia.

4) Anesthetic effects.

5) Surgical: instrumentation with manipulation.

6. How do anesthesia agents affect SSEP monitoring differently?

Keypoint:

1) Volatileanesthetics have the greatest effect among all anesthetics on EPs, causing dose-dependent decreases in wave amplitude and increases in latencies.

2) Intravenous aesthetics in clinical doses range generally have fewer effects on EPs compared to volatile agents, but in high doses they can also decrease amplitude and increase latencies.

3）Latency：the time from starting the stimulus to the point of recorded the maximum amplitude of a positive or negative peak（warning sign：latency prolong>10% normal）.

4）Amplitude：Maximum height of a positive or negative peak（warning sign：amplitude decreases>50% normal）.

7. Does $N_2O$ affect SSEP monitoring?

Keypoint：Yes，$N_2O$ also causes decreases in SSEP wave amplitude.

8. What are advantages and disadvantages using SSEP Monitoring?

Keypoint：

Advantages：

1）Provides continuous monitoring of the neurological sensory pathways during spine surgery as a result it reduces neurological and spinal cord injuries.

2）Decreases the risk for possible accidental extubation，anesthesia awareness，and pulmonary embolus（PE）that may occur with wake-up test.

Disadvantages：

1）Does not have a perfect correlation to the motor neurological pathways.

2）Expensive equipment.

3）Need for only trained personnel to perform neurophysiologic monitoring.

4）Needles must be placed into the patient（invasive procedure）.

5）Cortical recordings may be attenuated by certain anesthetics.

9. Sensory（dorsal spinal cord）evoked potential preservation does not guarantee normal motor（ventral spinal cord）function（false-negative）because of their different anatomic pathways. Why use SSEP? How well does SSEP monitoring detect an injury that may cause paralysis?

Keypoint：

1）Several studies have shown a good correlation of simultaneous changes in both sensory and motor pathways with mechanical cord changes from surgical manipulation & instrumentation.

2）Studies have shown that SSEP monitoring is predictive of neurological outcome in spinal surgery.

3）The Scoliosis Research Society performed a multi-center survey in 1995 in which they reviewed over 51,000 surgical spine cases. They found：

a）That patients with experienced SSEP monitoring teams had 50% fewer post-op neurological deficits than patients with inexperienced teams.

b）That the occurrence of a motor deficit without SSEP warning（false negative）was 0.63%. A SSEP change was seen in all other patients who experienced a post-op neurological deficit.

10. "Can I place a Foley catheter since the patient does not have sensation below T4?" One O.R. nurse asked you before inducing patient. What is your response? Why or why not?

Keypoint：No，the nurse is not allowed to place Foley catheter before inducing this patient for general anesthesia due to concern for autonomic hyperreflexia（AH）.

11. What is autonomic hyperreflexia（AH）?

Keypoint：

1）A syndrome characterized by acute generalized sympathetic hyper reactivity in response to triggering stimuli. It occurs primarily in patients with spinal cord injury（SCI）at or above T4 – T7. Its incidence among the SCI population ranges from 66% to 75%.

2）The triggering stimulus can be nearly any endogenous or exogenous stimulus occurring below the level of the cord lesion.The reflex most commonly occurs intraoperatively but has also been reported postoperatively following recovery from both subarachnoid block and general anesthesia.

3）Distension of the rectum or urinary bladder is the most common precipitant, but the reflex may occur from spasm or distension of other viscera or from tactile or thermal stimulation of the skin.

12. What are autonomic hyperreflexia（AH）signs and symptoms?

Keypoint:

1）Patients may experience sweating, flushing, nasal obstruction, severe headache, difficulty breathing, shivering, gooseflesh, and blurring of vision.

2）Clinical observations may include severe acute hypertension（HTN）, bradycardia, arrhythmias, profuse sweating, vasodilation above the level of SCI, pallor and vasoconstriction below the level of SCI.

3）Other changes: skin and rectal Temp., ischemia in EKG, mental status change, CVA, MI, and even death.

13. What is the possible pathophysiology of AH?

Keypoint: The lack of supraspinal inhibition allows the sympathetic outflow below the lesion to react to the stimulus unopposed.

14. How to prevent and treat AH?

Keypoint:

1）Spinal block can be as a reliable technique for prevention of AH when operative procedures are performed in the lower abdomen, pelvis, and lower extremity.

2）General anesthesia also appears to be reliable in the prevention of AH, when a good depth of anesthetic effect is achieved.

3）Epidural anesthesia is unreliable for urologic procedures because of incomplete anesthesia of the sacral roots.

4）Nitroprusside can be effectively in the treatment of hypertensive crisis associated with AH. AH is best terminated by removal of the inciting stimulus.

15. How do you induce this patient? What are the potential side effects to use succinylcholine in this patient?

Keypoint：

1）Midazolam，fentanyl，and propofol，then paralyzed with vecuronium 5 mg to facilitate endotracheal intubation and then prone positioning.

2）Potential succinylcholine-related side effects include：

a）Massive hyperkalemia：Patients at risk are CVA，SCI，unhealed 3° burns，crush injuries，etc.

b）Rhabdomyolysis：Patients with Duchenne's muscular dystrophy may develop rhabdomyolysis，hyperkalemia，and intractable cardiac arrest.

c）Malignant hyperthermia.

d）Cardiac arrhythmias.

e）Anaphylactic reactions.

f）Others：postoperative myalgia，increases in IOP（intraocular pressure），ICP（intracranial pressure）and IGP（intragastric pressure），etc.


16. How do you maintain the anesthesia? TIVA vs. inhalational anesthesia?

Keypoint：

1）TIVA（total intravenous anesthesia）or intravenous-inhalational combined anesthesia，including propofol with remifentanil，dexmedetomidine，fentanyland/or ketamine，and low dose desflurane.

a）Propofol $100 \sim 200$ mcg/kg/min，remifentanil $0.05 \sim 0.5$ mcg/kg/min，dexmedetomidine $0.2 \sim 0.7$ mcg/kg/hr.，fentanyl $1 \sim 2$ mcg/kg/hr.，and/or ketamine 10 mcg/kg/min.

b）Midazolam 1 mg/hr.

c）Desflurane $0.5 \sim 0.7$ MAC.

2）Monitoring urine output（UOP）and estimated blood loss（EBL）per hour.

3）Check eyes and pressure points every hour.

17. How about the muscle relaxant? How do SSEP, TcMEP and EMG monitoring affect your muscle relaxant use?

Keypoint:

1) If only monitoring SSEP applied:

a) During instrumentation placement — muscle relaxant to achieve 0/4 on TOF (train of four). I prefer 1/4.

b) After pedicle screw placement — muscle relaxation to achieve a minimum of 2/4 (4/4 preferred) on TOF. The pedicle screw stimulation lasts about 10~15 min.

c) After pedicle screw stimulation — muscle relaxant to achieve 0/4 on TOF. I prefer 1/4.

2) If monitoring SSEP and TcMEP applied: No muscle relaxant except succinylcholine (but contraindicated in this patient) for intubation (It is common practice to use TIVA & no relaxant in cervical spine or high level thoracic spine surgery).

3) If monitoring EMG: No muscle relaxant.


18. What are potential complications in the complex PSF (reconstruction) & instrumentation, if any?

Keypoint:

1) Substantial blood loss.

2) Visual loss.

3) Intraoperative anesthesia awareness.

4) Spinal cord ischemia (paraplegia or paraparesis).

5) DVT (deep venous thrombosis), PE (pulmonary embolism), venous air embolism (VAE).

6) Peripheral nerve injury.

7) Acute renal failure, ATN (acute tubular necrosis).

8) MI (myocardial infarction), CVA (cerebral vascular accident), etc.

19. How do you do to decrease blood loss and transfusion?

Keypoint:

1) Deliberate hypotensionmay be used in young healthy patients or patients without neurologic deficits or co-existing medical diseases, but the efficacy is not approved.

2) Antifibrinolytics: Tranexamic acid vs. aprotinin (the aprotinin has been discontinued in the spinal deformity surgery secondary to risk of acute renal failure by FDA).

3) Cell saving.

4) Hemodilution (ANH-acute normovolemic hemodilution): discontinued use.

5) Positioning: patients usually positioned prone on a Jackson table, Wilson frame or bolsters to free the abdomen to minimize epidural venous engorgement as a result to reduce bleed, and avoid decreasing venous blood return and cardiac output.

20. What are risk factors for visual loss during posterior spine surgery? Who are high risk patients?

Keypoint:

1) Preoperative anemia.

2) Vascular risk factors: HTN (hypertension), carotid artery disease, glaucoma, obesity, and DM (diabetes mellitus) may be associated with perioperative visual loss.

High risk patients includes:

3) 1 + 2 (above).

4) Undergoing prolonged procedures (exceed an average of 6.5 h in duration), having substantial blood loss (reaches an average of 45% of EBV-estimated blood volume), large volume crystalloid administration, or combinations.

21. ASA (Americansociety of anesthesiologists) Guidelines: How to prevent visual loss associated with spine surgery?

Keypoint:

1) BP Management:

a) BP should be continually monitored in high-risk patients.

b) Deliberate hypotension (in the patients without pre-op hypertension or other co-existing medical diseases) during the spine surgery NOT associated with periop visual loss. MAP should be within 20% of baseline MAP, or SBP should be greater than 100 mmHg.

2) IVF (intravenous fluid) management:

a) CVP monitoring should always be considered in high risk patients.

b) Colloids (albumin preferred) should be used along with crystalloids to maintain intravascular volume in patients who have substantial blood loss.

3) Management of anemia.

a) Hb or Hct levels should be periodically monitored during spine surgery at high risk patients.

b) Hb or Hct should be maintained at a minimum of 9.4 g/dL, or 28%, respectively.

4) Vasopressors: Insufficient evidence to provide guidance for the use of α-adrenergic agonists in high-risk patients but often used intraoperatively.

5) Patient positioning:

a) The high-risk patients should be positioned so that the head is level with or higher than the heart when possible.

b) The high-risk patient's head should be maintained in a neutral forward position when possible.

6) Surgical procedures. Consideration should be given the use of staged spine procedures in high-risk patients.

7) Postoperative management.

a) A high-risk patient's vision should be assessed when the patient becomes alert (e.g., PACU, ICU, or nursing floor).

b) If there is concern regarding potential visual loss, an urgent ophthalmologic consultation should be obtained to determine its cause.

22. Assuming 20 min into the case, the patient's $SpO_2$ was 85% on $FiO_2$ 100%, HR of 110 and PIP (peak inspiratory pressure) rises to 40 $cmH_2O$ from 20 $cmH_2O$. What is the most likely diagnosis? How to diagnose pneumothorax?

Keypoint: Most likely is Pneumothorax! Always keep in mind and be prepared for a pneumothorax intraoperatively.

1) Increased airway pressure.

2) Tracheal deviation.

3) Jugular venous distension (JVD).

4) Decreased breath sounds on the affected side.

5) Hypoxemia.

6) Hypotension.

23. Seven hours into the case, her UOP is (urine output) 15 mL/hour, and CVP is 20 $cmH_2O$. Foley catheter is still in place. What do you do now?

Keypoint:

1) Evaluate patient for evidence of hypovolemia or decreased cardiac output: check BP, pulse pressure and HR.

2) After ruled out post-renal causes, then consider pre-renal or renal cause, and administer colloid and crystalloid, if needed.

3) Review EBL (estimated blood loss) and check H/H (Hgb/Hct), and transfuse PRBC, if needed.

4) Review the patient's H&P (history and physical), and check electrolytes as needed.

24. $EtCO_2$ dropped from 32 to 13 mmHg suddenly. HR from 80 to 125 bpm, and BP begin to fall. How to manage this patient now?

Keypoint:

1) Notify the surgeon immediately of a possible PE (pulmonary embolism) or VAE (venous air embolism).

2) Administer 100% $O_2$.

3) Confirm the diagnosis, e.g. by $etCO_2$ and ABG (arterial blood gas), or TEE (it can detect air 0.02 mL/kg and the most sensitive).

4) If VAE is confirmed:

a) Flood the surgical field with NS (normal saline) or packed the wound with NS-soaked sponges;

b) Provide Valsalva maneuver by manual ventilation to prevent further air entering the heart;

c) Reposition the patient (left decubitus and Trendelenburg position);

d) Consider applying 5 $cmH_2O$ PEEP;

e) Support the circulation with vasopressors and inotropes as needed.

5) If hemodynamic compromise is severe: Call for help! Supine position-perform CPR if cardiac arrest occurs; Direct aspiration of air form CVP line. Internal cardiac massage may be required.

25. If the monitoring electrophysiologist (EP) told you that your patient lost all SSEP signals during instrumentation, what are your responses? Why?

Keypoint:

1) Quickly to rule out cause resulting from technical, physiologic or anesthetic factors (see the five main variables, refer to intraoperative question 4 above).

2) If the waveform does not return to normal, the surgeon should be notified immediately and release distraction on the cord.

3) Paraplegia is one of the most feared complications of spinal surgery. Therefore, it is so important that any intraoperative compromise of spinal cord function be detected as early as possible and reversed immediately.

4) The two methods well developed to accomplish this are the neurophysiologic

monitoring (SSEP, MEP and EMG), and the wake-up test.

5) The neurophysiologic monitoring such as SSEP assists in early diagnosis and intervention in situations of potential spinal cord compromise but there are some disadvantages (as discussed above).

6) The compromise may be the result of direct trauma, ischemia, compression, or hematoma.

26. What is the wake-up test? Why to perform intraoperative wake-up test? How to perform it intraoperatively?

Keypoint:

1) The wake-up test consists of the intraoperative awakening of the patient after completion of spinal instrumentation. The intraoperative wake-up test can be used to confirm neurologic dysfunction directly in the presence of changes in SSEP or MEP waveforms.

2) How to perform wake-up test: Open questions.

At about 17: 30 pm: the patient is turned to supine position, and has severe facial edema and swollen eyes, started spontaneous breathing, and appeared to have severe pain, restless associated with elevated BP and tachycardia (BP 200/100 mmHg, HR 120). Fentanyl 100 mcg, Hydromorphone (Dilaudid) 1 mg, Metoprolol 2 mg, and Midazolam 1 mg given.

19: 30 pm: VS are BP 150/90 mmHg, P 102, and SaO$_2$ 99%. Moving upper extremities and head involuntarily but confused and did not follow verbal commands to move lower extremities.

27. What is the most likely diagnosis? What are your differential diagnoses (DDX)? What do you do now?

Keypoint:

The most likely diagnosis is delayed emergence.

1) First address the life-threatening causes（ABCD）:

a) A for airway: Patent? Hypoxemia?

b) B for breathing: Adequate? Hypercarbia（$CO_2$ narcosis）? Hypocarbia (that removes the drive to breathe)?

c) C for circulation: Hypotension? Hypertensive? Arrythmia? Ischemia?

d) D for diabetic? Cirrhotic? R/O (rule out) hypoglycemia.

2) After that, consider other causes of the differential diagnoses（PMN）:

a) P for pharmacologic: premeds (scopolamine and droperidol), narcotics, benzodiazepines, muscle relaxants, residual anesthetics（inhalational vs. IV）, etc.

b) M for metabolic: Temp., pH, electrolytes, etc. Check ABG and BMP.

c) N for neurological: CVA (ischemic, hemorrhagic, or embolic), or post-seizures state? Head CT scan, and /or a neurological consult?

---

## > 术 中 管 理 <

患者现在在手术室,并准备全麻诱导。

1. 你将如何对该患者进行监测? 需要监测哪些特殊项目吗?

要点: 监测项目包括美国麻醉学会（ASA）标准监测项目（血压、心电图、氧饱和度 $SaO_2$、呼末二氧化碳和中心体温）,插尿管监测尿量、体感诱发电位（SSEP）、有创动脉压、中心静脉压（CVP）及脑电双频谱指数（BIS）。

2. 该患者术中是否真的需要任何有创监测吗?

是的,该患者术中的确需要有创动脉压和中心静脉压（CVP）监测。

要点:

1) 该患者在术中行有创动脉压监测时,动脉传感器应当放置什么位置调节零点? 为什么? 脊柱手术术中平均动脉压目标是什么?

a）动脉导管用来行有创动脉压连续监测。该患者在术中行有创动脉压监测时，动脉传感器应当放置于该患者外耳道水平，以确保重要脏器（脑、心脏、肾脏、脊髓和眼球等）的血流灌注及氧气输送。

b）术中动脉导管可方便地用于抽血化验，检查血气分析、电解质和血球压积。

c）脊柱手术术中平均动脉压目标：在健康年轻患者维持在 MAP＞60 mmHg。在老年人或者合并其他内科疾病的患者维持在 MAP＞85 mmHg。手术分离结束前更高的血压也是可以接受的。

2）为什么该患者中心静脉导管是必须的？在俯卧位如何监测 CVP？

a）除监测中心静脉压（CVP），评估血容量外，该患者还有放置中心静脉导管的多个适应证：复杂脊柱后路重建手术有大出血、气栓、肺栓塞、气胸、心梗式血管意外等风险，导致血流动力学不稳定，此时需要推注肾上腺素和去甲肾上腺素。此外中心静脉导管术后可用作静脉高营养。

b）在俯卧位时，CVP 可能会误导左心室和右心室舒张末期容积的读数。更重要的是监测 CVP 的趋势，而不是绝对数值。

3）该患者术中有必要放置 PA 导管吗？为什么/为什么不？

我不打算在该患者术前放置肺动脉导管，因为她只有轻度肺动脉高压，此外肺动脉导管测定楔压（wedge pressure）在俯卧位时，也不准确。

a）肺动脉导管在脊柱侧弯或者脊柱后侧突畸形该类患者中，并非常规放置，除非患者合并由于杜氏肌营养不良（Duchenne muscular dystrophy）所致的心肌病，中度或者重度肺动脉高压，或者右心功能不全，此时 PA 用于优化液体替代治疗。

b）放置肺动脉导管系有创手术，可合并严重并发症如肺动脉破裂。一旦肺动脉破裂，其死亡率为 50%，而且在合并肺动脉高压患者的死亡率更高，所以放置肺动脉导管时一定要考虑风险获益比。若有必要，术中可放置经食道超声（TEE）。

3. 脊髓监测有哪些选择？脊柱侧弯手术中神经并发症发生率是多少？脊柱手术中，哪些是截瘫高风险患者？

要点：

1) 包括：电神经生理学监测：体感诱发电位(SSEP)、运动诱发电位(MEP)如经颅运动诱发电位(TcMEP)、肌电图(EMG)和唤醒试验。

2) 脊柱侧弯研究会(The Scoliosis Research Society)2006 年进行的多中心研究回顾了超过 6 334 例脊柱手术病例,他们报道了截瘫或部分脊髓损伤的严重并发症为 0.26%。脊柱侧弯前后路联合融合手术及脊柱矫形器械置入的脊髓损伤并发症(1.12%),大大高于单独前路(0.0%)或后路脊柱手术(0.21%)。

3) 发生截瘫高风险患者为严重脊柱侧弯畸形>120°、脊柱后侧凸、神经纤维瘤病、先天性脊柱侧弯,或已存在神经缺陷,并且在脊柱手术中需要放置更多矫形器的患者。

4. 什么是诱发电位(EP)？ 什么是体感诱发电位(SSEP)？

要点：EP 监测是通过无创方式监测神经对感觉或运动刺激的神经生理学反应以测量诱发电位,评估神经功能,如 SSEP,经颅运动诱发电位(TcMEP)和肌电图(EMG)。SSEP 可以监测外周神经、脊髓背侧及感觉皮质的功能。在脊髓矫形器置入手术中应用可能更有益,且更广泛。

5. 哪些因素影响体感诱发电位(SSEP)？

要点：五大主要影响因素,包括：

1) 原发病及神经损伤。

2) 技术问题：神经生理监测人员经验不足,电信号干扰(假象或电刀)等。

3) 生理情况：三低(低温、缺氧、低血压)、弥漫性或局部神经缺血、贫血。

4) 麻醉药物的影响。

5) 外科手术：外科手术操作或矫形器械置入。

6. 麻醉药物是如何干扰体感诱发电位监测的?

要点：

1) 所有麻醉药物中,吸入麻醉药对 SSEP 影响最大,可引起剂量依赖性的波幅减低、潜伏期延长。

2) 相比吸入性麻醉药,临床剂量的静脉麻醉药对诱发电位的影响较小,但大剂量静脉麻醉药也可引起波幅减低、潜伏期延长。

3）潜伏期：从刺激开始到最大波幅度正或负峰值的时间（警告标志：潜伏期正常值延长＞10%）。

4）波幅或振幅：从波幅的最高点或最低点到基线的距离（警告标志：正常值振幅减小＞50%）。

7. 氧化亚氮对体感诱发电位是否有影响？

要点：是的，氧化亚氮也可引起 SSEP 变化，即波幅减低。

8. 体感诱发电位监测的优缺点？

要点：

SSEP 的优点：

1）提供术中感觉神经通路的连续监测，降低脊髓神经损伤的并发症。

2）可降低唤醒试验时患者意外拔管、术中知晓及肺栓风险。

SSEP 的缺点：

1）与运动神经通路相关性欠佳。

2）设备昂贵。

3）需受训的专职人员进行神经生理学监测。

4）需将探针刺入患者身体（有创）。

5）某些麻醉剂可能减弱皮层记录。

9. 由于解剖传导通路不同，感觉（脊髓背侧）诱发电位监测不能保证运动（脊髓腹侧）功能正常（假阴性）。为什么使用体感诱发电位监测？体感诱发电位监测如何发现可能引起瘫痪的损伤？

要点：

1）数项研究表明脊柱手术操作和器械置入使脊髓发生机械改变时，会同时出现运动及感觉通路的变化，两者具有良好的相关性；

2）研究表明 SSEP 监测对脊柱手术术后神经功能结果具有预测性；

3）脊柱侧弯研究会 1995 年进行的多中心研究回顾了超过 51 000 例脊柱手术

病例,研究发现:

a）术中进行 SSEP 监测的病例中,术后脊髓及神经功能受损的发生率在经验丰富的电神经生理学家组比经验不足的监测者组低 50%。

b）术后出现运动神经损伤但 SSEP 监测未发现（假阴性）的发生率为 0.63%,所有术后出现神经功能损伤的患者都出现了体感诱发电位改变。

10. "由于患者 T4 以下感觉丧失,我是否可置入 Foley 尿管"? 一名手术室护士在全身麻醉诱导前向你提出这个问题。你应如何作答? 为什么/为什么不?

要点:不行! 这个患者在全麻诱导之前,护士不可插尿管,因为可致自主反射亢进。

11. 什么是自主反射亢进（AH)?

要点:

1）由于触发刺激引起机体急性广泛交感神经反应性亢进所出现的综合征。常见于 T4～T7 节段或以上节段脊髓损伤患者(SCI),在脊髓损伤患者中其发生率范围是 66%～75%。

2）诱发刺激可以是发生在损伤平面以下任何内源性或外源性刺激,该反射最常见于手术中,但也有报道称术后腰麻和全麻恢复期出现该反射。

3）直肠或膀胱膨胀扩张是最常见的诱发因素,但其他脏器痉挛、扩张或皮肤触觉、温觉刺激均可能引起反射。

12. AH 有哪些症状和体征?

要点:

1）可能出现出汗、皮肤潮红、鼻塞、严重头痛、呼吸困难、寒战、皮疹和视物不清。

2）体征可能包括严重的急性高血压、心动过缓、心律失常、大量出汗、脊髓损伤节段以上部位血管扩张,损伤节段以下部位血管收缩皮肤苍白。

3）其他改变:皮肤及直肠温度改变、心电图示心肌缺血、精神症状、脑血管意外、心肌梗死,甚至死亡。

13. AH 可能的病理生理学是什么？

要点：损伤节段以下脊髓失去上位神经元的抑制作用，导致损伤平面下交感神经冲动过度释放。

14. 如何预防和治疗 AH？

要点：

1）若手术部位位于下腹部、盆腔或下肢，腰麻（SAB）是一种预防 AH 的可靠方法。

2）如果麻醉深度合适，全麻也是一种预防 AH 的可靠方法。

3）由于对骶神经根阻滞不完全，因而行泌尿外科手术时使用硬膜外麻醉对于预防 AH 效果不可靠。

4）硝普钠用于治疗 AH 引起的高血压危象最有效。终止 AH 的最佳办法是迅速停止刺激诱发因素。

15. 你如何实施全麻诱导？该患者使用氯琥珀胆碱可能出现哪些不良反应？

要点：

1）咪达唑仑、芬太尼和丙泊酚，然后给予肌松剂维库溴铵 5 mg，完成插管并俯卧位。

2）使用氯琥珀胆碱可能出现的不良反应：

a）严重高钾血症：脑血管意外、脊髓损伤、未治疗的三度烧伤、严重挤压伤等。患者易发生高钾血症。

b）横纹肌溶解：Duchenne 型肌营养不良患者可能出现横纹肌溶解、高钾血症、顽固性心脏骤停。

c）恶性高热。

d）心律失常。

e）过敏反应休克。

f）其他：术后肌痛、眼内压、颅内压和胃内压升高等。

16. 你如何实施全麻维持？全凭静脉麻醉 vs 吸入麻醉？

要点：

1）最常用的是全凭静脉麻醉（TIVA），或静脉-吸入复合麻醉（丙泊酚和镇痛药物输注如瑞芬、右美托咪定、芬太尼和/或氯胺酮和低剂量的吸入麻醉药，和苯二氮䓬类）。

a）丙泊酚 $100\sim200\ \mu g/(kg \cdot min)$，瑞芬 $0.05\sim0.5\ \mu g/(kg \cdot min)$，右美托咪定 $0.2\sim0.7\ \mu g/(kg \cdot h)$，芬太尼 $1\sim2\ \mu g/(kg \cdot h)$，和/或氯胺酮 $10\ \mu g/(kg \cdot min)$。

b）咪达唑仑 1 mg/h。

c）地氟烷 0.5～0.7 MAC。

2）监测每小时尿量及出血量。

3）每小时检查眼睛及压迫点情况。

17. 当监测体感诱发电位（SSEP）、经颅运动诱发电位（TcMEP）和肌电图（EMG）时，是否影响肌松药的使用？

要点：

1）如果仅监测体感诱发电位（SSEP）：

a）脊柱矫形器置入期间—肌松需达到 0/4，以 4 个成串刺激（train of four, TOF）监测，首选 1/4。

b）椎弓根螺钉放置完毕后—肌松至少应达到 2/4，以 TOF（首选 4/4）监测，椎弓根螺钉刺激持续约 10～15 min。

c）椎弓根螺钉刺激完成后—肌松维持在 0/4，以 TOF 监测，首选 1/4。

2）如果监测体感诱发电位（SSEP）和经颅运动诱发电位（TcMEP）：除了给予琥珀酰胆碱（该患者禁忌使用）完成插管外，不需给予肌松药（颈椎或高段胸段脊柱手术中经常应用全静脉麻醉且不使用肌松药）。

3）如果监测肌电图（EMG）：避免使用肌松剂。

18. 复杂后路脊柱融合术（重建）及脊柱矫形器械置入，可能出现哪些并发症？

要点：

1）大量失血。

2）视力丧失。

3）术中知晓。

4）脊髓缺血（截瘫或轻瘫）。

5）深静脉血栓、肺栓塞或静脉气栓。

6）外周神经损伤。

7）急性肾衰竭和急性肾小管坏死。

8）心肌梗死、脑血管意外等。

19. 你将采用何种措施减少出血及输血？

要点：

1）控制性降压：可用于接受多节段胸椎或腰椎手术的年轻患者，或没有神经损伤或合并其他内科疾病的患者，但是其效用尚未得到证实。

2）抗纤溶药：氨甲环酸 vs.抑肽酶（由于抑肽酶存在引起急性肾衰竭的风险，已经不再用于脊柱矫形手术）。

3）术中血液回收。

4）血液稀释（ANH-急性等容量血液稀释）：已经弃用。

5）体位：患者俯卧位于 Jakson 床、Wilson 架或垫枕上，有助于避免腹部受压，减小硬膜外静脉充盈，从而减少出血，避免回心血量及心输出量减少。

20. 后路脊髓手术中哪些是失明的危险因素？哪些是高危患者？

要点：

1）术前贫血。

2）血管危险因素：高血压、颈动脉疾病、青光眼、肥胖及糖尿病患者可能出现围术期视力丧失。

高危患者包括：

3）上述 1+2。

4）手术时间长（平均超过 6.5 h），大量失血（达到平均有效血容量的 45%），输注大量晶体液，或两者兼有。

21. 如何预防脊柱手术相关的失明?

要点:

1) BP 管理:

a) 高危患者应当连续监测血压。

b) 脊髓手术中实施控制性降压(术前无高血压或其他疾病的患者)与围术期失明无关,MAP 波动范围应控制在基础 MAP 的 20%之内,或者保证收缩压高于100 mmHg。

2) 液体管理:

a) 高危患者应考虑 CVP 监测。

b) 当患者出现大量失血时,胶体液(常用白蛋白)应与晶体液同时使用以维持血容量。

3) 贫血的管理:

a) 高危患者在实施脊髓手术过程中应当周期性监测血红蛋白(Hb)或血色素(Hct)水平。

b) 血红蛋白应保持在至少 94 g/L 以上,或血色素保持至少在28%以上。

4) 升压药:目前尚无充分的证据指导如何在高危患者使用 α 肾上腺素能激动剂治疗。但术中经常使用 α 肾上腺素能受体激动剂。

5) 患者体位。

a) 高危患者摆体位时应保证头部与心脏同一水平或高于心脏水平。

b) 高危患者头部需保持中立向前的位置。

6) 手术操作:高危患者应当考虑分期脊柱手术。

7) 术后管理:

a) 高危患者术后清醒后应当评估其视力(如在 PACU、ICU、护理楼层)。

b) 如果可能出现失明,应当立即请眼科会诊查明原因。

22. 假如手术 20 min 后,吸纯氧时患者的氧饱和度 99%降至 85%,心率 110 次/min,气道峰压 20 cmH₂O 增大至 40 cmH₂O,最可能的诊断是什么? 如何诊断气胸?

要点:最可能的诊断是气胸,时刻提防并随时准备应对可能发生的气胸。

1）气道压力升高。

2）气管偏移。

3）颈静脉扩张（JVD）。

4）气胸侧肺呼吸音降低。

5）低氧血症。

6）低血压。

23. 手术进行 7 个小时后，该患者尿量（UOP）15 mL/h，CVP 20 cmH$_2$O。Foley 尿导管仍在原处。你现在应该如何做？

要点：

1）评估患者有无低血容量或心输出量减少证据：检查血压，脉压和心率。

2）排除肾后性原因，然后考虑肾前性或肾性原因，如有需要，给予胶体和晶体补液。

3）评估出血量（EBL）和检查血红蛋白/血色素（H/H），如有需要，输血。

4）评估患者病史和体格检查，并检查电解质。

24. 呼末二氧化碳从 32 mmHg 突然降至 13 mmHg。心率从 80 次/min 升到 125 次/min，血压开始下降。你如何处理？

要点：

1）应立即通知外科医师可能发生肺栓（PE）或空气栓（VAE）。

2）给予 100% 氧气。

3）确定诊断，如呼末二氧化碳和血气分析，或经食道超声心动检查（TEE 最敏感，可以检测到 0.02 mL/kg 气泡）。

4）如果 VAE 确认：

a）外科手术区生理盐水灌洗或生理盐水浸湿海绵包裹伤口。

b）手控通气，防止气体进入心脏。

c）患者左侧卧位，取头低脚高位。

d）考虑应用 PEEP 5 cmH$_2$O。

e）循环支持：用升压药和正性肌力药物。

5)如果血流动力学严重不稳:立即求助! 如果心脏骤停,仰卧位进行 CPR;从中心静脉导管(CVP)直接回抽空气。可能需要进行心内按摩。

25.如果正在实施监测的电神经生理学家发现并通知你:矫形器置入期间,患者失去所有体感诱发电位(SSEP)数据,你如何处理? 为什么?

要点:

1)迅速分析原因是技术因素,生理因素或麻醉因素(见前述术中问题 4:五大主要影响因素)。

2)如果波形没有很快恢复正常,应当迅速告知外科医师,停止对脊髓的牵拉。

3)截瘫是脊柱手术最可怕的并发症,因此术中任何对脊髓功能有损伤的因素都应尽早发现和及时纠正。

4)充分利用已发展成熟、可满足要求的两种监测手段,包括电神经生理学监测(SSEP、MEP 和 EMG)和唤醒试验。

5)通过电神经生理学监测如体感诱发电位(SSEP)可以对潜在的脊髓损伤作出早期诊断和干预,但该监测也存在某些缺点(见前述)。

6)造成脊髓损伤的原因可能是直接创伤、缺血、压迫或血肿。

26.什么是唤醒试验? 为什么实施唤醒试验? 术中如何实施?

要点:

1)唤醒试验是指术中完成脊柱矫形器械置入后将患者唤醒,术中通过监测体感诱发电位(SSEP)或运动诱发电位(MEP)了解脊髓神经功能,如果波形出现变化,术中唤醒试验能够直接发现是否有脊髓神经功能障碍。

2)术中如何实施:开放性问题。

约在下午 17:30,患者改为仰卧位,出现严重颜面部水肿及眼睛肿胀,自主呼吸恢复,表现出严重疼痛和烦躁不安,伴高血压及心动过速(BP 200/100 mmHg,HR 120 次/min)。给予芬太尼 100 $\mu$g,盐酸氢吗啡酮 1 mg,美托洛尔 2 mg,咪达唑仑 1 mg。

下午 19:30:BP 150/90 mmHg,P 102 次/min,SaO$_2$ 99%,患者上肢和头部不自主活动,但意识不清,不能听从指令活动下肢。

27. 最可能诊断是什么？哪些鉴别诊断？你现在应该怎样做？

要点：

最可能的诊断是苏醒延迟。

1）首先考虑威胁生命的病因（ABCD）：

a）A 是气道：气道是否开放？低氧血症？

b）B 是通气：通气是否充分？高碳酸血症（$CO_2$ 昏迷）？低碳酸血症（引起呼吸驱动停止）？

c）C 是循环：循环—低血压？高血压？心律不齐？缺血？

d）D 是糖尿病：是否糖尿病引起的？肝硬化？排除低血糖。

2）考虑过上述因素后，全面分析其他可能的病因（PMN）：

a）P 是药物：包括术前用药（东莨菪碱和氟哌利多）、麻醉性镇痛剂、苯二氮䓬类、肌松药、残余麻醉剂（吸入 vs 静脉）等。

b）M 是代谢：包括检查体温、电解质（BMP）、血气（ABG）和肝肾功能是否正常等。

c）C 是神经：包括 CVA（脑缺血、出血、栓塞）或惊厥后状态？头颅 CT 和/或神经科会诊？

## > **Postoperative management** <

1. Is this patient ready for extubation? Why or why not?

Keypoint：No，she cannot be extubated because she has severe facial edema，possible airway edema，and does not follow commands. She cannot move her low extremities yet.

ACME Guideline for Extubation：

1）Adequate level of consciousness.

2）Airway reflexes intact（extubating someone who promptly aspirates is bad practice）.

3）The ETT tube is NOT acting as a "stent". The airway collapses after the "stenting" of the airway is removed by YOU (such as post-massive fluid resuscitation, and massive edema everywhere means massive edema in the airway. How do you confirm?).

4) Stable hemodynamics.

5) Vital capacity greater than 10 mL/kg, tidal volume greater than $3 \sim 6$ mL/kg, spontaneous respiration rate less than 30/min and negative inspiratory force greater than $-30$ cmH$_2$O.

6) Normal temperature, good pain control, SaO$_2$, ETCO$_2$, etc.


2. Patient should be sedated in ICU in order to tolerate the endotracheal tube (ETT), but easily arousable enough to be examined every hour for potential neurologic complications. Neurological sequelae probably remain to be the most feared complications, and it is very important to document postoperative neurologic exam findings. How are you going to sedate this patient?

Keypoint: I would like to use dexmedetomidine because it is a good choice for short-term analgesia and sedation in this type patient population. It offers potent synergy with opioids for analgesia, and it is easily titrated for frequent wake-up neurological examinations. My other choice would be a combination of fentanyl and midazolam infusion.


3. How are you going to manage this type patient's postoperative pain?

Keypoint:

1) Multimodal therapy: Most patients undergone scoliosis or kyphoscoliosis surgery use intravenous patient-controlled analgesia (PCA). Hydromorphone and morphine are commonly used opioids, and IV PCA is usually used until postoperative day 2. Preoperative methadone and perioperative ketamine can reduce postoperative opioid requirements and associated complications. Oral analgesics (e.g., oxycodone or hydrocodone with acetaminophen) should be

administered once the patient is awake enough to swallow pills. Antiemetics should be given prophylactically, starting in the operating room. Serotonin receptor antagonists (e.g., ondansetron) are the first-line treatment.

2) Neuraxial analgesia will reduce opioid requirements and associated a) complications such as PONV and itching, as well as shorten hospitalization. Epidural catheter can be placed intraoperatively. Opioids and /or local anesthetics can be infused. Local anesthetics may interfere with the postoperative neurologic exam so you have to discuss timing with the surgeon. b) Intrathecal preservative-free morphine has been shown to provide better pain relief than intravenous opioids in patients undergoing lumbar spine surgery.

3) Peri-incisional local anesthetics injection or infusion may reduce narcotic analgesic requirements postoperatively to reduce incidence of chronic pain and narcotics related complications such as PONV.

4. What complications may occur following scoliosis or kyphoscoliosis posterior corrective surgery? How to manage these complications, if any?

Keypoint: These complications include bleeding, pneumothorax, hemothorax, atelectasis, adynamic ileus, pleural effusion, neurologic injury and blindness.

Pneumothorax may occur due to central line placement and anterior or posterior surgical dissections. Chest radiography should be obtained upon arrival in the ICU or post-anesthesia care unit (PACU).

Atelectasis may occur because of the use of opioids and prolonged supine positioning. Incentive spirometry and deep breathing should be emphasized.

Delayed paraplegia in the first few days postoperatively has been reported, in addition to intraoperative neurological complications due to instrumentation or distraction of the spine.

Neurological complication probably remains the most feared one. Therefore, it is very important for continued neuromonitoring postoperatively.

Postoperative blindness is a rare with incidence of $0 \sim 0.1\%$, but devastating complication associated prone position. Risk factors include male, morbid obesity, Wilson frame, undergoing prolonged procedures (exceed an average of 6.5 h in duration), having substantial blood loss (reaches an average of 45% of EBV), large volume crystalloid administration, or any combinations.

5. How to optimize postoperative pulmonary status in this patient population?

Keypoint: Incentive spirometry (IS) should be taught preoperatively and should be used aggressively in the postoperative period. It is mandatory. Deep breathing and coughing should be always encouraged. Adequate analgesia should be achieved with opioids to allow coughing and incentive spirometry without excessive respiratory depression.

> 术 后 管 理 <

1. 该患者是否可以拔管？为什么/为什么不？

要点：患者意识不够清醒,有严重面部水肿,可能有气道水肿且不能活动下肢,所以不可以拔管。

ACME 拔管指南：

1）患者意识足够清醒。

2）气道反射完好（患者拔管时出现误吸是不应该的）。

3）气管插管并非"支架"。将"支架"移除后可能出现气道塌陷（大量液体复苏后,全身大面积水肿意味着气道可能存在水肿,你将如何判断?）。

4）血流动力学稳定。

5）潮气量大于 $3\sim6$ mL/kg,肺活量（VC）$>10$ mL/kg,自主呼吸频率$<30$次/min,吸气负压$>-30$ cmH$_2$O。

6）体温正常;疼痛控制良好;SaO$_2$和 etCO$_2$正常。

2. 患者拟在 ICU 中镇静以耐受气管内导管，但需要患者容易唤醒以配合每小时对神经系统潜在并发症的检查。神经系统后遗症是最恐怖的并发症，因此术后记录神经检查结果非常重要。你将如何镇静这个患者？

要点：我会使用右美托咪定，因为对于这类患者人群的短期镇静来说，它是良好的选择。它与阿片类药物协同达到强效镇痛，并且很容易满足频繁的神经系统体格检查。另外的选择是芬太尼和咪达唑仑的联合静脉输注。

3. 如何治疗这类患者的术后疼痛？

要点：

1) 多模式药物治疗方案：大多数行脊柱侧弯或脊柱后侧凸手术的患者，使用静脉内患者自控镇痛（PCA）。氢吗啡酮和吗啡是常用的阿片类药物，并且 PCA 通常使用到术后第 2 天。术前给予美沙酮及围术期给予氯胺酮都可以有效降低镇痛剂的用量及全身不良反应。一旦患者苏醒，可以吞服药片时，应当采用口服镇痛药（例如羟考酮或含有对乙酰氨基酚的氢可酮）。在手术室时就应当开始预防性给予止吐药。$5-HT_3$ 受体拮抗剂（例如昂丹司琼）是治疗术后恶心呕吐（PONV）的一线药物。

2) 轴索镇痛能减少阿片类药物的用量和相关并发症，如 PONV 和瘙痒技术；还能缩短住院时间。

a) 可于术中置入硬膜外导管，以给阿片类药物和/或局麻药。局麻药可能干扰术后神经功能检测，因此要和外科医师讨论给药时机。

b) 对于腰椎手术的患者，鞘内注射无防腐剂吗啡的止痛效果要好于静脉注射吗啡。

3) 手术切口注射或持续泵注射局麻药可减少术后麻醉性镇痛药的需要量，降低慢性疼痛的发生率，减少相关并发症，如术后恶心呕吐（PONV）。

4. 脊柱侧弯或脊柱后侧凸经后路手术，术后可能发生什么并发症？如何处理？

要点：这些并发症包括出血、气胸、血胸、肺不张、动力性肠梗阻、胸腔积液和神经损伤和失明。

气胸：中心静脉置管、胸段脊柱前路或后路外科操作均可能导致气胸发生。

一旦到达 ICU 或麻醉后监护室（PACU）就应当立即进行胸部 X 线检查。

肺不张：由于使用阿片类药物和长期仰卧位，可能会发生肺不张。应强调刺激性肺活量测定法和深呼吸。

迟发性截瘫：除了由于脊柱矫形器械置入或脊髓牵拉导致的术中神经系统并发症外，还有报道术后几天内的迟发性截瘫。因此，术后持续的神经监测非常重要。

术后失明：术后失明非常罕见（0～0.1%），但后果很严重，与俯卧位有关。其危险因素包含男性、病理性肥胖、Wilson 框架手术时间长（平均超过 6.5 个小时）、大量失血（达到平均有效血容量的 45%）、大量输晶体液，或两者兼有。

5. 如何改善这类患者的术后肺功能？

要点：应在术前教会患者刺激性肺活量测定法（IS），并在术后期间积极使用。这是强制性的措施。鼓励尽量深呼吸和咳嗽。应该使用阿片类药物达到足够的镇痛，以鼓励咳嗽和刺激性肺活量测定法，且不会出现过度的呼吸抑制。

**References**

[1] Spine Surgery, in Jaffe RA, Schmiesing CA and Golianu B (Eds)：Anesthesiologist's Manual of Surgical Procedures (5th edition). Wolters Kluwer. 2014.

[2] Spine Surgery, in Chu L and Fuller A (Eds)：Manual of Clinical Anesthesiology. Wolters Kluwer Health-Lippincott Williams & Wilkins. 2012.

[3] Spinal Surgery：Monitoring. The Anesthetized Patitent；and Anesthesia For Neurosurgery. In：Barash PG, Cullen BF, and Stoelting RK (eds)：Clinical Anesthesia (7th edition). Wolters Kluwer Lippincott-Raven. 2013.

[4] Pulmonary Hypertension-echocardiography：https：//lifeinthefastlane. com/ccc/pulmonary-hypertension-echocardiography/.

[5] Colomina MJ, Koo M, Basora M, et al. Intraoperative tranexamic acid use in major spine surgery in adults：a multicentre, randomized, placebo-controlled trial. Br J Anaesth. 2017；118(3)：380-390.

[6] The Postoperative Visual Loss Study Group. Risk factors associated with ischemic optic neuropathy after spinal fusion surgery. Anesthesiology. 2012；116(1)：15-24.

［7］Practice advisory for perioperative visual loss associated with spine surgery: a report by ASA Task Force on Perioperative Blindness. Anesthesiology. 2006; 104(6): 1319 - 1328.

［8］Karlsson AK. Autonomic dysreflexia. Spinal Cord. 1999; 37(6): 383 - 391.

［9］Cheng MA, Todorov A, Tempelhoff R, McHugh T, Crowder CM, Lauryssen C. The effect of prone positioning on introcular pressure in anesthetized patients. Anesthesiology. 2001; 95(6): 1351 - 1355.

［10］Cheng MA, Sigurdson W, Tempelhoff R, et al. Visual loss after surgery: A survey. Neurosurgery. 2000; 46(3): 625 - 631.

［11］Nuwer MR, Dawson EG, Carlson LG, Kanim LE, Sherman JE: Somatosensory evoked potential spinal cord monitoring reduces neurologic deficits after scoliosis surgery: results of a large multicenter survey. Electroencephalogr Clin Neurophysiol. 1995; 96(1): 6 - 11.

［12］Nuwer MR, Evoked Potential Monitoring in the Operating Room. Raven Press, New York, NY, 1986.

［13］Okubadejo GO, Bridewell KH, Lenke LG, et al. Aprotinin may decrease blood loss in complex adult spinal deformity surgery, but it increases the risk of acute renal failure, presented in the 81st International Anesthesia Research Society held on March 23 - 27, 2007 in Orlando, FL.

［14］Cole JW, Murray DJ, Snider RJ, et al. Aprotinin reduces blood loss during spinal surgery. Spine. 2003; 28(21): 2482 - 2485.

［15］Lentschener C, Cottin P, Bouaziz H, et al. Reduction of blood loss and transfusion requirement by aprotinin in posterior lumbar spine fusion. Aneth Analg. 1999; 89(3): 590 - 597.

［16］Urban MK, Beckman J, Gordon M, et al. The efficacy of antifibrinolytics in the reduction of blood loss during complex adult reconstructive spine surgery. Spine. 2001; 26(10): 1152 - 1156.

［17］Christopherson TJ: Succinylcholine Side Effects. In: Anesthesiology Review (2nd edition). Faust RJ (ed). Churchill Livingstone. Mayo Foundation, 135 - 138; 1994.

［18］Bishop ML: Autonomic Hyperreflexia. In: Anesthesiology Review (2nd edition). Faust RJ (ed). Churchill Livingstone. Mayo Foundation, 407 - 408; 1994.

［19］Coe JD, Arlet V, Donaldson W, et al. Complications in spinal fusion for adolescent idiopathic scoliosis in the new millennium. A report of the Scoliosis Research Society

Morbidity and Mortality Committee. Spine. 2006；31(3)：345 - 349.

[20] Weinzierl MR，Reinacher P，Gilsbach JM，et al. Combined motor and somatosensory evoked potentials for intraoperative monitoring：intra- and postoperative data in a series of 69 operations. Neurosurg Rev. 2007；30(2)：109 - 116.

[21] Hermanns H，Lipfert P，Meier S，et al. Cortical somatosensory-evoked potentials during spine surgery in patients with neuromuscular and idiopathic scoliosis under propofol-remifentanil anaesthesia. Br J Anaesth. 2007；98(3)：362 - 365.

Chris C. Lee

李成付

# 12 Perioperative care for intracranial aneurysm clipping

## 颅内动脉瘤夹闭术的围术期管理

> **Basic information** <

A 40 year-old 100 kg woman is going to undergo clipping of an anterior communicating artery aneurysm. She sustained a subarachnoid hemorrhage (SAH) 2 days ago but did not have consciousness and does not have cerebral vasospasm. A gastric stapling procedure was done 2 years ago resulted in 50 kg weight reduction.

Vitals: BP 160/100, P 100, R 24, SpO$_2$ 91% on 3 L/min nasal cannula O$_2$. Oral temp 37.5.

Medications: OTC (over the counter) vitamins.

Labs: Hgb 11 g/dL.

Echocardiography: None on the record.

Chest x-ray: None on the record.

> **基 本 信 息** <

病史：一名40岁中年女性患者，体重100 kg，2天前因蛛网膜下腔出血入院治疗,无意识丧失和脑血管痉挛,拟行前交通动脉动脉瘤夹闭术。既往史:2 年前曾行胃减容手术,成功减肥 50 kg。

生命体征:BP 160/100 mmHg,P 100 次/min,R 24 次/min,$SpO_2$ 91%,鼻导管吸氧 3 L/min。舌下温度 37.5℃。

用药:口服维生素。

实验室检查:血红蛋白 110 g/L。

超声心动图:无记录。

胸部 X 线:无记录。

---

> ## Preoperative management <

1. Neuro evaluation: What is her neurologic grade? Is it important? Why? How to diagnose an intracranial hypertension?

Keypoint: Understand different grading scales for SAH. Correlate the disease severity with prognosis and maybe perioperative risks.

2. BP management: Should the BP be treated? Why/why not? What is the goal of BP management? What is CPP (cerebral perfusion pressure)? What is TMP (transmural pressure)? Difference between CPP and TMP?

Keypoint: Understand the importance of BP control in patients with SAH. Differentiate the difference between CPP and TMP.

3. Cardiac abnormality: Will you order the test(s) for the heart? Which one(s)? EF = 30%, proceed? Run of v-tach albeit spontaneously resolved, proceed? Surgeon insists to proceed. Your response?

Keypoint: Understand the impact of SAH on the heart. Understand the cardiac signs and symptoms associated with SAH. Skills of communication. Ability in resolving different perspectives.

4. Pulmonary edema：Is SpO$_2$ concerning? Differential diagnosis? Intervention?

Keypoint：Understand the impact of SAH on the lungs.

5. Coiling vs. clipping：Difference between coiling and clipping? Anesthetic implications of coiling? Clipping?

Keypoint：Understand the basics of coiling and clipping. Understand the anesthetic implications of different interventions.

6. Timing of intervention：Surgeon insists to proceed with clipping on day 3 post-bleeding，agree? Concerns?

Keypoint：Be aware of the evidence related to the timing of clipping. Adopt evidence-based practice. An effective communication with the surgeon starts with the grasp of the cutting-edge evidence.

> 术 前 管 理 <

1. 神经系统评估：她的神经症状的分级是多少？是否重要？为什么？如何诊断患者是否有颅内高压？

要点：了解蛛网膜下腔出血的不同分级标准，疾病严重程度与预后和围术期风险相关。

2. 血压管理：这个患者的血压应该治疗吗？为什么/为什么不？血压管理的目标是什么？什么是脑灌流压（CPP）？什么是脑动脉瘤跨膜压（TMP）？CPP 和 TMP 之间的区别？

要点：了解血压控制对蛛网膜下腔出血患者的重要性，区分 CPP 和 TMP 之间的差异。

3. 心脏异常：你是否要求心脏检查？哪一个（些）？左心射血分数（EF）30%，

会坚持麻醉吗? 患者有短暂室性心动过速,尽管已自行消退,继续吗? 外科医师坚持要做手术,你的反应?

要点:了解蛛网膜下腔出血对心脏的影响。了解蛛网膜下腔出血伴有的心功能紊乱的体征和症状。沟通技巧。解决不同问题的能力。

4.肺水肿:是否担心患者的 $SpO_2$? 鉴别诊断? 干预?

要点:了解长期蛛网膜下腔出血对肺的影响。

5.脑动脉瘤金属圈介入栓塞和夹闭术:介入栓塞和夹闭术之间的差异? 脑动脉介入栓塞的麻醉方法? 与脑动脉夹闭的麻醉方法差异?

要点:了解脑动脉瘤金属圈介入栓塞和脑动脉手术夹闭的基础知识,了解两者麻醉方法的不同。

6.治疗时机:外科医师坚持在出血后第 3 天进行手术夹闭,同意吗? 你对这个患者的担心有哪些?

要点:了解与脑动脉瘤夹闭时机相关的循证医学,采取循证实践,与外科医师能有效地沟通,用证据说理。

## > **Intraoperative management** <

1. Monitoring:Is the arterial line required? Why? Is CVP (central venous pressure catheter) required? Why? Is PA (pulmonary arterial catheter) catheter indicated? Is $etCO_2$ an accurate estimate of $PaCO_2$? Do you need to monitor air emboli? How? Does the brain need to be monitored? How? MEP (motor evoke potentials)? SSEP (somatosensory evoke potentials)? EEG (electroencephalography)?

Keypoint:Be able to defend the choice of monitoring, such as arterial line. Be familiar with different neuro monitoring. The pros and cons of different neuro monitoring.

2. Anesthesia induction: Colleague believes rapid IV induction mandatory. Agree? Why? Methods to accomplish. Choice of agents? Succinylcholine?

Keypoint: Understand the pros and cons of rapid induction. Understand the impact of succinylcholine on neurological condition. Be flexible, especially when facing something that is outside of your confort zone. Proactively seek the needed evidence.

3. Anesthesia maintenance: How? Reason(s). Is nitrous oxide okay to use? Why? Which agents are ideal if MEP is placed?

Keypoint: Understand the pros and cons of different anesthetic agents. Understand the priorities of aneurysm clipping and the role the anesthesia plays in facilitating the surgery. Understand the impact of anesthetic technique on neuro monitoring.

4. Brain relaxation: Surgeon complains a bulging brain. Your response. Interventions? Mannitol? $CO_2$?

Keypoint: Understand the concept of brain relaxation. The difference between ICP and brain relaxation. The methods that can be implemented to relax a bulging brain.

5. Neuroprotection: Surgeon asks for hypothermia. Agree? How about burst suppression?

Keypoint: Understand the concept of neuroprotection. Be familiar with the current evidence related to this topic.

6. Deliberate hypotension or transient cardiac arrest: Plan is for profound hypotension at time of aneurysm clipping and moderate hypotension at other times. Method(s) to produce. How would you determine the safe lower limit for BP? Organs at risk. Management to prevent organ damage? Surgeon asks for

transient cardiac arrest. How to produce it?

Keypoint: Understand the rationale of intentional transient hypotension and cardiac arrest. The risks associated with hypotension and cardiac arrest. The method of achieving profound hypotension and cardiac arrest. The skills in communication. The habit and ability of seeking evidence and self-learning.

7. Management of ventilation: Airway pressure of 55 cmH$_2$O is required to deliver calculated tidal volume. Possible cause(s)? Is this hazardous? Why? Despite this usual tidal volume, PaO$_2$ 70 mmHg when FiO$_2$ 0.5 and PaCO$_2$ 46. Reason(s)? Your management? Should PEEP be applied? Why/why not?

Keypoint: Understand the impact of SAH on the lungs. Be familiar with the pulmonary complications. Understand respiratory physiology and apply the knowledge in patient care.

8. Intraoperative aneurysm rupture: Abruptly the surgeon notices and informs you that the aneurysm has ruptured and that a temporary clip will need to be placed. Your response? Burst suppression? How to accomplish it? How to monitor it? How to help the surgeon? Temporary clipping? Adenosine? Lower BP?

Keypoint: Know how to help the surgeon when the aneurysm is adversely ruptured. Maintain effective and timely communication with the surgeon. Understand the risks associated with the application of temporary clip. Understand the potential adverse consequences associated with burst suppression. Know how to use adenosine. Know the method of inducing transient hypotension.

> 术 中 管 理 <

1. 监测：是否需要放置有创动脉？为什么？是否需要置入中心静脉导管（CVP）？为什么？是否需要放置肺动脉导管（PAC）？呼气末二氧化碳（etCO$_2$）是

否可以准确估计动脉血中的二氧化碳分压（$PaCO_2$）？是否需要监测空气栓塞？怎么做？需要进行脑功能监测吗？怎么做？什么是脑电的运动诱发电位（MEP）？躯体感觉诱发电位（SSEP）？脑电图（EEG）？

要点：术中监测的选择，如有创动脉，熟悉不同的神经功能监测以及不同监测之间的优缺点。

2. 麻醉诱导：你的同事认为必须进行快速诱导，同意吗？为什么？采用什么方法，什么药？可以用琥珀酰胆碱吗？

要点：理解快速诱导的利弊，了解琥珀酰胆碱对已有神经系统疾病的影响。尤其是当你面对的状况超出你的常规范围时要灵活。主动去寻找所需的证据。

3. 麻醉维持：如何维持麻醉？理由。可以用氧化亚氮吗？为什么？如果术中监测运动诱发电位，哪些药物是理想的选择？

要点：了解不同麻醉药的利弊，了解脑动脉瘤夹闭手术的首选药和麻醉对手术的影响，了解麻醉技术对神经功能监测的影响。

4. 脑松弛：外科医师抱怨脑膨胀，你的反应，怎么干预？甘露醇？改变二氧化碳的水平（$CO_2$）？

要点：了解大脑松弛的概念，颅内压（ICP）和大脑松弛之间的差异，可以用于实施大脑松弛的方法。

5. 神经保护：外科医师要求术中低温，你是否同意？什么是脑电图梭状波的抑制？

要点：了解神经保护的概念，熟悉与此相关的当前证据。

6. 控制性降压或短暂性心搏骤停：事先的计划是在脑动脉瘤阻断时予以深度控制性降压，其他时间予以中度降压。方法是什么？如何确定血压的安全下限？其他器官是否有风险，如何防止其他器官损害。假如外科医师要求暂时性心搏骤停，如何实施？

要点：理解短暂性控制性低压和心搏骤停的理论基础；与低血压和心搏骤停

相关的风险;实现深度低血压和心搏骤停的方法;沟通技巧;寻求证据和自我学习的习惯和能力。

7. 机械通气管理:当需要 55 cmH$_2$O 的气道压力来达到预设的潮气量,可能的原因? 这会造成危险吗? 为什么? 在这样潮气量通气下和50% 的吸入氧浓度,患者的二氧分压(PaCO$_2$)是 46 mmHg,氧分压(PaO$_2$) 为 70 mmHg,原因是什么? 怎么处理? 是否应该应用呼气末正压(PEEP)? 为什么/为什么不?

要点:了解蛛网膜下腔出血对肺的影响,熟悉肺部并发症,了解呼吸生理学并将知识应用于患者。

8. 术中脑动脉瘤破裂:突然外科医师告诉你动脉瘤破裂了,需要放置一个临时钳闭夹,你怎么回应? 是否需要施行脑电梭状波的抑制? 如何完成? 如何监测? 如何在需要上临时钳闭夹的时候帮助外科医师? 静脉推注腺苷,还是降低 BP?

要点:知道当脑动脉瘤破裂时如何协助外科医师,保持与外科医师有效和及时的沟通,了解与临时钳闭夹相关的风险,了解与脑电梭状波抑制相关的潜在不良后果。了解如何使用腺苷。知道诱导短暂性低血压的方法。

## > Postoperative management <

1. Early and smooth emergence: Surgeon requests patient be awake in OR, your response? How do you decide whether to allow the patient to emergence after aneurysm clipping? What considerations prevail? After propofol-remifentanil anesthesia, patient does not wake up promptly, your response?

Keypoint: Understand the goals during emergence. Know how to achieve a smooth and rapid emergence.

2. Management of hypertension: Patient intubated and spontaneous breathing on the arrival in recovery room. BP is 200/100. Cause(s)? Risk(s)?

Colleague suggests chlorpromazine. Agree? Your management? Suggest extubation?

Keypoint：Master the differential diagnosis of post-craniotomy hypertension.

3. New postoperative neurological deficit：Six hours postoperatively，the now awake extubated patient develops paralysis of contralateral arm and leg without change in vital signs or level of consciousness. Differential diagnosis? Management?

Keypoint：Be familiar with differential diagnosis of focal neurological deficits. Be familiar with the interventions.

4. Delayed cerebral ischemia（DCI）：The patient did well until the evening of post-surgery day 4 when she is noted to no longer respond to voice or verbal command. Differential diagnosis? Delayed cerebral ischemia? Cerebral vasospasm? Management?

Keypoint：Understand the outcome importance of DCI. Differential diagnosis between DCI and vasospasm. Be familiar with the management of these complications.

> 术 后 管 理 <

1. 平稳和尽早苏醒：外科医师要求患者在手术室苏醒，你的反应？你如何决定是否让患者在脑动脉瘤切除术后及时苏醒？什么考虑优先？在丙泊酚-瑞芬太尼麻醉后，患者没能及时醒来，你的反应？

要点：理解麻醉苏醒期的目标，知道如何实现平稳和快速的苏醒。

2. 高血压的管理：患者自主呼吸入，带管麻醉恢复室。BP 为 200/100 mmHg，原因是什么？有什么风险？同事建议应用氯丙嗪，同意吗？你的治疗方法？建议拔管吗？

要点：掌握颅脑手术后高血压的鉴别诊断。

3.新发生的术后神经功能缺损：术后 6 个小时,患者清醒已拔管,此时患者出现了对侧手臂和腿的麻痹,生命体征和意识没有变化,鉴别诊断? 治疗?

要点：熟悉局部性神经功能障碍的鉴别诊断,熟悉治疗措施。

4.延迟性脑缺血：患者的手术很顺利,但是到了术后第 4 天的晚上,突发对语音或口头指令没有反应,鉴别诊断? 延迟性脑缺血? 脑血管痉挛? 治疗?

要点：了解延迟性脑缺血愈后的重要性,延迟性脑缺血与脑血管痉挛之间的鉴别诊断,熟悉这些并发症的治疗。

**Acknowledgement**

Dr. Shudong Fang, MD, PhD from Shanghai 9th People's Hospital translated the text to Chinese.

感谢上海交通大学附属第九人民医院方舒东医师的翻译。

**Suggested Reading**

Hunt WE, Hess RM. Surgical risk as related to time of intervention in the repair of intracranial aneurysms. J Neurosurg. 1968; 28(1): 14 - 20.

Report of world federation of neurological surgeons committee on a universal subarachnoid hemorrhage grading scale. J Neurosurg. 1988; 68(6): 985 - 986.

Fisher CM, Kistler JP, Davis JM. Relation of cerebral vasospasm to subarachnoid hemorrhage visualized by computerized tomographic scanning. Neurosurgery. 1980; 6(1): 1 - 9.

Rosen DS, Macdonald RL. Subarachnoid hemorrhage grading scales: a systematic review. Neurocrit Care. 2005; 2(2): 110 - 118.

Sakr YL, Ghosn I, Vincent JL. Cardiac manifestations after subarachnoid hemorrhage: a systematic review of the literature. Prog Cardiovasc Dis. 2002; 45(1): 67 - 80.

Behrouz R, Sullebarger JT, Malek AR. Cardiac manifestations of subarachnoid hemorrhage. Expert Rev Cardiovasc Ther. 2011; 9(3): 303 - 307.

Samuels MA. The brain-heart connection. Circulation. 2007; 116(1): 77 - 84.

Naidech AM, Kreiter KT, Janjua N, et al. Cardiac troponin elevation, cardiovascular morbidity, and outcome after subarachnoid hemorrhage. Circulation. 2005; 112 (18):

2851－2856.

Lee VH，Connolly HM，Fulgham JR，et al. Tako-tsubo cardiomyopathy in aneurysmal subarachnoid hemorrhage：an underappreciated ventricular dysfunction. J Neurosurg. 2006；105 (2)：264－270.

Boland TA，Lee VH，Bleck TP. Stress-induced cardiomyopathy. Crit Care Med. 2015；43 (3)：686－693.

Muroi C，Keller E. Treatment regimen in patients with neurogenic pulmonary edema after subarachnoid hemorrhage. J Neurosurg Anesthesiol. 2009；21(1)：68.

Macmillan CS，Grant IS，Andrews PJ. Pulmonary and cardiac sequelae of subarachnoid haemorrhage：time for active management? Intensive Care Med. 2002；28(8)：1012－1023.

Molyneux A，Kerr R，Stratton I，et al. International Subarachnoid Aneurysm Trial (ISAT) Collaborative Group. International Subarachnoid Aneurysm Trial (ISAT) of neurosurgical clipping versus endovascular coiling in 2143 patients with ruptured intracranial aneurysms：a randomised trial. Lancet. 2002；360(9342)：1267－1274.

Molyneux AJ，Kerr RS，Yu LM，et al. International Subarachnoid Aneurysm Trial (ISAT) Collaborative Group. International subarachnoid aneurysm trial (ISAT) of neurosurgical clipping versus endovascular coiling in 2143 patients with ruptured intracranial aneurysms：a randomised comparison of effects on survival，dependency，seizures，rebleeding，subgroups，and aneurysm occlusion. Lancet. 2005；366(9488)：809－817.

Molyneux AJ，Birks J，Clarke A，et al. The durability of endovascular coiling versus neurosurgical clipping of ruptured cerebral aneurysms：18 year follow-up of the UK cohort of the International Subarachnoid Aneurysm Trial (ISAT). Lancet. 2015；385(9969)：691－697.

Lanzino G，Murad MH，d'Urso PI，et al. Coil embolization versus clipping for ruptured intracranial aneurysms：a meta-analysis of prospective controlled published studies. AJNR Am J Neuroradiol. 2013；34(9)：1764－1768.

Kassell NF，Torner JC，Jane JA，et al. The international cooperative study on the timing of aneurysm surgery. Part 2：Surgical results. J Neurosurg. 1990；73(1)：37－47.

Kassell NF，Torner JC，Haley EC Jr，et al. The international cooperative study on the timing of aneurysm surgery. Part 1：Overall management results. J Neurosurg. 1990；73(1)：18－36.

Haley EC Jr，Kassell NF，Torner JC. The international cooperative study on the timing of aneurysm surgery. The North American experience. Stroke. 1992；23(2)：205－214.

Szelényi A，Langer D，Kothbauer K，et al. Monitoring of muscle motor evoked potentials during cerebral aneurysm surgery：intraoperative changes and postoperative outcome. J Neurosurg. 2006；105(5)：675 - 681.

Irie T，Yoshitani K，Ohnishi Y，et al. The efficacy of motor-evoked potentials on cerebral aneurysm surgery and new-onset postoperative motor deficits. J Neurosurg Anesthesiol. 2010；22(3)：247 - 251.

Lanier WL，Milde JH，Michenfelder JD. Cerebral stimulation following succinylcholine in dogs. Anesthesiology. 1986；64(5)：551 - 559.

Kovarik WD，Mayberg TS，Lam AM，et al. Succinylcholine does not change intracranial pressure，cerebral blood flow velocity，or the electroencephalogram in patients with neurologic injury. Anesth Analg. 1994；78(3)：469 - 473.

Manninen PH，Mahendran B，Gelb AW，et al. Succinylcholine does not increase serum potassium levels in patients with acutely ruptured cerebral aneurysms. Anesth Analg. 1990；70 (2)：172 - 175.

Chui J，Mariappan R，Mehta J，et al. Comparison of propofol and volatile agents for maintenance of anesthesia during elective craniotomy procedures：systematic review and meta-analysis. Can J Anaesth. 2014；61(4)：347 - 356.

Hemmer LB，Zeeni C，Bebawy JF，et al. The incidence of unacceptable movement with motor evoked potentials during craniotomy for aneurysm clipping. World Neurosurg. 2014；81 (1)：99 - 104.

Pasternak JJ，Lanier WL. Is the using of nitrous oxide appropriate in neurosurgical and neurologically at-risk patients? Curr Opin Anaesthesiol. 2010；23(5)：544 - 550.

Lo YL，Dan YF，Tan YE，et al. Intraoperative motor-evoked potential monitoring in scoliosis surgery：comparison of desflurane/nitrous oxide with propofol total intravenous anesthetic regimens. J Neurosurg Anesthesiol. 2006；18(3)：211 - 214.

Pelosi L，Stevenson M，Hobbs GJ，et al. Intraoperative motor evoked potentials to transcranial electrical stimulation during two anaesthetic regimens. Clin Neurophysiol. 2001；112(6)：1076 - 1087.

Li J，Gelb AW，Flexman AM，et al. Definition，evaluation，and management of brain relaxation during craniotomy. Br J Anaesth. 2016；116(6)：759 - 769.

Todd MM，Hindman BJ，Clarke WR，et al. Intraoperative hypothermia for aneurysm surgery trial (IHAST) investigators. Mild intraoperative hypothermia during surgery for intracranial aneurysm. N Engl J Med. 2005；352(2)：135 - 145.

Li LR，You C，Chaudhary B. Intraoperative mild hypothermia for postoperative neurological deficits in people with intracranial aneurysm. Cochrane Database Syst Rev. 2016；3：CD008445.

Hindman BJ，Bayman EO，Pfisterer WK，et al. IHAST Investigators. No association between intraoperative hypothermia or supplemental protective drug and neurologic outcomes in patients undergoing temporary clipping during cerebral aneurysm surgery：findings from the intraoperative hypothermia for aneurysm surgery trial. Anesthesiology. 2010；112(1)：86 - 101.

Hoffman WE，Wheeler P，Edelman G，et al. Ausman JI. Hypoxic brain tissue following subarachnoid hemorrhage. Anesthesiology. 2000；92(2)：442 - 446.

Hoffman WE，Charbel FT，Edelman G，et al. Thiopental and desflurane treatment for brain protection. Neurosurgery. 1998；43(5)：1050 - 1053.

Guinn NR，McDonagh DL，Borel CO，et al. Adenosine-induced transient asystole for intracranial aneurysm surgery：a retrospective review. J Neurosurg Anesthesiol. 2011；23(1)：35 - 40.

Bebawy JF，Zeeni C，Sharma S，et al. Adenosine-induced flow arrest to facilitate intracranial aneurysm clip ligation does not worsen neurologic outcome. Anesth Analg. 2013；117(5)：1205 - 1210.

Kim H，Min KT，Lee JR，et al. Comparison of dexmedetomidine and remifentanil on airway reflex and hemodynamic changes during recovery after craniotomy. Yonsei Med J. 2016；57(4)：980 - 986.

Pauls RJ，Dickson TJ，Kaufmann AM，et al. A comparison of the ability of the EEGo and BIS monitors to assess emergence following neurosurgery. Can J Anaesth. 2009；56(5)：366 - 373.

Schmidt U，Bittner E，Pivi S，et al. Hemodynamic management and outcome of patients treated for cerebral vasospasm with intraarterial nicardipine and/or milrinone. Anesth Analg. 2010；110(3)：895 - 902.

Lingzhong Meng

孟令忠

# 13 Perioperative care for carotid endarterectomy

## 颈动脉内膜剥脱术的围术期管理

> **Basic information** <

A 70 year-old 70 kg man is scheduled for a right carotid endarterectomy (CEA) because of recurrent transient ischemic attacks (TIA). He has had two myocardial infarctions, the most recent heart attack was four months ago. He is taking propranolol 40 mg t.i.d. for hypertension and occasional sublingual nitroglycerin.

Vitals: BP ranges from 130/90 to 180/105, P 60, R 14, Oral temp 37.0.

Medications: See above.

Labs: Hct 50.

Echocardiography: Never.

Chest X-ray: None within last 5 years.

> 基 本 信 息 <

病史: 一名年龄 70 岁, 体重 70 kg 的老年患者, 因短暂性脑缺血反复发作, 拟择期行右颈动脉内膜剥脱术。既往及治疗史: 4 个月前心肌梗死 2 次, 规律服用普萘洛尔 40 mg，每天 3 次控制血压，偶尔舌下含服硝酸甘油。

生命体征：BP 130/90 mmHg 至 180/105 mmHg，P 60 次/min，R 14 次/min，口温 37.0℃。

药物：见病史。

实验室：Hct 50%。

超声心动图：没做。

胸部 X 线：过去 5 年内没有。

> **Preoperative management** <

1. Hypertension：Is BP adequately controlled? At what range are you satisfied? What are the hazards of acute BP reduction?

Keypoint：Master the management of hypertension and hypertensive disease. Understand the side effects of acute BP reduction. Understand the association between preoperative hypertension and perioperative outcomes.

2. Cardiac evaluation：Any studies needed for the heart? Which one? Why? What is the importance of the recent MI to the perioperative risks? Significance of occasional angina? Would you postpone CEA for further cardiovascular evaluation? If cardiology recommends drug-eluting coronary artery stents ×2, when would be the proper time window to proceed with CEA after percutaneous coronary intervention（PCI）? How do you manage dual antiplatelet therapy （DAPT）?

Keypoint：Cardiac evaluation is a key component before CEA. Be specific about the studies and interventions needed before surgery. Understand the risks of myocardial ischemia and infarction. Understand the indications for PCI. Know the management of DAPT in the perioperative period. Skill of literature search and ability of knowledge self-update on the evolving issues.

3. Neuro evaluation：How to evaluate this patient's neurologic status? How to evaluate the carotid artery? How to evaluate neurovascular anatomy? What is the importance of the circle of Willis?

Keypoint：Be aware of the importance of neuro exams. Understand neuroanatomy. Understand the importance of collateral flow including the circle of Willis.

4. Endarterectomy vs stenting：The patient family members ask for your opinion on the treatment options：endarterectomy vs. stenting. Your response? Risks associated with endarterectomy? Risks associated with stenting?

Keypoint：Skills of communication. Be aware of the evidence comparing CEA and CAS. Understand the differences of the risks associated with CEA and CAS，respectively.

5. Timing of endarterectomy：In the afternoon of the day before surgery，the patient had an episode of TIA（transient ischemia attack），with worse symptoms and longer duration compared to the previous episodes. Proceed or not? The surgeon insists to proceed. Your response? During the night before surgery，the patient had an acute anterior circulation ischemic stroke which，fortunately，responded favorably to tPA. Is it still okay to proceed urgently for CEA?

Keypoint：Ability and skills of dealing with the conflicts between medical professionals with different perspectives. Be aware of the recent evidence related to the timing of CEA. Foster a habit of seeking evidence throughout the career.

> **术 前 管 理** <

1. 高血压：血压是否得到充分控制？在什么范围你满意？急性血压降的太低

的危害是什么？

要点：掌握高血压和高血压疾病的管理，了解急性血压降低的不良反应，了解术前高血压与围术期预后之间的关系。

2. 心脏评估：心脏还需要什么检查？哪一个？为什么？患者有近期心肌梗死，对围术期风险的重要性是什么？偶尔心绞痛的意义？你会推迟颈动脉内膜剥脱术而做进一步的心血管评估吗？如果心脏科医师建议行经皮冠状动脉介入（PCI）放 2 根药物洗脱冠状动脉支架，PCI 后何时是行 CEA 的合适时间？如何管理患者的双重抗血小板治疗（DAPT）？

要点：心脏评估是 CEA 手术的关键组成部分，具体了解手术前的检查和干预措施，了解心肌缺血和梗死的风险，了解 PCI 的适应证，了解围术期 DAPT 的管理。具有熟悉近期的文献以及知识不断更新的能力。

3. 神经系统评估：如何评估这位患者的神经系统的状况？如何评估颈动脉的病变？如何评估神经血管解剖？Willis 环的重要性是什么？

要点：了解神经检查的重要性，了解神经解剖学，包括 Willis 环在内的侧支血流的重要性。

4. 颈动脉内膜剥脱术与颈动脉支架：患者家属询问你对治疗的意见，颈动脉内膜剥脱术与颈动脉支架，哪一个更好。你的回应是？颈动脉内膜剥脱术相关的风险？颈动脉支架植入相关的风险？

要点：沟通技巧。了解和比较颈动脉内膜剥脱术和颈动脉支架的循证医学，且了解颈动脉内膜剥脱术和颈动脉支架各自所相关的特殊的风险。

5. 颈动脉内膜剥脱术的时机：在手术前一天的下午，患者曾有短暂性脑缺血（TIA）发作，与先前发作相比，症状更严重，持续时间更长，是否继续？外科医师坚持继续。你的反应是？在手术前一天的晚上，患者发生了大脑前动脉的急性循环缺血性卒中，幸运的是，对组织血浆纤溶酶（tPA）有良好的反应。是否同意行紧急进行颈动脉内膜剥脱术？

要点：以不同的角度处理医学专业人士之间的冲突的能力和技能。了解有关颈动脉内膜剥脱术手术时间最新证据，培养在整个职业生涯中寻找证据的习惯。

-------- > **Intraoperative management** < --------

1. Anesthetic techniques: Are there any advantages of cervical plexus block over general anesthesia? Disadvantages? How would you manage patient if he became restless and confused during carotid cross-clamping? The patient requests general anesthesia. Which agents will you choose for induction? Maintenance? Should muscle relaxants be used?

Keypoint: Skills of resolving the conflicts between different professionals with different perspectives. Understand the difference between CEA and CAS. Be aware of the recent evidence related to the effects of different anesthetic techniques on the outcomes. Be confident during the decision making while adopting the most recent quality evidence.

2. Anesthetic monitors: Is invasive arterial blood pressure monitoring necessary? Why? How to improve the diagnostic value of ECG monitoring? Which ECG lead has the best diagnostic value for myocardial ischemia? Why?

Keypoint: Be familiar with the reasons of different monitors. Be able to defend why choosing invasive arterial blood pressure monitoring.

3. Neurological monitors: Should the brain be monitored? How? The best neuro monitor? Is EEG monitoring has a diagnostic value for cerebral ischemia? How about BIS (Bispectral index)? SSEP (somatosensory evoked potentials) vs. MEP (motor evoked potentials)? How about cerebral tissue oxygen saturation monitor?

Keypoint: Understand the risks of cerebral ischemia during cross clamp and balloon occlusion. Be aware of the technologies available for neuro monitoring. Understand the pros and cons of different monitors.

4. BP（blood pressure）management：BP dropped to 130/90 mmHg（the patient's baseline）five mins after endotracheal intubation. Your response? How about 120/80 mmHg? What is the goal of intraoperative BP management? Why? Which drugs are to be chosen? Why?

Keypoint：Be skillful in decision making of BP management. Be able to defend your decision. Understand the pros and cons of different approaches. Skills of communication. Be aware of the recent evidence related to BP management during CEA. Be able to use the evidence to defend the decision.

5. CBF（cerebral blood flow）regulation and importance of collateral flow：How does the brain compensate for the flow-restrictive stenosis? Is CBF robustly regulated in patients with severe carotid stenosis? Autoregulation? $CO_2$ reactivity? Collateral flow to the ipsilateral brain perfused by the stenotic ICA（internal carotid artery）? Without collateral flow，what is the consequence of ICA clamping?

Keypoint：Understand the physiology of CBF regulation. Understand the mechanisms of cerebral autoregulation，$CO_2$ reactivity，$CMRO_2$（cerebral metabolic rate of oxygen）-CBF coupling，and anesthetic effects on CBF. Understand the importance of collateral flows. Understand the impact of cross clamp on the CBF. Understand the different ways of CBF monitoring. Be aware of the recent evidence related to BP，$CO_2$，and anesthetic depth management during CEA.

6. The conflicts between the brain and the heart：Between the brain and the heart，which organ should be prioritized? What is the conflicting interest between the brain and the heart? How to balance it?

Keypoint：This is an important question. A higher BP is good for the brain. However，it also increases the workload of the heart. It may be a balance. The evidence may be lacking. However，it is an opportunity for critical thinking.

7. Decision of shunting：What is the purpose of shunting? How to determine if shunting is needed or not?

Keypoint：This is an important question for both surgeons and anesthesiologists. Understand how the decision is normally made.

8. Management of complications：During surgery，the patient's heart rate drops from 75 to 40/bpm，are you going to treat it? Why? What might be the etiology? Now BP drops from 170/100 to 90/60. Are you going to treat it? How?

Keypoint：Be the master of crisis management. Be aware of the potential complications during CEA.

9. Neuroprotection：The significance of ICA cross-clamping? Measures to protect the brain during carotid cross-clamping? Drugs? Hypothermia? Evidence of effectiveness?

Keypoint：Be aware of the evidence related to neuroprotection during CEA.

> 术 中 管 理 <

1. 麻醉方式：颈丛神经阻滞较全身麻醉有什么优点和缺点？如果患者在颈动脉钳闭阻断期间突然变得躁动、意识模糊，你如何处理？患者要求全身麻醉，你将选择哪些麻醉药进行诱导和维持？是否应使用肌肉松弛剂？

要点：应用不同的观点解决不同专业人士之间冲突的技巧。了解颈动脉内膜剥脱术和支架置入术之间的区别。关注最近有关不同麻醉技术对结局影响的证据，采用最新高质量证据自信的做出决策。

2. 麻醉监测：是否需要有创动脉血压监测？为什么？如何提高心电图监测的诊断价值？哪个心电图导联对心肌缺血有最好的诊断价值？为什么？

要点：熟悉不同监测的原因，能够解释为什么选择有创性动脉血压监测。

3. 神经系统监测：应该进行脑的功能监测吗？怎么做？什么是最好的神经系统监测？脑电图监测是否有诊断脑缺血的价值？BIS 怎么样？诱发的躯体感觉电位还是运动诱发电位（SSEP 与 MEP）？脑氧饱和度监测如何？

要点：了解夹闭和球囊阻塞颈动脉期间发生脑缺血的危险。了解不同的神经监测的技术，熟悉它们之间的优缺点。

4. 血压管理：气管插管后 5 min 血压降至 130/90 mmHg（该患者的基础血压），你的反应？如果降至 120/80 mmHg，你的反应是？术中血压管理的目标是什么？为什么？选择哪些药物？为什么？

要点：熟练掌握血压管理利于决策，了解不同方法的利弊，具有良好的沟通技巧。了解最近有关颈动脉内膜剥脱术血压管理的证据，能够使用证据应用于决策。

5. 脑血流调节和侧支血流的重要性：大脑如何代偿血流限制性狭窄？在严重颈动脉狭窄患者中脑血流是否得到稳定的调节？自动调节？对二氧化碳的反应性？侧支血流通过狭窄的颈内动脉（ICA）灌注同侧脑部？假如没有侧支血流，ICA 夹闭的后果是什么？

要点：了解脑血流调节的生理学，了解脑血流自动调节、二氧化碳反应性、脑氧代谢-脑血流（$CMRO_2$- CBF）耦合和麻醉对脑血流的影响的机制。了解侧支血流的重要性，了解钳闭对脑血流的影响，了解不同的脑血流监测方法。了解最近的有关血压、二氧化碳和麻醉深度管理在颈动脉内膜剥脱术期间的证据。

6. 脑和心脏之间的冲突：在脑和心脏之间，应该优先保护哪个器官？脑和心脏之间的冲突是什么？如何平衡？

要点：这是一个很重要的问题，血压高对脑是有益的，但它也增加了心脏的工作负荷，这可能是一个平衡，可能缺乏证据，但这是一个思考的关键。

7. 分流的决定：分流的目的是什么？如何确定是否需要分流？

要点：这对于外科医师和麻醉医师来说都是一个重要的问题，了解这个决定是如何做出的。

8. 并发症的管理：在手术期间，患者的心率从 75 次/min 下降到 40 次/min，需要处理吗？为什么？大概的病因是什么？现在 BP 从 170/100 mmHg 下降到 90/60 mmHg，需要处理吗？怎么做？

要点：紧急情况的处理，注意颈动脉内膜剥脱术期间的潜在并发症。

9. 神经保护：颅内动脉夹闭的意义？在颈动脉夹闭期间的脑保护措施？药物？低温？有效性的证据？

要点：注意颈动脉内膜剥脱术期间神经保护相关的证据。

------------------------->  **Postoperative management**  <-------------------------

1. Hypertension and tachycardia：In the immediate postoperative period，BP is 220/120，P 110 bpm. Dangers of this? Treatment?

Keypoint：Understand the mechanism of hypertension after CEA. Understand the potential risks associated with postoperative hypertension.

2. Fail to wake up：Differential diagnosis? Would you administer naloxone and/or physostigmine? How to decide?

Keypoint：Be familiar with the differential diagnosis of delayed awakening.

3. Strider：Over a 60-min period，an inspiratory strider developed，possible causes? Treatment? Suppose you are unable to intubate the patient，what would you do?

Keypoint：Be familiar with the differential diagnosis of airway complications after CEA.

4. Hyperperfusion syndrome：3 days later，the patient complains headache，followed by vomit and mental status change. Differential diagnosis? Management?

Keypoint：Understand the mechanism and potential adverse outcomes associated with hyperperfusion syndrome. Be familiar with the clinical signs and symptoms and diagnosis. Treatment options. The Importance of continuous BP monitoring and management.

5. Outcomes：What is the 30 day mortality rate of CEA? What are the common causes of mortality after CEA? Which is more common，cardiac or cerebral complications?

Keypoint：Be familiar with the complications and outcomes after CEA.

> 术 后 管 理 <

1. 高血压和心动过速：在术后很短的时间内，BP 220/120 mmHg，HR 110 次/min，有危险吗？如何治疗？

要点：了解颈动脉内膜剥脱术后高血压的机制，了解与术后高血压相关的潜在风险。

2. 苏醒延迟：鉴别诊断？你会应用纳洛酮和/或毒扁豆碱吗？如何决定？
要点：熟悉苏醒延迟的鉴别诊断。

3. 喘鸣（吸气困难）：在 60 min 内，发展为吸气性喘鸣。可能的原因是？如何治疗？假设你无法给患者插管，你会怎么做？
要点：熟悉颈动脉内膜剥脱术术后呼吸道并发症的鉴别诊断。

4. 脑血流高灌注综合征：术后 3 天,患者主诉头痛,伴有呕吐和精神状态变化。鉴别诊断？如何治疗？

要点：了解与高灌注综合征相关的机制和潜在的不良后果,熟悉临床体征和症状、诊断和治疗选择。持续血压监测和管理的重要性。

5. 预后：颈动脉内膜剥脱术后 30 天的死亡率是多少？死亡的常见原因是什么？心脏或大脑并发症哪个更常见？

要点：熟悉颈动脉内膜剥脱术后的并发症和预后。

**Acknowledgement：**

Dr. Shudong Fang, MD, PhD from Shanghai 9th People's Hospital translated the text to Chinese.

感谢上海交通大学附属第九人民医院方舒东医师的翻译。

**Suggested Reading**

Stefanini GG, Holmes DR Jr. Drug-eluting coronary-artery stents. N Engl J Med. 2013；368(3)：254‐265.

Levine GN, Bates ER, Bittl JA, et al. 2016 ACC/AHA guideline focused update on duration of dual antiplatelet therapy in patients with coronary artery disease：A report of the American College of Cardiology/American Heart Association Task Force on Clinical Practice Guidelines. J Am Coll Cardiol. 2016；68(10)：1082‐1115.

Boulanger M, Camelière L, Felgueiras R, et al. Periprocedural myocardial infarction after carotid endarterectomy and stenting：Systematic review and meta-analysis. Stroke. 2015；46(10)：2843‐2848.

Brott TG, Hobson RW 2nd, Howard G, et al. Stenting versus endarterectomy for treatment of carotid-artery stenosis. N Engl J Med. 2010；363(1)：11‐23.

Brott TG, Howard G, Roubin GS, et al. Long-Term Results of Stenting versus Endarterectomy for Carotid-Artery Stenosis. N Engl J Med. 2016；374(11)：1021‐1131.

Patterson BO, Holt PJ, Hinchliffe RJ, et al. Urgent carotid endarterectomy for patients with unstable symptoms：systematic review and meta-analysis of outcomes. Vascular. 2009；17

(5): 243 - 252.

Bruls S, Van Damme H, Defraigne JO. Timing of carotid endarterectomy: a comprehensive review. Acta Chir Belg. 2012; 112(1): 3 - 7.

Loftus IM, Paraskevas KI, Naylor AR. Urgent Carotid Endarterectomy Does Not Increase Risk and Will Prevent More Strokes. Angiology. 2016 Aug 16. pii: 0003319716664286. [Epub ahead of print]

Rantner B, Schmidauer C, Knoflach M, et al. Very urgent carotid endarterectomy does not increase the procedural risk. Eur J Vasc Endovasc Surg. 2015; 49(2): 129 - 136.

Ferrero E, Ferri M, Viazzo A, et al. A retrospective study on early carotid endarterectomy within 48 hours after transient ischemic attack and stroke in evolution. Ann Vasc Surg. 2014; 28(1): 227 - 238.

Koraen-Smith L, Troëng T, Björck M, et al. Wahlgren CM; Swedish vascular registry and the riks-stroke collaboration. Urgent carotid surgery and stenting may be safe after systemic thrombolysis for stroke. Stroke. 2014; 45(3): 776 - 780.

Yong YP, Saunders J, Abisi S, et al. Safety of carotid endarterectomy following thrombolysis for acute ischemic stroke. J Vasc Surg. 2013; 58(6): 1671 - 1677.

Chou EL, Sgroi MD, Chen SL, et al. Influence of gender and use of regional anesthesia on carotid endarterectomy outcomes. J Vasc Surg. 2016; 64(1): 9 - 14.

Leichtle SW, Mouawad NJ, Welch K, et al. Outcomes of carotid endarterectomy under general and regional anesthesia from the American College of Surgeons' National Surgical Quality Improvement Program. J Vasc Surg. 2012; 56(1): 81 - 88.

Schechter MA, Shortell CK, Scarborough JE. Regional versus general anesthesia for carotid endarterectomy: the American College of Surgeons National Surgical Quality Improvement Program perspective. Surgery. 2012; 152(3): 309 - 314.

Kfoury E, Dort J, Trickey A, et al. Carotid endarterectomy under local and/or regional anesthesia has less risk of myocardial infarction compared to general anesthesia: An analysis of national surgical quality improvement program database. Vascular. 2015; 23(2): 113 - 119.

Vaniyapong T, Chongruksut W, Rerkasem K. Local versus general anaesthesia for carotid endarterectomy. Cochrane Database Syst Rev. 2013; (12): CD000126.

GALA Trial Collaborative Group, Lewis SC, Warlow CP, et al. General anaesthesia versus local anaesthesia for carotid surgery (GALA): a multicentre, randomised controlled trial. Lancet. 2008；372(9656)：2132 - 2142.

Hye RJ，Voeks JH，Malas MB，et al. Anesthetic type and risk of myocardial infarction after carotid endarterectomy in the carotid revascularization endarterectomy versus stenting trial (CREST). J Vasc Surg. 2016；64(1)：3 - 8.

Dellaretti M，de Vasconcelos LT，Dourado J，et al. The importance of internal carotid artery occlusion tolerance test in carotid endarterectomy under locoregional anesthesia. Acta Neurochir (Wien). 2016；158(6)：1077 - 1081.

Choi BM，Park SK，Shin S，et al. Neurologic derangement and regional cerebral oxygen desaturation associated with patency of the circle of Willis during carotid endarterectomy. J Cardiothorac Vasc Anesth. 2015；29(5)：1200 - 1205.

Sharbrough FW， Messick JM Jr， Sundt TM Jr. Correlation of continuous electroencephalograms with cerebral blood flow measurements during carotid endarterectomy. Stroke. 1973；4(4)：674 - 683.

Sundt TM Jr，Sharbrough FW，Anderson RE，et al. Cerebral blood flow measurements and electroencephalograms during carotid endarterectomy. J Neurosurg. 1974；41（3）：310 - 320.

Beese U，Langer H，Lang W，et al. Comparison of near-infrared spectroscopy and somatosensory evoked potentials for the detection of cerebral ischemia during carotid endarterectomy. Stroke. 1998；29(10)：2032 - 2037.

Perez W，Dukatz C，El-Dalati S，et al. Cerebral oxygenation and processed EEG response to clamping and shunting during carotid endarterectomy under general anesthesia. J Clin Monit Comput. 2015；29(6)：713 - 720.

Sussman ES，Kellner CP，Mergeche JL，et al. Radiographic absence of the posterior communicating arteries and the prediction of cognitive dysfunction after carotid endarterectomy. J Neurosurg. 2014；121(3)：593 - 598.

Pennekamp CW，van Laar PJ，Hendrikse J，et al. Incompleteness of the circle of Willis is related to EEG-based shunting during carotid endarterectomy. Eur J Vasc Endovasc Surg. 2013；46(6)：631 - 637.

Mergeche JL，Bruce SS，Sander Connolly E，et al. Reduced middle cerebral artery velocity during cross-clamp predicts cognitive dysfunction after carotid endarterectomy. J Clin Neurosci. 2014；21(3)：406 - 411.

Ringelstein EB, Sievers C, Ecker S, et al. Noninvasive assessment of $CO_2$-induced cerebral vasomotor response in normal individuals and patients with internal carotid artery occlusions. Stroke. 1988; 19(8): 963 - 969.

Müller M, Schimrigk K. Vasomotor reactivity and pattern of collateral blood flow in severe occlusive carotid artery disease. Stroke. 1996; 27(2): 296 - 299.

Powers WJ. William M. Feinberg award for excellence in clinical stroke: hemodynamics and stroke risk in carotid artery occlusion. Stroke. 2014; 45(10): 3123 - 3128.

Reinhard M, Müller T, Guschlbauer B, et al. Dynamic cerebral autoregulation and collateral flow patterns in patients with severe carotid stenosis or occlusion. Ultrasound Med Biol. 2003; 29(8): 1105 - 1113.

Reinhard M, Roth M, Müller T, et al. Cerebral autoregulation in carotid artery occlusive disease assessed from spontaneous blood pressure fluctuations by the correlation coefficient index. Stroke. 2003; 34(9): 2138 - 2144.

Reinhard M, Roth M, Müller T, et al. Effect of carotid endarterectomy or stenting on impairment of dynamic cerebral autoregulation. Stroke. 2004; 35(6): 1381 - 1387.

Tang SC, Huang YW, Shieh JS, et al. Dynamic cerebral autoregulation in carotid stenosis before and after carotid stenting. J Vasc Surg. 2008; 48(1): 88 - 92.

Plessers M, Van Herzeele I, Vermassen F, et al. Neurocognitive functioning after carotid revascularization: a systematic review. Cerebrovasc Dis Extra. 2014; 4(2): 132 - 148.

Pennekamp CW, Immink RV, den Ruijter HM, Kappelle LJ, Bots ML, Buhre WF, et al. Near-infrared spectroscopy to indicate selective shunt use during carotid endarterectomy. Eur J Vasc Endovasc Surg. 2013; 46(4): 397 - 403.

Sato K, Abe K, Kosaka Y, et al. [A case of cardiac arrest caused by coronary spasm related to induction of general anesthesia before carotid endarterectomy]. No Shinkei Geka. 2016; 44(7): 591 - 598.

Candela S, Dito R, Casolla B, et al. Hypothermia during carotid endarterectomy: A safety study. PLoS One. 2016; 11(4): e0152658.

Bouri S, Thapar A, Shalhoub J, et al. Hypertension and the post-carotid endarterectomy cerebral hyperperfusion syndrome. Eur J Vasc Endovasc Surg. 2011; 41(2): 229 - 237.

Nouraei SA, Al-Rawi PG, Sigaudo-Roussel D, et al. Carotid endarterectomy impairs blood pressure homeostasis by reducing the physiologic baroreflex reserve. J Vasc Surg. 2005; 41(4):

631 - 637.

Sigaudo-Roussel D, Evans DH, Naylor AR, et al. Deterioration in carotid baroreflex during carotid endarterectomy. J Vasc Surg. 2002; 36(4): 793 - 798.

van Mook WN, Rennenberg RJ, Schurink GW, et al. Cerebral hyperperfusion syndrome. Lancet Neurol. 2005; 4(12): 877 - 888.

Lieb M, Shah U, Hines GL. Cerebral hyperperfusion syndrome after carotid intervention: a review. Cardiol Rev. 2012; 20(2): 84 - 89.

Maas MB, Kwolek CJ, Hirsch JA, et al. Clinical risk predictors for cerebral hyperperfusion syndrome after carotid endarterectomy. J Neurol Neurosurg Psychiatry. 2013; 84(5): 569 - 572.

Ogasawara K, Sakai N, Kuroiwa T, et al. Intracranial hemorrhage associated with cerebral hyperperfusion syndrome following carotid endarterectomy and carotid artery stenting: retrospective review of 4494 patients. J Neurosurg. 2007; 107(6): 1130 - 1136.

Matsumoto S, Nakahara I, Higashi T, et al. Near-infrared spectroscopy in carotid artery stenting predicts cerebral hyperperfusion syndrome. Neurology. 2009; 72(17): 1512 - 1518.

Pennekamp CW, Immink RV, den Ruijter HM, et al. Near-infrared spectroscopy can predict the onset of cerebral hyperperfusion syndrome after carotid endarterectomy. Cerebrovasc Dis. 2012; 34(4): 314 - 321.

Zhou W, Baughman BD, Soman S, et al. Volume of subclinical embolic infarct correlates to long-term cognitive changes after carotid revascularization. J Vasc Surg. 2017; 65(3): 686 - 694.

Hitchner E, Baughman BD, Soman S, et al. Microembolization is associated with transient cognitive decline in patients undergoing carotid interventions. J Vasc Surg. 2016; 64 (6): 1719 - 1725.

Lingzhong Meng

孟令忠

# 14 Complicated obstetric case

合并多种疾病的临产妇的麻醉管理

--------------------------------- > **Basic information** < ---------------------------------

A 37 years old parturient with painful contraction and hypertension.

The patient is a 37 years old Caucasian female，G2P1001，34-week gestation with premature rapture of membrane（PROM）. She has a VAS（visual analog scale）pain score of 4/10 during regular uterine contractions at 3 ～ 4 minutes apart. She has been admitted for preterm labor. Fetal heart rate （FHT）is 140 s/minute with good variability.

She presented complaints of elevated blood pressure（BP）and shortness of breath over the last month. She received corticosteroids a week ago. Her platelet account was 105,000/mm$^3$ at her last office visit，two weeks ago.

Her past medical history was also remarkable for hypertension（HTN），retinopathy，hypercholesterolemia, diabetes mellitus type I（DMI）class H，hypothyroidism，gatroesophageal reflux disease，and smoking. She was diagnosed with antithrombin Ⅲ deficiency due to an episode of deep venous thrombosis（DVT）at 19-week gestation. She has been placed on lovenox （enoxaparin）60 mg SQ bid since then and her last injection was 24 hours ago. Four years earlier，she experienced a myocardial infarction （MI） with subsequent placement of a single sirolimus-elutung stent (SES) (Cypher TM Cordis) in the proximal left anterior descending coronary artery that was 70% stenosed.

On physical examination, she is noted to be a morbid obese (Wt. 93.6 kg, Ht. 152 cm, BMI 40.5). The admission BP 191/107 mmHg. The patient is having increased swelling in her upper and lower extremities; Airway: Malampatti Ⅱ.

Admission medication included levothyroxine, famotidine, and insulin via a Paradigm 7 000 series indwelling pump (Medtronic). She had been taking clopridogrel 75 mg and aspirin 81 mg for 1-year post the placement of DES.

The significant initial laboratory results are platelet 107,000, HbA1c 6.7%, glucose 246 mg/dL, and three plus proteinuria. Cardiac enzymes are negatives.

Electrocardiogram is normal sinus rhythm.

Echocardiogram shows a normal left ventricle (LV) systolic function, LV ejection fraction (EF) 65%, normal wall motion, and a mild mitral regurgitation.

Initial treatments include: intravenous (IV) labetalol, hydralazine, and magnesium infusion.

Her BP has been reduced and maintained at 150 s/90 s mmHg. HR 84 次/min, RR 18/min, Hct 35%. Cervix is dilated at 2 cm.

> 基 本 信 息 <

37 岁临产妇,有疼痛性宫缩和高血压。

患者是 37 岁的白人妇女,G2P1001,孕 34 周,胎膜早破,在间隔 3~4 min 的规律宫缩中,她的疼痛程度按照视觉模拟评分系统(VAS)评分是 4/10。她被诊断为早产,胎心率为 140 次/min,变异佳。

现病史:在近 1 个月里,她的血压逐渐升高并伴有呼吸急促,1 周前服用了皮质类固醇药物,2 周前最后一次去诊所看病时,测得血小板计数为 105×10⁹/L。

既往史：高血压、视网膜病变、高胆固醇血症、1 型糖尿病 H 级、甲减、食管反流性疾病，并有抽烟史。在孕 19 周的时候，因为抗凝血酶Ⅲ缺乏而发作过一次深静脉血栓。此后开始注射依诺肝素钠注射液，一次皮下注射 60 mg，每天 2 次。最近一次注射是在 24 个小时之前。4 年以前她曾因心肌梗死，在已经有 70% 狭窄的冠状动脉左前降支的近端放置了一个西罗霉素药物洗脱支架（sirolimus eluting stent，SES）。

入院体检：病理性肥胖（体重 93.6 kg，身高 152 cm，体重指数 40.5），入院血压 191/107 mmHg。该患者上、下肢水肿明显。气道：Mallampatti 气道分类Ⅱ级。

入院后用药：左甲状腺素、法莫替丁、胰岛素（通过含有 7 000 个单位的胰岛素泵注射使用）。在放置西罗霉素药物洗脱支架后，她曾经服用氯吡格雷 75 mg 约 1 年，阿司匹林 81 mg 持续至今。

重要的入院实验室结果：血小板计数 $107 \times 10^9$/L，糖化血红蛋白（HbA1c）6.7%，血糖 13.67 mmol/L，尿蛋白（+++）。心肌酶谱正常。

心电图：窦性心律，正常心电图。

超声心动图：左室收缩功能正常，左室射血分数 65%，正常的室壁运动和轻微的二尖瓣反流。

入院后治疗及病情进展：静脉注射拉贝洛尔、肼屈嗪和镁离子溶液。

血压下降，基本维持在 150/90 mmHg 左右，心率 84 次/min，呼吸 18 次/min。血细胞比容 35%。宫口约 2 cm。

## > **Preoperative management** <

1. What is the classification of hypertensive disorders in pregnancy?

Keypoint：

1) This question is to test the knowledge.

2) The suggestive answer：Hypertension disorder in pregnancyis one of the most common medical problems encountered during pregnancy，complicating

2%~8% of pregnancies. Hypertensive disorders during pregnancy are classified into 4 categories, as recommended by the National High Blood Pressure Education Program Working Group on High Blood Pressure in Pregancy: ① gestational hypertension (transient hypertension of pregnancy or hypertension identified after 20 week of pregnancy and resolved within 12 weeks postpartum); ② preeclampsia; ③ chronic hypertension; and ④ preeclampsia superimposed on chronic hypertension. This terminology is preferred over the older but widely used term pregnancy-induced hypertension (PIH) because it is more precise.

3) Preparing direction: read reference 6.

2. Did this patient have preeclampsia?

Keypoint:

1) This question is to test clinical application of knowledge.

2) The suggestive answer: the patient has pre-eclampsia.

3) Preparing direction: read reference 1, 4, and 6.

3. What is the clinical significance of DM HbA1c?

Keypoint:

1) This question is to test knowledge.

2) The suggestive answer: the hemoglobin A1c test may be used to screen for and diagnose diabetes and prediabetes in adults. Hemoglobin A1c, also glycated hemoglobin or HbA1c, is formed in the blood when glucose attaches to hemoglobin. The higher the level of glucose in the blood, the more glycated hemoglobin is formed. The HbA1c test, however, should not be used for screening for cystic fibrosis-related diabetes, for diagnosis of gestational diabetes in pregnant women, or for diagnosis of diabetes in children and adolescence, people who have had recent severe bleeding or blood transfusions, those with chronic kidney or liver disease, or people with blood disorders such as iron-deficiency anemia, vitamin $B_{12}$ deficiency anemia, and some hemoglobin

variants (e.g., patients with sickle cell disease or thalassemia). In these cases, a fasting plasma glucose or oral glucose tolerance test should be used for screening or diagnosing diabetes. Only HbA1c tests that have been referenced to an accepted laboratory method. The HbA1c test is also used to monitor the glucose control of diabetics over time. The goal of those with diabetes is to keep their blood glucose levels as close to normal as possible. This helps to minimize the complications caused by chronically elevated glucose levels, such as progressive damage to body organs like the kidneys, eyes, cardiovascular system, and nerves. The HbA1c test result gives a picture of the average amount of glucose in the blood over the last $2 \sim 3$ months. This can help diabetics and their healthcare providers know if the measures that are being taken to control their diabetes are successful or need to be adjusted.

3) Preparing direction: JAMA. 2017; 317(4): 379 - 387.

4. What are the factors that contribute to an increased risk of epidural hematoma?

Keypoint:

1) This question is to test clinical knowledge.

2) The suggestive answer: The epidural hematoma may occur after trauma, lumbar puncture, epidural anesthesia, operation, coagulopathy, vascular malformation, neoplasm, hypertension, diabetes mellitus, pregnancy, anticoagulative medication, etc. Some authors reported spinal epidural hematoma without obvious cause as spontaneous epidural hematoma.

3) Preparing direction: Lancet. 1996; 347(8994): 131.

5. What would you conduct her cardiac evaluation?

Keypoint:

1) This question is to test clinical application of knowledge.

2) The suggestive answer: this patient's cardiac function is within normal

limit.

6. What is other information needed to formulate your anesthetic plan?

Keypoint:

1) This question is to test clinical application of knowledge and communication ability.

2) The suggestive answer: assess respiratory function, evaluate risks and benefits of different anesthetic techniques, and multi-disciplinary communication.

3) Preparing direction: Br J Anaesth. 2011; 107 (S1): i90 - i95.

7. Can the regional techniques be used for this patient's labor analgesia? If so, when?

Keypoint:

1) This question is to test clinical application of knowledge.

2) The suggestive answer: neuraxial anesthesia/analgesia can be safely administrated in this patient now.

3) Preparing direction: reference 1.

Labor Analgesia

After discussion among obstetricians, anesthesiologists, and pediatricians, epidural labor analgesia was chosen.

8. Why choose vaginal delivery over cesarean delivery?

Keypoint:

1) This question is to test clinical application of knowledge.

2) The suggestive answer: talk about the advantages of vaginal delivery.

3) Preparing direction: reference 1.

9. Do you consider using anti-acid therapy? Why?

Keypoint：

1）This question is to test clinical application of knowledge.

2）The suggestive answer：We should consider it，since the patient has risk of being full stomach.

3）Preparing direction：Indian J Anaesth. 2010；54（5）：415 - 420.

10. Which spinal vertebral space should be used for the epidural catheter placement? Why?

Keypoint：

1）This question is to test clinical knowledge.

2）The suggestive answer：lower lumbar intervertebral space.

3）Preparing direction：BJA Education. 2016；16（7）：213 - 220.

11. After placement of the epidural catheter，would you use the "testing dose"? Why?

Keypoint：

1）This question is to test clinical knowledge.

2）The suggestive answer：yes，to avoid serious complications. Do what is correct thing.

3）Preparing direction：Anesth Analg. 2006；102（3）：921 - 929.

12. Which dermatome level should be blocked in order to achieve good labor analgesia?

Keypoint：

1）This question is to test clinical knowledge，clinical application of knowledge，and communication skills.

2）The suggestive answer：T10 - L1 for stage Ⅰ and T10 - S2 for stage Ⅱ.

3）Preparing direction：Anesth Analg. 2006；102（3）：921 - 929.

13. How would you monitor this patient for the symptoms and signs of epidural hematoma?

Keypoint：

1）This question is to test clinical knowledge，clinical application of knowledge，and communication skills.

2）The suggestive answer：regular neural function check. Do what is the right thing.

3）Preparing direction：Lancet. 1996(8994)；347：131.

14. When the anticoagulation therapy is re-started?

Keypoint：

1）This question is to test clinical knowledge，clinical application of knowledge.

2）The suggestive answer：it depends on the type of the methods/medications.

3）Preparing direction：ASRA. 2016；41(2)：181‑194.

## > 术 前 管 理 <

1. 妊娠期高血压疾病的分类是什么？

要点：

1）这是知识测试问题。

2）参考答案：高血压是妊娠期间最常见问题之一，2%～8%妊娠患者受其影响。据全国妊娠期高血压知识教育项目工作组的意见，妊娠期间的高血压被分为四类：① 妊娠期高血压（妊娠 20 周之后出现的暂时高血压并于产后 12 周之内消失）。② 子痫前期。③ 慢性高血压。④子痫前期合并慢性高血压。目前的共识是，上述分类更加贴切。而妊娠高血压综合征（pregnancy-induced hypertension，PIH）这个曾被广泛使用的名称，已逐渐被取代。

3）请阅读参考文献 6。

2. 该患者是否可诊断为子痫前期？

要点：

1）这是知识测试题。

2）参考答案：该患者属于子痫前期。

3）请阅读参考文献 1,4 和 6。

3. 糖尿病中糖化血红蛋白的临床意义是什么？

要点：

1）这是知识测试题。

2）参考答案：A1c 血红蛋白可作为筛查成人糖尿病和糖尿病前期的指标,也叫作糖化血红蛋白或 A1c。它由糖与血红蛋白在血液中结合而形成。血糖越高,糖化血红蛋白生成越多。A1c 检测不适用于以下情况：囊性纤维化相关性糖尿病的筛查,妊娠期糖尿病的诊断,儿童和青少年糖尿病的诊断,近期有严重出血、贫血或输血,慢性肝肾疾病患者,某些血液病患者如缺铁性贫血、维生素 $B_{12}$ 缺乏性贫血及血红蛋白变形（如镰状细胞疾病或地中海贫血）。对于上述情况,空腹血糖和口服糖耐量测量可用于糖尿病的筛选和诊断。HbA1c 测定已被认为是一个公认的实验室方法。HbA1c 检测也可用于监测某段时间的血糖控制情况。糖尿病控制的目标是血糖水平尽量接近正常,这有助于尽量减少长期血糖升高所致的并发症,如机体器官包括肾、眼、心血管系统和神经受到的进行性损害。A1c 检测结果反映近 2～3 个月的平均血糖水平。这有助于糖尿病患者及其医务人员判断血糖控制治疗是否成功或是需进一步调整治疗。

3）请参考：JAMA. 2017；317（4）：379 - 387.

4. 什么因素会导致发生硬膜外血肿的风险增大？

要点：

1）这是知识测试题。

2）参考答案：硬膜外血肿可发生于下列情况之后：创伤、腰椎穿刺、硬膜外麻醉、手术、凝血功能异常、血管畸形、肿瘤新生物、高血压、糖尿病、妊娠和抗凝治疗等。无明显诱因下出现的椎管硬膜外血肿被称为自发性硬膜外血肿。

3）请参考：Lancet. 1996；347（8994）：131.

5. 你对该患者的心脏功能如何评价？

要点：

1）这个问题测试知识的临床运用。

2）参考答案：心功能在正常范围内。

6. 在制订麻醉方案之前，还需要了解哪些信息？

要点：

1）这个问题测试麻醉知识的临床应用和沟通能力。

2）参考答案：了解患者呼吸功能，评估各种麻醉技术的利与弊。不同学科医师之间的交流。

3）请参考：Br J Anaesth. 2011；107（S1）：i90－i95.

7. 在该患者分娩镇痛过程中能应用椎管内麻醉吗？如果能，什么时候用比较合适？

要点：

1）这问题测试知识的临床运用。

2）参考答案：椎管内阻滞技术可安全用于该例患者。

3）请见参考文献1。

分娩镇痛

经过产科医师、麻醉医师、儿科医师之间的互相讨论，最后决定采用硬膜外分娩镇痛。

8. 为什么选择阴道分娩而不考虑剖宫产？

要点：

1）这个问题测试知识的临床运用。

2）参考答案：讨论经阴道分娩的好处。

3）请见参考文献 1。

9. 你是否考虑使用抗酸剂？为什么？

要点：

1）这个问题测试知识的临床运用。

2）参考答案：可考虑使用抗酸药物，因为该患者可能是个饱胃患者。

3）请参考：Indian J Anaesth. 2010；54(5)：415-420.

10. 硬膜外导管应在哪个腰椎间隙置入为佳？为什么？

要点：

1）这个问题测试临床知识。

2）参考答案：低位腰椎间隙。

3）请参考：BJA Education. 2016；16 (7)：213-220.

11. 放置硬膜外导管后，你是否考虑使用试验剂量？为什么？

要点：

1）这个问题测试临床知识。

2）参考答案：为了避免严重并发症，必须常规先使用试验剂量。坚持做正确的事。

3）请参考：Anesth Analg. 2006；102(3)：921-929.

12. 为达到良好的分娩镇痛，阻断平面应维持在多大范围之内为宜？为什么？

要点：

1）这个问题测试临床知识及运用，还有沟通技巧。

2）参考答案：第一产程为：T10-L1，第二产程为 T10-S2。

3）请参考：Anesth Analg. 2006；102(3)：921-929.

13. 如何监护该患者才能及时发现可能出现的硬膜外血肿的症状与体征？

要点：

1) 这个问题测试临床知识及运用，还有沟通技巧。

2) 参考答案：必须定时检查神经功能。该做的必须做。

3) 请参考：Lancet. 1996；347(8994)：131.

14. 什么时候重新开始抗凝血治疗？

要点：

1) 这个问题测试临床知识及运用。

2) 参考答案：依患者用药情况及麻醉/手术方法而定。

3) 请参考：ASRA. 2016；41(2)：181 - 194.

## > **Intraoperative management** <

Nine hours later，obstetricians noticed a fetal bradycardia which was determined as late decelerations. Despite promptly intra-uterus resuscitation，the fetal bradycardia during each contraction progressively worsened，so a stat C-section was called.

1. What is a late deceleration?

Keypoint：

1) This question is to test clinical knowledge.

2) The suggestive answer：Late decelerations don't begin until the peak of a contraction or after the uterine contraction is finished. They're smooth，shallow dips in heart rate that mirror the shape of the contraction that's causing them. Late decelerations can be a sign in some cases that the baby isn't getting enough oxygen. Late decelerations that occur along with a fast heart rate（tachycardia）and very little variability can mean that the contractions may be harming the baby by depriving them of oxygen.

3）Preparing direction：Am Fam Physician. 1999；59（9）：2487 – 2500.

2. How to administer intra-uterus resuscitation?

KeyPoint：

1）This question is to test clinical knowledge，clinical application of knowledge.

2）The suggestive answer：Syntocinon off；full left or right lateral or knee elbow for possible cord compression；continue the same position for transfer and on the operating table；tocolysis：terbutaline 0.25 mg subcutaneous，alternatively for immediate action GTN sublingual spray，2 puffs initially，repeat after 1 minute until contractions stop，maximum 3 doses；oxygen；maximum flow（15 litre/min）via tight fitting Hudson mask with reservoir bag；fluid；and vasoactive medications.

3）Preparing direction：Int J Obstet Anesth. 2002；11（2）：105 – 116.

3. What is your anesthetic plan?

Keypoint：

1）This question is to test clinical knowledge，clinical application of knowledge.

2）The suggestive answer：general anesthesia，if cannot achieve quick epidural anesthesia.

3）Preparing direction：Am J Perinatol. 2009；26（3）：221 – 226.

After negative aspiration of epidural catheter，a five mL of 1.5% lidocaine was injected via epidural catheter. A few minutes later，the patient complained that she could not move both of her legs and difficulty to breath.

4. What was happening?

Keypoint：

1）This question is to test clinical application of knowledge.

2) The suggestive answer: epidural catheter migration.

3) Preparing direction: Anaesthesia. 2002; 57: 418.

5. What would be your anesthetic plan now?

Keypoint:

1) This question is to test clinical application of knowledge.

2) The suggestive answer: change to general anesthesia.

3) Preparing direction: Am J Perinatol. 2009; 26(3): 221 - 226.

6. What is the incidence of epidural catheter migration?

Keypoint:

1) This question is to test knowledge.

2) The suggestive answer: about 0.1%.

7. How to communicate with patient and her family during stat cesarean delivery?

Keypoint:

1) This question is to test clinical application of knowledge and communication skills.

2) The suggestive answer: tell the truth.

3) Preparing direction: Surgery. 2014; 155(5): 841 - 850.

8. How to perform analgesia after a stat cesarean delivery?

Keypoint:

1) This question is to test clinical application of knowledge.

2) The suggestive answer: Post-op pain control: PCIA; PCEA can be used. Same dose as labor analgesia, PO pain meds; Nerve block; and alternative medicine.

3) Preparing direction: https://www.healthgrades.com/procedures/5-

ways-to-manage-pain-after-a-c-sectionand Clin Perinatol. 2013；40(3)：443 - 455.

## 〉 术 中 管 理 〈

9 个小时后产科医师发现胎心缓慢的现象，并诊断为晚期减速。尽管采用胎儿宫内复苏，但是在每次宫缩的时候胎心减速的情况变得越来越严重，因此决定实施剖宫产。

1. 什么是晚期减速？

要点：

1）这个问题测试临床知识。

2）参考答案：宫缩最强时或宫缩结束后才可能出现晚期减速。表现为心率变化基线少许缓慢下沉，随宫缩状态而变化。晚期减速有时是胎儿缺氧的征象。如伴有心动过速且心率变异小，意味着宫缩引起胎儿缺氧。

3）请参见：Am Fam Physician. 1999；59(9)：2487 - 2500.

2. 如何实施胎儿宫内复苏？

要点：

1）这个问题测试临床知识及运用。

2）参考答案：停用缩宫素；完全左或右侧卧位，或膝肘卧位以缓解可能存在的脐带压迫，无论转移患者过程中还是在手术台上均保持该体位；抑制宫缩：特布他林，0.25 mg，皮下注射，或速效硝酸甘油舌下喷撒，先喷 2 次，1 min 后可再次使用至宫缩停止，最多 3 次；氧疗：扣紧氧气面罩，氧流量开到最大，15 L/min；液体治疗；血管活性药物治疗。

3）请参考：Int J Obstet Anesth. 2002；11(2)：105 - 116.

3. 此时你的麻醉方案是什么？

要点：

1) 这个问题测试临床知识及运用。

2) 参考答案：如果不能快速建立硬膜外麻醉,使用全麻。

3) 请参考：Am J Perinatol. 2009；26(3)：221 - 226.

硬膜外导管负压吸引无脑脊液后,经硬膜外导管注入 5 mL 1.5%利多卡因,几分钟后,患者立即觉得她的双腿动弹不得,而且感到呼吸困难。

4. 患者病情发生了什么变化?

要点：

1) 这个问题测试知识的临床运用。

2) 参考答案：硬膜外导管移位了。

3) 请参考：Anaesthesia. 2002；57：418.

5. 现在你的麻醉方案又将如何?

要点：

1) 这个问题测试知识的临床运用。

2) 参考答案：改为全身麻醉。

3) 请参考：Am J Perinatol. 2009；26(3)：221 - 226.

6. 硬膜外导管移位发生率是多少?

要点：

1) 这个问题考查麻醉知识。

2) 参考答案：大约 0.1%。

7. 紧急剖宫产时后,如何与患者和家属沟通?

要点：

1) 这个问题考验知识的临床运用及沟通技能。

2) 参考答案：会见家属,说实话。

3) 请参考：Surgery. 2014；155(5)：841 - 850.

8. 急诊剖宫产后如何镇痛？

要点：

1）这个问题考验知识的临床运用。

2）参考答案：患者控制的静脉镇痛；患者控制的硬膜外镇痛神，剂量和分娩镇痛相似；口服镇痛药、神经阻滞和整合医学。

3）请参考：https://www.healthgrades.com/procedures/5-ways-to-manage-pain-after-a-c-section.和 Clin Perinatol. 2013；40(3)：443 - 455.

## > **Postoperative management** <

At the end of the surgery，epidural catheter aspiration was positive for CSF. Post-operatively，the patient remained hemodynamically stable throughout her hospitalization without any cardiac or neurological issues.

1. What could be done to manage her post-operative pain?

Keypoint：

1）This question is to test clinical application of knowledge.

2）The suggestive answer：multimodal approach.

3）Preparing direction：Clin Perinatol. 2013；40(3)：443 - 455.

2. How is the possibility of acute coronary syndrome in this patient after surgery?

Keypoint：

1）This question is to test clinical application of knowledge and communication skills.

2）The suggestive answer：Increased.

3）Preparing direction：Mayo Clin Proc. 2009；84(10)：917 - 938.

3. How to help the patient to stop smoking?

Keypoint：

1）This question is to test knowledge of preventive medicine and community service.

2）The suggestive answer：physicians only focus on their own specialties. They often ignore their social and community responsibility.

3）Preparing direction：MMWR. 2016；65(6)：1 - 180.

4. What is the risk of pre-eclampsia if the patient becomes pregnant again?

Keypoint：

1）This question is to test knowledge of preventive medicine.

2）The suggestive answer：yes.

3）Preparing direction：Reference 1，2，3，4，5.

## ＞ 术 后 管 理 ＜

手术结束时硬膜外导管负压吸出脑脊液。手术结束后,在整个住院期间,患者维持稳定的血流动力学,无心脏与神经方面的并发症。

1. 针对该患者的术后疼痛,你能做些什么?

要点：

1）这个问题测试知识的临床运用。

2）参考答案：多模式镇痛。

3）请参考：Clin Perinatol. 2013；40(3)：443 - 455.

2. 该患者术后,发生急性冠状动脉综合征的可能性有多大?

要点：

1）这个问题测试知识的临床运用及沟通技能。

2）参考答案：增加。

3）请参考：Mayo Clin Proc. 2009；84（10）：917－938.

3. 如何帮助患者戒烟？

要点：

1）这个问题测试预防医学及社区服务知识。

2）参考答案：医师可能只关注自己的专业，他们往往缺乏对社会和社区的责任感。

3）请参考：MMWR. 2016；65（6）：1－180.

4. 如果该患者今后再次怀孕，子痫前期发生的危险性是否会增加？

要点：

1）这个问题测试预防医学知识。

2）参考答案：是。

3）请参考：Reference 1，2，3，4，5。

**Acknowledgement：**

Qinqing Fan，MD，Xijing Hospital，Xi'an. Dr. Fan helps translate the text into Chinese. 感谢西安西京医院范秦晴医师的翻译。

**Reference**

［1］Bateman BT and Polley LS. Hypertensive Disorders. In：Obstetric Anesthesia，Principles and Practice 5th edition（Editors：Chestnut，Wong，Tsen，Kee，et al）. pp 825－859. 2014.

［2］Alkema L，Chou D，Hogan D，et al. Global，regional，and national levels and trends in maternal mortality between 1990 and 2015，with scenario-based projections to 2030：a systematic analysis by the UN Maternal Mortality Estimation Inter-Agency Group. Lancet. 2016；387（10017）：462－474.

［3］Main EK& Menard MK. Maternal mortality：time for national action. Obstet Gynecol. 2013；122（4）：735－736.

［4］Sibai BM. Hypertension. In：Obstetrics：Normal and Problem Pregnancies（Editors. Gabbe

S., et al). pp 779 - 824. 2012.

[5] Powers RW, Catov JM, Bodnar LM, Gallaher MJ, Lain KY, Roberts JM. Evidence of endothelial dysfunction in preeclampsia and risk of adverse pregnancy outcome. Reprod Sci. 15(4): 374 - 381.

[6] Xia Y. Progress in Preeclampsia. Chinese Journal of Practical Gynecology and Obstetrics. 2007; 3(7): 573 - 574.

Yun Xia

夏云

# 15 Elective C-section for a term pregnancy with placenta previa

## 足月妊娠合并前置胎盘的剖宫产麻醉

> **Basic information** <

30 years old pregnant woman，G3P1 37 weeks of gestation，was diagnosed as placenta previa and scheduled for elective cesarean delivery.

> **基 本 信 息** <

30 岁女性，孕 3 产 1，宫内妊娠 37 周，诊断为前置胎盘，计划实施剖宫产分娩。

> **Preoperative management** <

1. How do you assess this woman's intravascular volume status?

Keypoint：Focus on objective parameters such as HR，BP，UOP（urine output），dry mouth，etc.

2. Should you assess her intrawascular volume status by orthostatic

hypotension?

Keypoint：Left uterine displacement concept：Yes or no either way，explain why it is the most important. It is a very typical example of no matter what to answer but the importance of knowing the key concept and expressing it in a certain way.

3. Do you use the same standard as for a non-pregnant women, why or why not?

Keypoint：No right answer, but know that full term pregnant women have different intravascular volume.

4. What else of preoperative information do you need to proceed this case?

Keypoint：Other medical problems related to PPH（postpartum hemorrhage），such as where is the position of placenta? Complete placenta previa or incomplete? Placenta percreta? Coagulation profile? Prepared agents for uterine atony? How big the IV accesses are? These information are very useful for preoperative preparation and intraoperative patient safety.

5. How do you explain to the patient and her family members that what is placenta previa and what risk involved in peri-operatively?

Keypoint：The types will affect management：front partial is the bloodiest case.

6. Do you need to have her typing & cross or typing and screen, why?

Keypoint：Important to answer yes rather than which one due to different systems.

7. What is her anesthesia plan for the cesarean delivery, spinal, epidural, CSE（combined spinal and epidural），general anesthesia with ETT（endotracheal tube）or LMA（laryngeal mask airway）?

Keypoints：CSE or general should be OK. The matter is to have a backup plan. Your score would not be discounted unless you choose general anesthesia with LMA because it has not been well accepted for clinical use but at research stage.

8. Peripheral IV access? Arterial line? CVP（central venous catheter）? PA （pulmonary artery）catheter?

Keypoint：Other than PA catheter，they are reasonable. Arterial line is useful for not only blood pressure monitor but also frequent blood sample draws for labs. Central line is rather a big intravenous access than monitoring CVP.

9. What do you want to know from obstetricians，and what kind of obstetrical information that could potentially change your mind for her anesthetic plans?

Keypoint：Cutting through placenta is not fun. Posterior one would be not bad.

10. What would you say when the obstetrician tells "you go ahead for induction" while he is dressing up?

Keypoint：Have to have a knife on hand otherwise the baby may have more anesthetics if do so.

## > 术 前 管 理 <

1. 你怎样对产妇的血容量进行评估？

要点：关注客观临床指标的变化，如心跳、血压、尿量和黏膜脱水问题等。

2. 你能用直立性低血压判断她是否存在低血容量吗？

要点：子宫左侧移位的概念。回答是或否都无妨，重要的是解释为什么。这是一个典型的例子，无论如何回答，最重要的是知道核心的概念，并能用合适的方法表达。

3. 可以用非妊娠妇女相同的标准来对她进行评估吗，为什么？

要点：没有正确的答案，但只要知道足月妊娠的妇女血管内容量不一样。

4. 需要什么其他的术前信息，才能开始剖宫产？

要点：与产后出血有关的情况，比如胎盘的位置在哪里？前置胎盘是完全性还是部分性？有否胎盘植入？有没有凝血功能障碍？备有子宫收缩乏力的药物吗？胎盘的位置在子宫前壁还是后壁？是否准备了粗的静脉通道？这一系列问题对于术前准备和患者术中的安全非常有用。

5. 你如何告知患者及其家属什么是前置胎盘，以及手术前后的风险？

要点：前置胎备的类型不同会影响处理方案，腹侧的前置性胎盘出血量很大。

6. 你需要血型血交叉吗？还是血型血抗体筛选？

要点：这个问题的关键是答"是"，而不是回答"哪一个"，因为每个医院有不同的规定。

7. 对于这个产妇的剖宫产，你会选择什么样的麻醉方法，腰麻、硬膜外麻醉、腰硬联合麻醉、气管插管全麻，还是喉罩全麻？

要点：腰硬联合麻醉或是全麻都可以，关键是有后续方案。只要不选喉罩全麻，你就不会被扣分，因为喉罩全麻至今还处于研究阶段，是没有被广泛认可的临床方法。

8. 需要准备外周静脉通路、动脉穿刺、中心静脉压或者漂浮导管吗？

要点：除了漂浮导管，其他都是合理的。动脉导管不仅用于血压监测，还可以定期抽血检验。中心静脉导管更多的只作为大静脉通道，而不是监测中心静脉压。

9. 你需要从产科医师那里了解什么信息，什么产科信息可能改变你的麻醉方案？

要点：切开胎盘不是儿戏（腹侧前置胎盘需要切开胎盘取出胎儿，这种情况出血量多，更加凶险）。子宫后壁前置胎盘却不是那么凶险（可能出现产后子宫下段收缩乏力,需要子宫腔内填塞;因为这部分没有太多子宫肌,对各类收缩子宫的药物都不太敏感)。

10. 当产科医师穿好无菌衣告诉你,"你可以进行诱导了",你会告诉他们什么?

要点:让他把手术刀拿在手里后,再开始全麻诱导,否则胎儿暴露在麻醉药物的时间太久。

## > **Intraoperative management** <

1. After the baby delivered, the surgical team was busy and quiet, what should you ask to them?

Keypoint:Keep in mind that the most common problem is miscommunication between teams. It might be the time when bleeding is very extensive and surgeons are working on stopping bleeding. Initiating a conversation is very important at this situation. Discussions should include the current issues, the plans, and next couples of steps to take care of any emergent situations with patient centered.

2. After you found the patient's hemodynamics is unstable, what is your first action?

Keypoint:As always, maintaining hemodynamics stable is the first, then find its etiology.

3. This patient is current under combined spinal and epidural anesthesia. Do you want to convert to general anesthesia?

Keypoint:Yes, I want to convert the case to general anesthesia ...

In general, if the diagnosis is certain and bleeding is out of control, general anesthesia may be a good choice. However, if the bleeding is under control and hemodynamics is stable，there is no need to do so. Once again，stating your answer and giving your reasons are the way to answer these questions. Do not ask the examiner about current situations but you can assume patient's situations and then give your answers.

## > 术 中 管 理 <

1. 当婴儿娩出时,外科医师团队非常忙碌和安静,你需要询问什么?

要点:牢牢记住,沟通不畅是团队医疗中最常见的问题。很可能出血很广泛,产科医师正在忙于止血。而没有顾上和我们交流。这时我们应该积极地和他们交流,以患者为中心,讨论目前情况、救治方案以及紧急情况下的一些处理步骤,共同努力抢治患者。

2. 发现血流动力学不稳定的时候,你的第一反应是什么?

要点:首先是维持血流动力学稳定,其次是寻找原因。

3. 此产妇采用的是腰硬联合麻醉,你需要改为全麻吗?

提示:对,我会把患者变为全麻⋯⋯

一般来说,如果诊断明确,出血未得到控制,全麻可能是一个好的选择。但如果出血已经控制,血液动力学也稳定,则没有必要这样做。持续采用现有的腰硬联合也是可以的。再次强调,回答这类问题的方法是说出你的答案并给出理由。不要追问考官患者现在的情况,你要假设患者的情况并给出相应答案。

## > Postoperative management <

1. The patient has been intubated in the middle of case，bleeding is under control at the end of surgery，and the patient received cell salvaged blood and 4

packed red blood cell，are you going to extubate this patient?

Keypoint：The answer could be either extubating or keeping intubation. The same approach：preparing for reasons of your answer.

2. The patient received spinal Duramorph for her postoperative pain control，because of her postpartum hemorrhage，the obstetrician did not want to give her NSAIDs. What will you do if the patient complaints pain 5/10 postoperatively?

Keypoint：The answer should address how to deal with potential airway obstruction，hypoventilation，and hypoxemia with combination of neuroaxial morphine and systemic opioid administration.

3. The patient still has her epidural catheter in place. Do you want to pull it out right after surgery? Why?

Keypoint：This patient may have coagulopathy issues after massive blood transfusion due to either dilution or consuming，or even DIC. Pulling the epidural catheter without checking laboratory profile may result in potential epidural hematoma. Keeping it in for postoperative neuroaxial analgesia to prevent the patient's ambulation generally is not a good explanation or choice due to risk of deep venous thrombosis and pulmonary embolism，which has been one of top etiologies of maternal mortality in many countries.

## > 术 后 管 理 <

1. 手术中，患者转为了全麻，术中她输了的自体血和 4 个单位的异体红细胞，出血得到了控制，你会拔管吗?

要点：可以回答拔管或保留插管。同样的方法，为你的回答准备好理由。

2. 该患者已经使用了蛛网膜下腔的吗啡作为术后镇痛。产科医师由于顾虑产后出血,不主张使用非甾体类抗炎药。患者主诉腹部疼痛 5/10,你怎么处理?

要点:回答时需要阐明蛛网膜下腔吗啡联合静脉阿片类药物时,可能导致的气道阻塞、通气不足和低氧血症。

3. 患者的硬膜外导管仍然在位,你会马上将导管拔除吗? 为什么?

要点:大量输血后,可能出现稀释性、消耗性甚至 DIC 所导致的凝血功能障碍。没做凝血检查就拔除硬膜外导管可能导致硬膜外血肿。保留导管用于术后镇痛通常不是一个很好的解释或选择,可能因为限制了产后的下床行走,有引起深静脉血栓的形成和肺栓塞的风险。这已经成为很多国家产妇死亡的主要原因。

**Reference**

[1] 2016 美国麻醉医师学会/产科与围产医学会《产科麻醉指南——剖宫产部分》. J NPLD - GHI. 2016;3(2):26.

[2] 剖宫产——全身麻醉 VS 椎管内麻醉. J NPLD-GHI. 2015;2(4):2.

[3] 全麻剖宫产——喉罩还是插管? J NPLD-GHI. 2015;2(3):29.

[4] Bateman BT,Mhyre JM,Ehrenfeld J,et al. The risk and outcomes of epidural hematomas after perioperative and obstetric epidural catheterization:a report from the Multicenter Perioperative Outcomes Group Research Consortium. Anesth & Analg. 2013;116(6):1380 - 1385.

[5] Mhyre JM,Riesner MN,Polley LS,et al. A series of anesthesia-related maternal deaths in Michigan,1985 - 2003. Anesthesiology. 2007;106(6):1096 - 1104.

[6] Mhyre JM. Maternal mortality. Curr Opin in Anesthesiol. 2012;25(3):277 - 285.

Lingqun Hu

胡灵群

# 16 Anesthesia management for aortic valve replacement

## 主动脉瓣置换术的麻醉管理

--------------------> **Basic information** <--------------------

A 71 year-old gentleman with history of hypertension，dyslipidemia and diabetics presented to our office on July 4，2016 with complaints of progressive weakness，short of breath for 3 months and new onset syncope and substernal burning pain of 6 week duration. This pain was worse with exertion and was relieved by rest. Patient would have pain on walking even around 100 yards. 6 weeks ago，the patient could walk 2 blocks on level ground without shortness of breath or chest pain. Patient denied any history of radiation or referral of pain. It was not related to breathing or positional changes.

On examination，Blood pressure was 140/90 mmHg and Pulse was regular at 60 beats per minute. Cardiovascular exam revealed a Grade 4/6 ejection systolic murmur best heard in the right second intercostal region radiating bilaterally to the neck.

Other significant medical problems included：hypertension，dyslipidemia，TIA.

Vitals：BP 140/90 mmHg，HR 60，RR 12，Temp 36.8℃，Wt 80 kg，Ht 178 cm.

Medications：Atenolol and statins.

Labs：Glucose 196 mg/dL，Na 141 mEq/L，K 4.9 mEq/L，creatinine 1.9 mg/dL，HCO₃⁻ 26 mEq/L.

ABG：pH 7.34，$PCO_2$ 49 mmHg，$PO_2$ 81 mmHg，$HCO_3^-$ 30 mEq/L.

ECG revealed left ventricular hypertrophy (LVH) with nonspecific ST‐T wave changes in inferior leads.

Echocardiography：Echocardiography (ECHO) revealed aortic valve (AV) area of 0.6~0.7 cm², mean gradient：48 mmHg and ejection fraction (EF) of 65%. AV was heavily calcified. AV peak velocity (AV Vmax) 4.66 m/s. ECHO also revealed 1⁺AI，2⁺TR and 1⁺MR. Thickened LV wall.

Heart catheterization：Hemodynamic measurement revealed LV pressure 240/0 with LV end diastolic pressure (LVEDP) of 10. Central aortic pressure was 166/59. There was a 55 mmHg mean gradient across the aortic valve. Pulmonary artery wedge pressure (PAWP)，mean of 24 mmHg，right atrium (RA) mean of 8 mmHg，right ventricle (RV) 60/10 with a right ventricular end diastolic pressure (RVEDP) of 14 mmHg，pulmonary artery (PA) 60/17 mmHg. The aortic valve area was calculated at 0.6 cm²，which was similar from ECHO.

Left ventriculogram revealed normal LV systolic motion and EF of 60%. Left main coronary artery revealed a common ostium-giving rise to the left anterior descending (LAD) and the circumflex. Right coronary artery (RCA) revealed a 99% ostial narrowing. LAD revealed a 50% narrowing in its proximal segment and a 40% ostial diagonal narrowing. Circumflex coronary artery had a 30% stenosis.

## > 基 本 信 息 <

男性,71岁,既往高血压、血脂紊乱、糖尿病病史,因进行性乏力和气短3个月,胸骨下烧灼痛6个月,伴新发的晕厥,于2016年7月4日至我院就诊。劳力后疼痛加重,活动后可缓解。患者行走约100码(约91.44 m)后即出现疼痛。6周前,患者可以平地行走两个街区,无气短和胸痛的症状。患者否认接受射线和发生牵涉痛的经历。疼痛与呼吸和体位改变无关。

查体:血压 140/90 mmHg,脉搏规律,60 次/min。心脏听诊发现,胸骨右缘第二肋间可闻及 4/6 级喷射性收缩期杂音,向两侧颈部放射。

其他显著的并发症包括:高血压、血脂紊乱、短暂性脑缺血发作(TIA)。

生命体征:血压 140/90 mmHg,心率 60 次/min,呼吸 12 次/min,体温36.8℃,体重 80 kg,身高 178 cm。

服用药物:阿替洛尔和他汀类。

实验室检查:血糖 10.89 mmol/L,Na 141 mmol/L,K 4.9 mmol/L,肌酐 167.96 $\mu$mmol/L,$HCO_3^-$ 26 mmol/L。

血气分析:pH 7.34,$PCO_2$ 49 mmHg,$PO_2$ 81 mmHg,$HCO_3^-$ 30 mmol/L。

心电图提示左室肥大,下壁导联非特异性 ST - T 改变。

超声心动图:主动脉瓣面积 0.6~0.7 $cm^2$,平均压力梯度 48 mmHg,射血分数 EF 65%。主动脉瓣(AV)钙化严重。主动脉瓣峰值流速(AV Vmax)4.66 m/s。还发现 $1^+$ 主动脉瓣关闭不全(AI),$2^+$ 三尖瓣反流(TR),$1^+$ 二尖瓣反流(MR),左室(LV)增厚。

心导管检查:血流动力学检测发现左室压力 240/0 mmHg,左室舒张末期压力(LVEDP)10 mmHg,中心动脉压力 166/59 mmHg,主动脉瓣平均跨瓣压 55 mmHg,平均肺动脉楔压(PAWP)24 mmHg,平均右房压 8 mmHg,右室(RV)压力 60/10 mmHg,右室舒张末期压力(RVEDP)14 mmHg,肺动脉(PA)压力 60/17 mmHg。主动脉瓣面积计算为 0.6 $cm^2$,与 ECHO 结果一致。

左室造影提示左室收缩运动正常,EF 60%。左冠状动脉主干同时发出左前降支(LAD)和回旋支。右冠状动脉(RCA)开口部狭窄 99%;左前降支近端狭窄 50%,开口部对角线狭窄 40%;回旋支狭窄 30%。

> **Preoperative management** <

1. What other tests before starting the anesthesia do you want? Why/why not?

Keypoint: this is an open question, it asks the candidate to have a good assessment for this patient, and any other condition should be optimized prior to surgery.

2. Your choice for the intraoperative monitoring, why?

Keypoint: the candidate should know the application and limitation of each monitor (invasive and noninvasive), know how to place an invasive monitor and associated complications.

3. Is a pulmonary artery catheter (PAC) indicated in the patients? Why?

Keypoint: this is to test whether the candidate knows how to place a PAC and complications during such a placement, how to interpret the data during different phases of surgery.

4. Is an awake arterial catheter indicated? Why/why not?

Keypoint: asking the risk assessment of significant hemodynamic changes during induction, extra preparation, rescue plan, pharmacologic base of each agent and its effect on the heart.

5. What you want to see from ECHO? Why?

Keypoint: this is to test the candidate's basic knowledge for echo and specifics for aortic stenosis.

6. What you want to see from cardiac catheterization report? Why?

Keypoint: this is to test the candidate's basic knowledge of CAD.

7. What kind of IV access do you need before induction?

Keypoint: this is practical question for bypass surgery, the access should include the peripheral and central, plus infusion lines.

8. Should the surgeon perform a CABG for RCA stenosis? Or should the cardiologist stent the RCA? Explain.

Keypoint：This is to test the candidate's extended knowledge on PCI and CABG.

> 术 前 管 理 <

1. 麻醉前你还准备做些什么检查？为什么或为什么不？

要点：这是一个开放的问题，要求应试者对这个患者做出正确的评估，术前应该将所有条件达到最优状态。

2. 关于术中监测，你的选择是什么？为什么？

要点：应试者应该知道每项监护（包括有创的和无创的）的使用方法和他们的局限之处，应该知道如何放置有创监测以及它们的并发症。

3. 肺动脉导管（PAC）是否适用于这个患者？为什么？

要点：这个问题考察应试者如何放置 PAC 以及相关并发症，如何在手术不同阶段解释相关数据。

4. 是否进行清醒动脉置管吗？为什么或为什么不？

要点：要求回答诱导期血流动力学剧烈波动的风险评估，需要做哪些额外准备、应急措施、每种药物的药理学基础以及对心脏的影响。

5. 你希望从 ECHO 中看到什么？为什么？

要点：这个问题考察应试者关于 ECHO 的基本知识和主动脉狭窄的特征。

6. 你希望从心导管报告中看到什么？为什么？

要点：这个问题考察应试者关于 CAD 的基本知识。

7. 诱导前你需要什么类型的静脉通路?

要点：这是体外手术中的一个切实问题，通路应该包括外周的和中心的，加上灌注的管道。

8. 对于 RCA 狭窄，外科医师需要进行 CABG 手术吗? 还是请心脏科医师放置支架? 解释这个问题。

建议：这个问题考察应试者关于 PCI 和 CABG 方面扩展的知识。

## > **Intraoperative management** <

1. What kind of anesthesia you choose to use?
Keypoint：this is to test the candidate's patient care and anesthesia knowledge.

2. What kind of induction agents you are going to use and why?
Keypoint：this is test the candidate's basic knowledge of general anesthesia.

3. What would be your role in the operating room（OR）before induction? Why?
Keypoint：This is to test the candidate's system-based practice.

4. During induction，the systolic blood pressure dropped from 140 to 100 mmHg，are you going to treat it? Why/why not?
Keypoint：This is to test the candidate's medical knowledge and practice-based learning and improvement on AS（aortic stenosis）hemodynamics.

5. Heart rate increased from 60 to 100 BPM，do you concern? Why/Why not?
Keypoint：This is to test the candidate's practice-based learning and improvement.

6. What is the hemodynamic goal you wish to achieve for this case?

Keypoint: This is to test the candidate's medical knowledge on AS hemodynamics.

7. Is intraoperative transesophageal echocardiography (TEE) indicated for this case? Why/Why not?

Keypoint: This is to test the candidate's medical knowledge on TEE indications.

8. If a TEE is used during surgery, what cardiac structures are you going to evaluate?

Keypoint: This is to test the candidate's medical knowledge and patient care.

9. If you find a patent foramen ovale (PFO), what will you do?

Keypoint: This is to test the candidate's interpersonal and communication skills.

10. What other monitors are you going to use? Why/Why not?

11. Is central venous access needed for this patient? Why/Why not?

12. If a PAC is used, what information you are looking for from it?

Keypoint: The above 3 questions are used to test the candidate's medical knowledge and system-based practice.

13. What anesthetics you are going to use for maintenance? Why/Why not?

Keypoint: this is to test the candidate's basic knowledge of anesthesia.

14. From your evaluation, what medications you are going to prepare to facilitate weaning off bypass? Why/Why not?

Keypoint: This is to test the candidate's practice-based learning and improvement.

After weaning off bypass, the blood pressure was about 90/56 mmHg, CI: 1.9, mixed venous $O_2$ saturation: 60%. Patient is on norepinephrine 0.05 mcg/kg/min, NTG 0.2/mcg/kg/min.

15. How are you going to manage this and why?

Keypoint: This is to test the candidate's knowledge and patient care.

16. Patient blood glucose was 220 mg/dL at the time of coming off bypass. Are you going to treat it and how? And what is your target?

Keypoint: The above question is to test the candidate's patient care, practice-based learning and improvement.

> 术 中 管 理 <

1. 你选择什么麻醉?
要点:这个问题考察应试者的患者监护和麻醉方面的知识。

2. 你准备使用什么类型的诱导药物? 为什么?
要点:这个问题考察应试者关于全身麻醉的基本知识。

3. 在诱导前,在手术室中你想成为什么角色? 为什么?
要点:这个问题考察应试者基于全局系统的实践理念。

4. 在诱导过程中,收缩压从 140 mmHg 降到 100 mmHg,你准备进行处理吗? 为什么处理或者为什么不处理?
要点:这个问题考察应试者关于主动脉狭窄的医学知识和基于实践的学习和改进能力。

5. 心率从 60 次/min 上升到 100 次/min,你怎么考虑？为什么处理或者为什么不处理？

要点：这个问题考察应试者基于实践的学习和改进能力。

6. 对于这个病例,你期望达到的血流动力学目标是什么？

要点：这个问题考察应试者关于主动脉狭窄的医学知识。

7. 术中给患者使用 TEE 有指征吗？为什么？

要点：这个问题考察应试者关于 TEE 适应证的医学知识。

8. 如果术中使用了 TEE,你准备评估哪些心脏的结构？

要点：这个问题考察应试者的患者监护和医学知识。

9. 如果你发现卵圆孔未闭,你将做什么？

要点：这个问题考察应试者的人际沟通技巧。

10. 你准备使用什么其他的监护设备？为什么使用或为什么不使用？

11. 这个患者需要开放中心静脉通路吗？为什么开放或为什么不开放？

12. 如果使用了 PAC,你期望从中得到什么信息？

要点：以上 3 个问题考察应试者的医学知识和基于全局系统的实践理念。

13. 麻醉维持你准备使用什么药物？为什么使用或为什么不使用？

要点：这个问题考察应试者关于麻醉的基本知识。

14. 根据你的评估,为了帮助终止体外,你准备使用什么药物？为什么使用或为什么不使用？

要点：这个问题考察应试者基于实践的学习和改进能力。

终止体外后,血压大约 90/56 mmHg,心指数 1.9,混合静脉氧饱和度 60%。去甲肾上腺素 0.05 $\mu$g(kg·min),硝酸甘油 0.2 $\mu$g(kg·min)。

15. 你打算如何管理呢？为什么？

要点：这个问题考察应试者的患者监护和医学知识。

16. 在终止体外时,患者血糖 12.22 mmol/L。你准备进行处理吗？如何处理？目标是什么？

要点：这个问题考察应试者的患者监护和基于实践的学习和改进能力。

## > **Postoperative management** <

Patient was extubated 2 hours after surgery in the intensive care unit（ICU）. When you went to exam the patient，you found the patient was disoriented.

1. How do you decide what is the appropriate time to extubate?

Keypoint：This question is to test the candidate's practice-based learning and improvement.

2. How do you evaluate patient's postoperative cognitive function?

Keypoint：The above question is to test the candidate's knowledge and patient care.

3. What is the incident of postop cognitive dysfunction?

Keypoint：The above question is to test the candidate's knowledge and system based learning.

4. How do you prevent it?

Keypoint：The above question is to test the candidate's knowledge and patient care，professionalism and patient care.

---

> 术 后 管 理 <

术后 2 个小时，患者在 ICU 内拔除气管导管。当你去查房的时候，你发现患者出现了定向力障碍。

1. 你如何决定拔除气管导管的合适时机？

要点：这个问题考察应试者基于实践的学习和改进能力。

2. 你如何评估患者术后的认知功能？

要点：以上问题考察应试者的患者监护和医学知识。

3. 术后认知功能障碍发生是多少？

要点：这个问题考察应试者的知识和基于全局系统的学习能力。

4. 如何预防？

要点：以上问题考察应试者的医学知识和患者监护以及专业素质。

**References**

[1] Nishimura RA，Otto CM，Bonow RO，et al. 2014 AHA/ACC guideline for the management of patients with valvular heart disease：a report of the American College of Cardiology/American Heart Association Task Force on Practice Guidelines. Circulation. 2014；129(23)：e521‐643.

[2] Szabo TA，Toole JM，Payne KJ，et al. Management of aortic valve bypass surgery. Semin Cardiothorac Vasc Anesth. 2012；16(1)：52‐58.

[3] Lester L. Anesthetic Considerations for Common Procedures in Geriatric Patients. Anesthesiol Clin. 2015；33(3)：491‐503.

[4] American Geriatrics Society Expert Panel on Postoperative Delirium in Older Adults. Postoperative delirium in older adults: best practice statement from the American Geriatrics Society. Am Coll Surg. 2015; 220(2): 136 - 148.

Hong Liu

刘虹

# 17 Anesthesia management for ascending aortic aneurysm surgery

## 升主动脉瘤手术麻醉管理

58 years old 92 kg, 170 cm male patient is scheduled to operation room for surgical repairing of ascending aortic aneurysm.

HPI: The patient was admitted 2 hours ago with severer back pain. Vital signs have been stable but workup demonstrates a 5.6 cm ascending aortic aneurysm, Cardiac catheterization at time revealed a 70% RCA (right coronary artery) stenosis and normal LV (left ventricle) ejection fraction.

MEDs: Metoprolol, enalapril, Nimodipine, flurosemide.

PMH: poorly controlled hypertension and obesity for more than 20 years.

Occasional angina 3 years ago. Type Ⅱ diabetes mellitus for 5 years treated with insulin.

PE: P: 76 bpm, BP 165/97 mmHg, RR 22, SaO₂ 96%, Temp: 37.1℃. Obese, looks very nervous male with back pain.

Airway: full dentition, uvula visible to tip, TMJ mobile, C-spinal extension mildly limited. Others within normal level.

CXR/CT scans: 5.6 cm ascending aortic aneurysm, LV concentric hypertrophy, RV prominence, increased pulmonary vascular markings.

Echo：HLV（hypertrophic left ventricle），moderated AI（aortic insufficiency）. EF 50%，RV（right ventricle）enlarged.

Labs：Hgb 12.9 gm/dL，platelet count 216 000/mL，Na 142 mEq/L，K 3.7 mEq/L，creatinine 1.8 mg/dL，BUN 32 mg/dL，blood sugar 226 gm/dL，PT，aPTT，INR WNL.

On arrival to the operation room，a 20 gauge IV catheter right arm. The patient is extremely anxious.

> 基 本 信 息 <

患者,58 岁,男性,92 kg,170 cm,拟行升主动脉瘤修复手术。

病史：患者入院 2 小时前,突发严重的背部疼痛。生命体征平稳,但是检查显示升主动脉瘤5.6 cm,同时心导管显示 70%的右冠状动脉狭窄,左心室射血分数正常。

用药史：美托洛尔、依那普利、尼莫地平和呋塞米。

既往史：高血压控制欠佳,肥胖超过 20 年。3 年前开始偶发心绞痛。2 型糖尿病 5 年,用胰岛素治疗。

体格检查：心率 76 bpm,血压 165/97 mmHg,呼吸 22 次/min,氧饱和度96%,温度 37.1℃。肥胖,神情非常紧张伴背部疼痛。

气道：全牙列,可见到悬雍垂尖,颞下颌关节移动好,颈椎伸展轻度受限。其他在正常水平。

胸片/CT 检查：5.6 cm 升主动脉瘤。左心室向心性肥厚,右室突出,肺血管纹理加重。

超声检查：左心室肥厚,中度主动脉瓣关闭不全。射血分数 50%,右室增大。

实验室检查：血红蛋白 129 g/L,血小板 216 ×10⁹/L,钠 142 mmol/L,血钾 3.7 mmol/L,肌肝 159.12 μmol/L,尿素 5.70 mmol/L(尿素氮 11.39 mmol/L),血糖 12.56 mmol/L。凝血酶原时间、活化部分凝血活酶时间和国际标准化比值均正常。

到达手术室时，右臂 20 号静脉留置针。患者极度焦虑。

## > **Preoperative management** <

1. Hypertension：What is the implication of hypertension to anesthetic management? What if BP 180/100，how do you management? What are the poor controlled HTN and obesity implied you?

Keypoint：know the definition of hypertension，the treatment indication prior anesthesia induction，and the balance to preserve vital organ perfusion. Also to understand that the uncontrolled hypertension is an independent perioperative risk. Obese patients with poorly controlled hypertension suggests that sleep apnea and airway obstruction syndrome，hypercapnia，pulmonary hypertension and dysfunction of right heart.

2. Cardiac status：history of CAD（coronary artery disease），surgeon asking what cardiac evaluation is needed，your respond? Would EF 50% affect your plan? RV enlarged? Concerns if aortic stenosis is present?

Keypoint：Mechanism of myocardial ischemia in patients with coronary artery disease. Knows anesthesia management for difference valvular diseases.

3. Base line ABG：Should ABG be ordered? Why/why not? What specific information do you seek? Why is it an important consideration pre-operation?

Keypoint：knowledge of arterial blood gas and interpretations，possible impact on anesthesia management.

4. Airway：What are airway assessments for obese patient? What are predictors of difficult laryngoscopy? Is it critical for airway management? Is the body mass index a reliable predictor?

Keypoint: definition of obese, the associated pathophysiological changes; how to evaluate the airway and preparation for the challenge, the practical skills and experience.

The following factors are predictitve of difficult intubation:

1) Thyromental distance<3 finger breadths (approximately 6.5 cm).

2) Neck circumference>43 cm (17 inches).

3) Inter-incisor distance<4.5 cm.

4) Mallampati 3 or 4.

Body mass index in isolation is not a reliable predictor of the difficulty of visualizeation.

5. Blood typing and cross match: Blood bank informs you, this patient has an unknown antibody, so the cross match has to wait for at least 45 min, would you postpone the surgery, if so, for how long? Surgeon asks you to start the case immediately since he will have a very important meeting late. Would you? Why/why not?

Keypoint: concept and principle of blood match (type and cross), some difficult scenarios, the impact of blood products availability to this surgery.

6. Pre-operative medications: What medication would you continue/discontinue pre-op? Why, for each? If extremely anxious, would you provide sedation? Why/why not?

Keypoint: the pharmacology of various pre-medications, the purpose and side effects, and the practical objective goals-anxiety, vital signs, etc.

7. Chest pain: The patient in preoperative section had a sudden onset of severe chest pain, nausea and vomiting, what would be your response? If his BP is 186/110? or BP is 76/42?

Keypoint: to exam the ability of crisis recognition and action, also be able to differentiate the different causes，acute aortic dissection vs. acute myocardial infarction，and their managements.

## > 术 前 管 理 <

1. 高血压：高血压对麻醉管理的影响是什么？如果 BP 180/100 mmHg，你如何处理？什么是控制不佳的高血压，肥胖症暗示你什么？

要点：高血压的定义，麻醉诱导前高血压的治疗指征，以及如何保证重要脏器的灌注。控制不佳的高血压是围术期独立的危险因素。肥胖伴有控制不佳的高血压的患者提示睡眠气道梗阻综合征、高碳酸血症、肺动脉高压和右心功能异常。

2. 心脏状态：因为冠心病病史，外科医师询问你需要如何进一步心脏评估，你的反应是什么？EF 50%，右室增大，是否影响您的计划？如果有主动脉瓣狭窄？

要点：冠心病患者心脏缺血的机制以及不同瓣膜疾病的麻醉管理。

3. 基础血气分析：应该测量基础血气吗？为什么/为什么不？你想要寻求什么特殊的信息？为什么它是术前需要着重考虑的问题？

要点：动脉血气分析的知识和解读，以及对麻醉管理的影响。

4. 气道：什么是肥胖患者气道评估标准？困难气管插管的预测指标是什么，是否对于气道管理至关重要？体重指数是不是独立的困难气道预测指标？

要点：肥胖的定义，以及相关的病理生理改变。如何评估气道，困难气道的处理、实际技巧和经验。

下述因素提示插管困难：

1) 颌甲间距（下颌至甲状软骨之间的距离）<3 横指（约 6.5 cm）。

2) 颈部周长>43 cm。

3) 门齿间距（张口度）<4.5 cm。

4) Mallampati 3 级或 4 级。

体重指数本身并不是困难气道的独立预测指标。

5. 血型和交叉配血：血库通知你,患者有不明抗体需要进一步检查,且交叉配血将至少等待 45 min。你是否要推迟手术？推迟多久？外科医师要求你立即开始,因为他晚些时候有非常重要的会议。你要开始吗？为什么/为什么不？

要点：配血的概念和原则,以及一些困难情况的处理。血液制品是否到位对该手术的影响。

6. 术前用药：什么药物会在术前继续或停止？为什么,每个吗？如果患者极度焦虑你会在入手术室前提供镇静吗？为什么/为什么不？

要点：不同麻醉前用药的药理学、用药目的、不良反应和具体想要达到的药理作用。

7. 胸痛：术前患者突然胸痛,恶心呕吐,你的反应是什么？BP：186/110 mmHg？BP：76/42 mmHg？

要点：危机鉴别和处理的能力。鉴别不同的原因,是急性主动脉夹层剥离还是急性心肌梗死以及处理原则。

# Intraoperative management

1. Monitoring：Radial arterial line? If so, which side, why/why not? Would you choose a CVP (central venous catheter)/PA (pulmonary arterial) catheter in this patient? How about TEE (transesophageal echocardiography)? Explain your choice. Would the EEG (electroencephagraphy) monitoring have any value for this patient? SSEPs (somatosensory evoke potentials)? Why/why not? Cerebral Oximetry? How will you use information from those monitors?

Keypoint：basic concept for common invasive monitoring, the knowledge, indication, and limitations; specific knowledge of brain monitoring and the new technology.

2. Airway management and induction: when and how would you perform the airway evaluation? What position? Would you choose intravenous induction followed by fiberoptic intubation acceptable? Why/why not? What is your plan? How will you minimize hemodynamic swing?

Keypoint: the practical skill for airway management, also pay attention to the importance of smooth hemodynamic during induction.

3. Post-induction bradycardia and hypotension: Prior to chest incision, BP 80/50, P 50. Etiology? Assume this is nodal rhythm, do you need to treat? Why/why not? If this were sinus bradycardia, would you treat? How do you rule out this is caused by ischemia?

Keypoint: basic knowledge of normal cardiac rhythm and arrhythmia, the causes of various bradycardia and the indication of treatment, specific measures.

4. Hypothermia: What is controlled hypothermia? Classification? Effect of hypothermia? What is circuit arrest? Why dose profound hypothermia protects the CNS (central nervous system)? Effect of hypothermia on hemostasis?

Keypoint: know the definition of controlled hypothermia and classification; the physiological effect of hypothermia and its effect on the CNS and hemostasis.

5. CPB management: 5 min after giving 1 mg/kg heparin, ACT 320 sec. Why, and what are your plan? After circle arrest, Hct is 18%, treat? Why? How?

Keypoint: understand the pharmacology of heparin, the principle of monitoring in the OR; the indication of safe start bypass; know the definition of circle arrest, the application for various cardiac surgery, and the effect bypass and circle arrest on hemostasis.

6. Hyperglycemia: Glucose 320 mg/dL, treat? Why/why not? If so, how would you treat? The potential complications of hyperglycemia?

Keypoint: understand the causes of intraoperative hyperglycemia and associated complications, the practical management approaches.

7. Inotropes: How do you determine the need for inotropic support prior to separation from CPB? Explain? What type inotrope will benefit if the patient also has a significant pulmonary hypertension (PHTN) with elevated CVP? Would the intraoperative TEE be helpful?

Keypoint: understand the cardiac bypass effect on the heart, ischemia and reperfusion injury; the indication of inotropic treatment, the choice of various agents and their pharmacological properties; specific agent indicated for the existing of pulmonary hypertension, the possible findings by intraoperative TEE.

8. Coagulopathy: What type lab tests will help you to differentiate coagulation disorder? How would you know the patient need more protamine? What is platelet dysfunction? What is factors deficiency? When would you start transfusion of FFP? Cryoprecipitate? Platelet? Fibrinogen? Factor Ⅷ? RBC? Why/ why not?

Keypoint: understand the causes and incidence of bypass associated coagulation disorder, specific tests, and the indication for specific component transfusion.

9. Fluid management: How much fluid will you administer before on CPB? Why? What type of fluid will you chose? Crystal/colloid intravenous fluid, why? To

minimize the blood loss? Your colleague suggests you limiting administer fluid after CPB? Do you agree? Why/why not? Does urine output matter?

Keypoint: understand the principle of fluid administration during cardiac surgery; know the new concept on volume restrict to improve outcome; know the limited indication of urine output for volume assessment.

## > 术 中 管 理 <

1. 监测: 桡动脉监测? 哪一边,为什么/为什么不? 你会选择放置/监测 CVP 和 PAP 吗? TEE 如何? 解释你的选择。EEG 监测对这个患者是否有价值? SSEP? 为什么/为什么不? 脑血氧饱和度如何? 您将如何使用和分析这些信息?

要点: 常用侵入性监测的基本概念、相关知识、适应证和局限性。脑功能监测的知识和新技术。

2. 气道管理和麻醉诱导: 你何时采用什么方法进行气道评估? 体位? 是否选择静脉诱导后纤维支气管镜插管? 为什么/为什么不? 你的计划是什么? 如何减少插管对血流动力学的影响?

要点: 气道管理的实用技巧;麻醉诱导时如何尽量保持血流动力学平稳。

3. 诱导后心动过缓和低血压: 胸部切开之前,BP 80/50 mmHg,P 50 bpm,原因? 假设窦性心律,你要治疗吗? 为什么/为什么不? 如果窦性心动过缓,怎么治疗? 你如何排除心肌缺血所致?

要点: 正常心脏节律和心律失常的基础知识,心动过缓的原因、治疗的指征和措施。

4. 低温: 什么是控制性低体温? 分级? 低温对机体的影响? 什么是循环停止? 为什么极度深低温能保护中枢神经系统? 低温对凝血的影响?

要点: 控制性低体温的定义和分级;低体温的生理影响,及其对中枢神经系统和凝血功能的影响。

5. 心肺转流管理：给予 1 mg/kg 肝素 5 min 后，ACT 320 s。为什么，你的计划是什么？循环停止后，Hct 为 18%，治疗？为什么？怎么样处理？

要点：理解肝素的药理学，在手术室内监测 ACT 的原则。安全的开始体外转流的指征，循环停止的定义及其在不同心脏手术的应用。体外转流和循环停止对凝血功能的影响。

6. 高血糖：血糖 17.78 mmol/L，是否治疗？为什么/为什么不？你会怎么治疗？高血糖所致的潜在并发症？

要点：术中高血糖的原因及相关并发症，以及实用的处理方法。

7. 正性肌力药：你如何确定患者是否在脱机之前需要正性肌力药物支持？说明？如果患者的 CVP 和 PAP 升高，哪种正心力药会受益？TEE 会有帮助吗？

要点：体外转流对心脏的影响，以及缺血再灌注损伤；心肌正性肌力药治疗的指征、不同药物的选择和药理学特性；用于治疗已经存在的肺动脉高压的特效药物。术中 TEE 可能的发现。

8. 凝血功能障碍：什么实验室检测会帮助你鉴别凝血障碍？你如何知道患者需要更多的鱼精蛋白？什么是血小板功能障碍？什么是凝血因子缺乏？你何时开始输血，FFP？干冷沉淀？血小板？纤维蛋白原？因子Ⅶ还是红细胞？为什么/为什么不？

要点：体外转流相关的凝血功能紊乱的原因和发生率、特殊的实验；成分输血的适应证。

9. 输液管理：你在心肺转流之前输入多少液体？为什么？你会选择什么类型的液体？晶体/胶体？为什么？为减少失血，你的同事建议你在脱机后限制液体输入？你同意吗？为什么/为什么不？尿量的多少有影响吗？

要点：心脏手术的输液原则。掌握限制容量有助于改善预后，以及尿量对于判断容量状态的局限性。

> **Postoperative management** <

1. AV block: patient becomes hypotensive on the arrival to ICU. BP 86/52 mmHg, differential diagnosis? ECG shows HR 40 with PVCs, treat? How would you reset the his pacemaker?

Keypoint: know the common dysrhythmias after cardiac surgery and the indication for urgent/emergent intervention; know how to reset the temporary pacemaker.

2. Surgical bleeding/coagulopathy: in the ICU, the chest tubing continues to put out bloody like drainage great 250 mL/hr for last two hours. What specific test would help you to tell this is a surgical bleeding or acquired coagulation dysfunction? How would you decided to transfuse more RBC vs, FFP, platelet? When would you call the surgeon to evaluate the patient for possible bring the patient back to OR for surgical re-exploration? Would the presence or absence of hypotension, normotensive, hypertensive affect your decision?

Keypoint: familiar with the common postoperative cardiac and surgical complications, knows the priority of surgical vs medical management.

3. Oliguria: During first 3 hours in ICU, his urine output is only 35 mL, adequate? Why/why not? Causes? Is a bedside TTE needed? His PAP (pulmonary arteria pressure) is 14 mmHg, and CO (cardiac output) is 4.0 L/min, should the fluids be administered? Which one? How much fluid is appropriate? The surgeon recommends furosemide, agree/disagree? Explain? Therapy if oliguria continuous?

Keypoint: familiar with the common causes of oliguria after cardiac surgery, the diagnosis approaches and management for general and specifics.

4. Failure to awaken: 6 hours post-OP in ICU, patient has not yet shown any signs of awakening, concerned? Possible causes? How will you investigate delayed emergence?

Keypoint: delayed emergence or slow awakening, the causes, diagnosis, and management; how to prioritize your approaches.

5. Left hand ischemia (arterial catheter location): Later in the evening, the nurse notifies you that his left hand is discolored and pale, differential diagnosis and management plan? Would it be helpful by infiltrating local anesthetic at the wrist indicated? Why/why not? Explain your plan?

Keypoint: be able to make a diagnosis of anesthesia complication and management solutions.

## > 术 后 管 理 <

1. 房室阻滞：患者在到达 ICU 时低血压。BP 86/52 mmHg,诊断/鉴别诊断? ECG 显示 HR 40 伴有室性早搏,治疗? 如何设置起搏器?

要点：心脏手术后的常见心律失常,需要紧急干预的指征。如何设置临时起搏器。

2. 手术出血/凝血病：到 ICU 后 2 个小时里,胸管引流出血性液体,超过 250 mL/h。什么实验室特殊检测能告诉你这是外科出血还是获得性凝血功能障碍? 你如何决定是否输注更多的红细胞,还是新鲜冰冻血浆和血小板? 你何时通知外科医师来估计患者是否需要返回手术室行手术探查? 如果患者是低血压,血压正常,是高血压,处理有什么区别?

要点：掌握心脏手术后的心脏和外科并发症,以及如何选择保守治疗还是再次手术。

3. 少尿：在 ICU 的前个 3 小时内，尿量为 35 mL。适量吗？为什么/为什么不？病因是？需要床边 TTE？肺动脉压为 14 mmHg，CO 为 4.0 L/min，是否补充液体？哪一种，多少液体适当？外科医师推荐呋塞米。同意不同意？解释说明？持续少尿的治疗对策？

要点：心脏手术后少尿的常见原因和诊断方法，常规处理和特殊的处理方法。

4. 苏醒延迟：术后到达 ICU 6 个小时，患者还没有表现出任何苏醒的迹象，担心吗？可能的原因？如何调查苏醒延迟？

要点：苏醒延迟和苏醒慢的原因、诊断和处理。如何优先考虑处理顺序？

5. 左手缺血（动脉导管位置）：半夜，护士通知你患者的左手冰冷苍白。诊断/鉴别诊断？治疗？手腕上局部麻醉药物注射浸润是否有用？为什么/为什么不？为什么？你会怎么做？

要点：麻醉并发症的诊断和处理。

**Reference**

[1] Joel A Kaplan，David L Reich，Joseph S Savino. Kaplan's Cardiac Anesthrsia. 6th ed. Elsevier Saunders；2011.

[2] Apfelbaum JL，Hagberg CA，Caplan RA，et al. Practice guidelines management of the difficult airway：an updated report by the American Society of Anesthesiologists Task Force on Management of Difficult Airway. Anesthesiology. 2013；118（2）：251-570.

[3] Sheff SR，May MC，Carlisle SE，et al. Predictors of a difficult intubation in bariatric patient：dose preoperative body mass index matter? Surg Obes Relat Dis. 2013；9（3）：344-349.

[4] Hagberg CA. Airway management in adult. Miller's Anesthesia. 8th ed. Elsevier Saunders；2015.

Shaofeng Zhou

周少凤

# 18 Anesthetic management of coronary artery bypass graft

## 冠状动脉搭桥术的麻醉

The patient was a 59 year-old female, who has newly onset chest pain. Her medical history is significant for hypertension, hyperlipidemia, chronic obstructive lung disease (COPD), obesity and obstructive sleep apnea (OSA).

Her medications are Metformin, Lipitor, Aspirin, Metoprolol, Lisinopril, Albuterol inhaler, Coumadin, as well as CPAP (continue positive airway pressure) for sleep apnea over years.

ECG shows ST segments depression and T wave inversion in anterior and anterolateral leads and atrial fibrillation.

A stress test was positive.

TTE (transthoracic echocardiography) revealed regional wall motion abnormality (RWMA) including severe hypokinesis in anterior and anterolateral wall, akinesis of inferior wall with EF 40%, but normal valvuar functions (aortic, mitral, tricuspid and pulmonic valves).

The coronary angiography demonstrated coronary artery disease (CAD) with triple vessels diseases with coronary stenosis of $> 70\%$ involving left anterior descending (LAD), circumflex (Cx) and right coronary arteries (RCA).

Laboratory results of CBC（complete blood count）and metabolic panel were within normal limits.

She had a cardiac arrest during the coronary angiography but successfully resuscitated. She is on heparin intravenous infusion. A coronary artery bypass graft（CABG）is scheduled semi-urgent.

> 基 本 信 息 <

患者，59 岁女性，近期出现胸痛。她的病史有高血压、高血脂、慢性阻塞性肺病（COPD）、肥胖与阻塞性睡眠呼吸窒息（OSA）。

用药：二甲双胍、立普妥、阿司匹林、美托洛尔、赖诺普利、沙丁胺醇吸入剂、华法林，及持续呼吸道正压（CPAP）多年以防止睡眠呼吸窒息。

心电图显示：前外侧导联 ST 段降低和 T 波倒置，及心房纤颤。

心电图负荷试验阳性。TTE 显示左心室（LV）局部室壁运动异常（RWMA），包括前壁和前外侧壁心肌运动严重减弱和下壁无收缩运动，射血分数为 40%，但各瓣膜功能正常，包括主动脉瓣、二尖瓣、三尖瓣功能和肺动脉瓣。

冠状动脉造影证实：三条血管冠状动脉疾病（CAD），冠状动脉狭窄＞70% 累及左前降支（LAD），回旋支（Cx）和右冠状动脉（RCA）。

实验室结果：血液常规检查（CBC）、电解质和肾功能指标均在正常范围内。

她在冠状动脉造影术中心跳骤停，但成功复苏。已安排行冠状动脉搭桥术（CABG）。

> **Preoperative management** <

**Assessment**

1. Based on her medical history what other information do you need before

starting this case?

Keypoint: the examinee should be able to recognize that the patient has multiple comorbidities. Her chronic obstructive lung disease, a pulmonary function should be assessed for severity to formulate a perioperative ventilator strategy. For obesity and abstractive sleep apnea, the airway should be carefully evaluated to determine a possible airway difficulty; whether she should use CPAP for postoperative airway and ventilation support.

2. Based on her medicines, what laboratory study you would like to order?

Keypoint: the patient took Coumadin, the examinee need to know how long the Coumadin has been stopped and the current coagulation function. A same day coagulation tests are required and based on the result blood product, e.g., FFP may need to be ordered.

3. Which medication you think the patient should stop or continue? Why/ why not?

Keypoint: besides the Coumadin, Lisinopril need to stop; β-blocker, metoprolol, need to be continued.

**Preparation**

4. How would you formulate the anesthetic plan based on this patient condition?

Keypoint: a comprehensive anesthesia plan in terms of pre-, intra- and post-operative care should be carefully formulated, including but not limited to, explanation of the anesthesia plan/goal/benefit/risk to the patient and her family, preoperative medication, induction agents, intubation, maintenance of the general anesthesia (GA), safe transportation, postoperative sedation, extubation, airway and ventilatory support.

5. What would your OR preparation to get ready before moving the patient

to the operative theater?

Keypoint：The anesthesia machine，monitors，infusion pumps，and blood warmer should all be checked before the patient arrives. Drugs-including anesthetic and vasoactive agents-should be immediately available.

6. How would you premedicate the patient in the preoperative holding area? What are the medications you would like to administer，and why?

Keypoint：Benzodiazepine，a sedative-hypnotics（diazepam，5～10 mg orally），alone or in combination with an opioid（morphine，5～10 mg intramuscularly or hydromorphone，1～2 mg intramuscularly），were popular in the past. Longer acting pre-medication agents（e.g.，lorazepam）are avoided by most practitioners to permit "fast tracking" of the patient through their recovery. A short acting agent，e.g.，Midazolam along or combined with a low dose fentanyl may be sufficient.

> 术 前 管 理 <

## 评估

1. 根据她的病史，在开始这个麻醉之前你还需要其他什么信息？

要点：考生应该能够认识到，患者有多种并发症。例如：针对 COPD，应评估肺功能受损严重程度，以便制定围术期的通气策略；针对肥胖和阻塞性睡眠窒息，应仔细检查气道明确插管的困难性；术后她是否要用 CPAP 行气道和通气支持。

2. 根据她的用药史，你还想做什么实验室检查？

要点：患者服用华法林，考生需要知道华法林已停用多久和当前的凝血功能。手术当天凝血试验是必需的，基于化验结果，可能需要准备血液制品，例如 FFP。

3. 你希望患者停止或继续使用什么药物？为什么？

要点：除了华法林，赖诺普利需要术前停止；而 β 受体阻断剂、美托洛尔，需要继续。

## 准备

4. 如何根据患者的情况制订麻醉计划？

要点：麻醉前、全面周密计划处理方案，包括术前、术中和术后处理方案。包括但不限于，对患者和家属解释麻醉计划/目标/优点/风险、术前用药、诱导药、气管插管、全麻维持、安全转运、术后镇静、拔管、气道和呼吸支持。

5. 在把患者送到手术室前，你如何准备手术室？

要点：麻醉机、监视仪、输药泵和液体加温设备在患者到来之前都要检查；药物，包括麻醉药物和血管活性药物应准备到位，随手可用。

6. 你怎样术前用药？用什么药，为什么？

要点：安定类镇静催眠药（地西泮 5～10 mg，口服），单独或与阿片类药物组合（吗啡 5～10 mg 或氢吗啡酮 1～2 mg，肌注），在过去经常使用的。目前，大多数医师避免用长效术前药物（如劳拉西泮），以便术后"快通道处理"。短效剂，例如，咪达唑仑和/或小剂量芬太尼已足够。

------------------- > **Intraoperative management** < -------------------

The patient is now in OR and you and your colleagues move the patient to the operative table.

1. Are you going to place an arterial line and what type venous access would you prefer? Why?

Keypoint：pre-induction arterial line in a moderately impaired LV（left ventricle) function is a safe measure. At least 2 venous accesses are required and one should be a central venous access.

2. Is a pulmonary artery catheter (PAC) indicated for this patient? What kind information from the PAC would be most useful?

Keypoint: the cardiac surgery could cause impairment of the cardiac function is anticipated, PAC is necessary for monitoring the heart. This not only applies to a patient with impaired LV function, but even for a normal LV function patient. PAC provides preload, cardiac performance and afterload information in a constant and timely manner, which may be helpful continuing to manage this patient in acuity unit.

3. Which site would you choose for the central venous access? Why? Would you use the ultrasound guidance for the central line placement?

Keypoint: right internal jugular vein commonly is the first choice due its clear anatomic landmark and straight line entering to SVC (superior vena cava) and right atrium. Ultrasound guided central line placement is the standard care in USA.

4. Are you going to use TEE (transesophageal echocardiography) and what are the most important applications of intraoperative TEE examination?

Keypoint: ASA/SCA (American society of anesthesiologists/society of cardiac anesthesia association) recommends using TEE for all cardiac and major vascular surgery. TEE provides valuable information about cardiac anatomy and function during surgery. Two-dimensional TEE can detect regional and global ventricular abnormalities, chamber dimensions, valvular anatomy, and the presence of intracardiac air. Three-dimensional TEE provides a more complete description of valvular anatomy and pathology. TEE can also be helpful in confirming cannulation of the coronary sinus for cardioplegia. Multiple views should be obtained from the upper esophagus, mid-esophagus, and transgastric positions. The two views most commonly used for monitoring during cardiac surgery are the four-chamber view and the transgastric midpapillary short axis views.

After the monitors have been placed to the patient and $O_2$ was supplied via a nasal cannula, an arterial line has also placed in the right radial artery. The patient was induced and anesthetized. Under GA, a pulmonary artery catheter was then inserted through the right internal jugular vein.

5. What anesthetic agents would you choose for induction for this patient? How do you use them?

Keypoint: induction should be performed in a smooth, controlled fashion with incremental and small doses often referred to as a cardiac induction. Agents with less myocardial depression and vasodilation should be selected. Sometime, the selection of an agent is generally less important than the way they are used.

6. What would you choose for the anesthetic maintenance? (inhalational or intravenous)? Why?

Keypoint: In recent years, total intravenous anesthesia with short-acting agents and combinations of intravenous and volatile agents has become most popular. Total intravenous anesthesia: the drive for cost containment in cardiac surgery is a major impetus for development of anesthesia techniques with short-acting agents. Large economic benefits resulted from earlier extubation, decreased ICU stays, earlier ambulation, and earlier hospital discharge ("fast-track" management). Mixed intravenous/inhalation anesthesia: renewed interest in volatile agents came about following studies demonstrating the protective effects of volatile agents on ischemic myocardium and an increased emphasis on fast-track recovery of cardiac patients.

A midsternotomy was performed, a sternal retractor applied to open the wound. The left internal mammary artery (LIMA) was now successfully isolated. The surgeon decided an on-pump CABG and asked you to give heparin.

7. What would the dose and route to administrate heparin? How would you monitor its anticoagulative effect?

Keypoint: Heparin, $300 \sim 400$ units/kg, is usually given. It should be administered through a reliable access, usually through central intravenous line. The activated clotting time (ACT) should be measured $3 \sim 5$ min later and ACT longer than $400 \sim 480$ sec is considered adequate.

8. After the first dose of heparin, the ACT was 200 sec, what would be your response?

Keypoint: Additional heparin, 100 units/kg.

9. After the 2nd dose of heparin, the ACT was 220, what would you think of this and to do in next?

Keypoint: Resistance to heparin is occasionally encountered; many such patients have antithrombin Ⅲ deficiency (acquired or congenital). Antithrombin Ⅲ is a circulating serine protease that irreversibly binds and inactivates thrombin (as well as the activated forms of factors Ⅹ, Ⅺ, Ⅻ, and Ⅻ). When heparin binds and formed the complexes with antithrombin Ⅲ, the anticoagulant activity of antithrombin Ⅲ is enhanced 1 000 - fold. Patients with antithrombin Ⅲ deficiency will achieve adequate anticoagulation following infusion of 2 units of fresh frozen plasma or antithrombin Ⅲ concentrate. Alternatively, recombinant human antithrombin Ⅲ may be administered.

After heparinization, the ascending aorta was cannulated first, then a two-stage cannula inserted into the right atrium and inferior vena cava for venous drainage. In addition, an anterograde cardioplegia catheter is placed via the ascending aorta and a retrograde coronary sinus cannula inserted through right atrium, respectively.

10. During cannulation of the right atrium, hypotension and sustained atrial tachycardia developed, what would be the etiology and your management?

Keypoint: Hypotension from impaired venous return may occur during manipulation of the venae cava and the heart. Venous cannulation frequently precipitates atrial arrhythmias, e.g., supraventricular tachycardia, which leads to hemodynamic deterioration. This may be treated pharmacologically, electrically, or by immediate initiation of bypass. Mal-positioning of the venous cannulas can interfere with venous return or impede venous drainage from the head and neck (superior vena cava syndrome).

11. Why the cardioplegia solution is perfused via both anterograde and retrograde?

Keypoint: in CAD patients, the coronary arteries may have diffused and lengthy diseases and, therefore, cardioplegia through anterograde infusion may not be evenly distributed in the myocardia; adding a retrograde infusion can effectively perfuse cardioplegia throughout the heart.

The cardiopulmonary bypass (CPB) has been established. The ascending aorta is clamped and cardioplegia has been given. The body temperature has been cooled down to 32 degree centigrade. A triple vessels CABG has been performed with the left internal mammalian artery (LIMA) anastomosed to the left anterior descending artyer (LAD), and saphenous venous grafts are employed to bypass circumflex artery (Cx) and right coronary artery (RCA) to the ascending aorta, respectively. Rewarming then started. Before removing the aortic cross clamp, lidocaine 100 mg and magnesium sulfate 2 g have been given via CPB.

12. Why lidocaine and magnesium should be given at this point?

Keypoint: Through rewarming process the blood and body temperature is normalized however the heart may still cold (lower than core temperature). Removing aortic cross clamp may cause ventricular fibrillation. Administration of lidocain and magnesium sulfate is a common protocol and may decrease the likelihood of ventricle fibrillation.

13. What is your check list for the preparation of weaning off CPB?

Keypoint: General guidelines for separation from CPB include the following:

The core body temperature should be at least 37℃.

A stable rhythm must be present. Atrioventricular pacing is often used and confers the benefit of a properly timed atrial systole. Persistence of atrioventricular block should prompt measurement of serum potassium concentration. If hyperkalemia is present, it can be treated with calcium, $NaHCO_3$, furosemide, or glucose and insulin.

The heart rate must be adequate (generally 80~100 beats/min). Slow heart rates are generally treated by pacing. Many inotropic agents will also increase heart rate. Supraventricular tachycardia generally requires cardioversion.

Laboratory values must be within acceptable limits. Significant acidosis (pH<7.20), hypocalcemia (ionized), and hyperkalemia (>5.5 mEq/L) should be treated; ideally the hematocrit should exceed 22%; however, a hematocrit< 22% should not by itself trigger transfusion of red blood cells at this time. When CPB reservoir volume and flow are adequate, ultrafiltration may be used to increase the hematocrit.

Adequate ventilation with 100% oxygen must have been resumed.

All monitors should be rechecked for proper function and recalibrated if necessary.

CPB is gradually discontinued. However，the patient is hypotensive.

14. What would be your differentiation for the low blood pressure? How would you treat the condition?

Keypoint：please see the attached table of "Post-CPB hypotension differentiation：hemodynamic subgroups".

Based on the causes of hypotension，you treat the hypotension accordingly using volume，inotrope，vasopressor and/or combined managements.

The hypotension has been adequately treated and the patient is hemodynamically stable. The surgeon requests a reversal of heparin.

15. What is the pharmacology of protamine and what are the adverse effects of the drug? How would you check the heparin is adequately reversed?

Keypoint：after coming off CPB，the patient remain stable，heparin activity is reversed with protamine. Protamine is a highly positively charged protein that binds and effectively inactivates heparin（a highly negatively charged polysaccharide）. Heparin-protamine complexes are then removed by the reticuloendothelial system. The reversal adequacy is judged by measuring ACT $3 \sim 5$ min after protamine infusion. Additional incremental doses of protamine may be necessary.

Protamine administration can result in a number of adverse hemodynamic effects，some of which are immunological in origin. Protamine given slowly（$5 \sim 10$ min）usually has few effects；when given more rapidly it produces vasodilation that is easily treated with volume and small doses of phenylephrine.

Catastrophic protamine reactions often include myocardial depression and marked pulmonary hypertension. Diabetic patients previously maintained on protamine-containing insulin（such as NPH）may be at increased risk for adverse reactions to protamine.

> **术 中 管 理** <

患者现已运送到手术室,你和你的同事将患者移动到手术台。

1. 你要放置动脉导管吗? 你要建立什么样的静脉通路? 为什么?

要点:在中度 LV 功能受损患者,诱导前放置动脉导管是安全的措施。至少要有两条静脉入路,其中一条为中心静脉。

2. 该患者有指征使用肺动脉导管(PAC)吗? 从 PAC 可得到什么有用的数据?

要点:心脏手术可能导致心脏功能受损,使用 PAC 是有必要的。PAC 不仅适用于 LV 功能受损的患者,而且也适用于 LV 功能正常的患者。PAC 可以持续及时地提供前负荷、心脏排血量和后负荷的数据,这些信息在处理一个重症患者可能是有帮助的。

3. 你选择哪条静脉行中心静脉穿刺? 为什么? 你会使用超声辅助中心静脉穿刺吗?

要点:右颈内静脉通常是首选,因其明确的解剖标志,以及与上腔静脉和右心房是一条直线。在美国,超声指导中心静脉置管是标准技术。

4. 你打算使用经食道超声心动图(TEE)吗? 术中 TEE 的最重要的应用是什么?

要点:ASA/SCA(美国麻醉医师学会/美国心脏麻醉协会)推荐在所有的心脏和大血管手术使用 TEE。TEE 在手术过程中提供宝贵的心脏解剖和功能信息。

二维 TEE 可以检测区域和整体心室异常、心室内径、瓣膜解剖和心腔内空气的存在。三维 TEE 提供更完整的瓣膜解剖和病理学信息。TEE 也可用以确定心脏停搏液冠状窦插管放置位置。TEE 图像应该从食管上段、食管中段和经胃数个位置(窗口)采集。最为常用的心脏手术中两个监测图像是食管中部四腔观和经胃乳头肌中部短轴图。

在各种无创监测下,鼻导管给氧,动脉导管放置在右桡动脉。此后,对患者行麻醉诱导。在全麻下,经右颈内静脉置入肺动脉导管。

5. 你将什么选择哪些麻醉药物诱导这个患者? 你如何使用它们?

要点:诱导应以平滑、可控的方式进行,分次小剂量推药通常称为心脏诱导。应选择心肌抑制和血管扩张都较弱的药物。对药物的选择没有比如何使用诱导药物更重要。

6. 你会选择什么麻醉维持技术(吸入或静脉)? 为什么?

要点:近年来,应用短效药物行全凭静脉麻醉和静脉药物加吸入性麻醉药物是最为流行的两种麻醉技术。全凭静脉麻醉:在心脏手术中控制成本是驱动应用短效药物麻醉技术的主要动力;从早期拔管,减少 ICU 住院时间、下床时间早、早出院("快通道"处理)可获取明显的经济效益。混合性静脉加吸入麻醉:吸入性药物对缺血性心肌的保护作用使人们对使用吸入性药物产生新兴趣;此外,不断增加地使用"快通道"术后处理也增加了这一技术的使用。

胸骨正中切口后,胸骨牵开器使切口张开。左乳内动脉(LIMA)被成功分离。外科医师决定应用体外循环,让你给肝素。

7. 你使用肝素的剂量和给药途径是什么? 你将如何监测肝素抗凝作用?

要点:肝素剂量通常是 300～400 U/kg。肝素应该通过可靠的静脉入路注射(通常是中心静脉)。肝素注射 3～5 min 后,测量 ACT。行体外循环,ACT 应在400～480 s。

8. 第一剂量肝素后，ACT 为 200 s，你怎样处理？

要点：额外追加肝素，100 U/kg。

9. 在你处理之后，ACT 是 220 s，你如何考虑和处理？

要点：偶尔你会遇到抗肝素患者。在许多患者是由于抗凝血酶Ⅲ缺乏（先天或后天性）。抗凝血酶Ⅲ是一个血液循环中的丝氨酸蛋白酶，其不可逆地与凝血酶结合将其灭活（它还和活性形式凝血因子 10，11，12，和 13 结合将这些因子灭活）。肝素与抗凝血酶Ⅲ结合形成复合物，可使抗凝血酶Ⅲ的抗凝活性提高 1 000 倍。对抗凝血酶Ⅲ缺乏的患者输注两个单位的 FFP 或抗凝血酶Ⅲ浓缩制品可达到充分抗凝。此外，也可使用重组的人抗凝血酶Ⅲ。

肝素化后，先行升主动脉插管，然后经右心房插入两级导管进入右房和下腔静脉行静脉血液引流。此外，前向性心停液灌注导管通过升主动脉插入；逆行性心停液灌注导管经右心房放入冠状静脉窦。

10. 右心房插管期间，发生低血压及持续性房性心动过速，病因是什么和怎样处理？

要点：在心房插管时，对下腔静脉和心脏的操作会阻碍静脉回流，从而引起低血压。腔静脉插管常常诱发房性心律失常，例如室上性心动过速，导致血流动力学恶化。对此可用药物治疗、电转心律或立即启动体外循环。静脉插管位置不当会影响静脉回流或妨碍头颈部静脉回流（上腔静脉综合征）。

11. 为什么心停液要顺行和逆行双向灌注？

关键点：冠心病患者的冠状动脉狭窄可以是广泛和冗长的，因此，单纯顺行灌注心停液往往不能均匀地分布整个心肌；添加一个逆行灌注能有效地使心停液均匀地灌注心肌，从而提高心肌保护效果。

体外循环（CPB）启动，用钳闭钳阻断升主动脉，然后给予停搏液。体温降低到 32℃。左乳内动脉与左前降支吻合，大隐静脉用于回旋支和右冠状动脉与升主动脉搭桥。然后开始复温,去除升主动脉钳闭钳以前,通过 CPB 输给患者利多卡因 100 mg 和硫酸镁 2 g。

12. 为什么在此时给予利多卡因和硫酸镁?

要点:通过复温过程,血液和体温逐渐正常,但心肌可能还冷(低于中心体温)。去除主动脉钳闭钳可引起心室颤动。因此给利多卡因和硫酸镁是常规用药,降低室颤发生的可能性。

13. 你认为脱离 CPB 的标准是什么?

要点:脱离 CPB 的总体原则包括以下几点:

中心体温至少应为 37℃。

必须有稳定的心律。通常采用房室起搏,有助于定时的心房收缩。持续性房室传导阻滞时应及时测定血清钾浓度。如果存在高钾血症,可给予钙、碳酸氢钠、呋塞米或葡萄糖和胰岛素治疗。

必须有足够的心率(一般 80~100 次/min)。心率过缓通常采用起搏处理;许多正性肌力药也会增加心率;室上性心动过速一般需电复律。

实验室数据必须在可接受的范围内。明显的酸中毒,pH<7.20,低钙血症(离子钙)和高钾血症(>5.5 mmol/L)应及时处理;血细胞比容最好大于 22%;但是血细胞比容<22%并不一定需要输红细胞。当 CPB 容量和流量适当,超微过滤可增加红细胞压积。

用 100%纯氧通气。

再次检查所有监护设备,确保功能正常。如有必要,再次校正。

患者逐渐脱离 CPB。然而她出现低血压。

14. 你如何鉴别诊断低血压?你如何治疗低血压?

要点:鉴别诊断低血压详见附表"CPB 后低血压的鉴别诊断:血流动力学亚组"。

根据低血压的原因,对症治疗低血压,可补充血容量、使用正性肌力药、血管收缩药和/或联合使用这些方法。

你适当地处理了低血压,患者血流动力学稳定,外科医师要求你拮抗肝素。

15. 鱼精蛋白的药理学和不良反应是什么? 你如何确定肝素充分逆转?

要点:脱离 CPB 后,患者血流动力学稳定,用鱼精蛋白拮抗肝素活性。鱼精蛋白是有大量正电荷的蛋白质,能够结合并有效灭活肝素(有大量负电荷的黏多糖)。肝素-鱼精蛋白复合物被网状内皮系统清除。逆转是否适当可在鱼精蛋白注射 3~5 min 后,测量 ACT 来判断。通常需要追加鱼精蛋白。

鱼精蛋白会产生一系列不良的血流动力学效应,其中一些属于免疫源性的。缓慢(5~10 min)静注鱼精蛋白通常不良反应较少;如快速静注会导致血管扩张,可通过补液或小剂量去氧肾上腺素纠正。

灾难性的鱼精蛋白反应通常包括心肌抑制和严重的肺动脉高压。以前使用含鱼精蛋白的胰岛素(如中性鱼精蛋白胰岛素,NPH)维持治疗的糖尿病患者,鱼精蛋白不良反应的风险增加。

## Postoperative management

1. How you would prepare to transport the patient from OR to ICU?

Keypoint:Transporting such a critically ill patient from the operating room to ICU is a complicated process, should consider all possibilities, such as monitor failure, overdose or interruption of drug infusions, and hemodynamic instability en route. Portable monitoring equipment, infusion pumps, and a full cylinder of oxygen with a self-inflating bag for ventilation should be ready prior to the end of the operation. Minimum monitoring during transportation includes the ECG, arterial blood pressure, and pulse oximetry. A spare endotracheal tube, laryngoscope, succinylcholine, and emergency resuscitation drugs should also accompany the patient.

2. How would you sedate this patient during transportation and in ICU?

Keypoint: the drugs used most common sedation may be maintained by a propofol or dexmedetomidine infusion.

3. If the chest tube drainage in the first 2 hours>250~300 mL/h (10 mL/kg/h), what do you think and what you need prepare to do?

Keypoint: Chest tube drainage in the first 2 h of more than 250~300 mL/h (10 mL/kg/h)-in the absence of a hemostatic defect-is excessive and may require surgical reexploration. Subsequent drainage that exceeds 100 mL/h is also worrisome. Intrathoracic bleeding at a site not adequately drained may cause cardiac tamponade, requiring immediate reopening of the chest.

4. If the patient developed hypertension despite analgesia and sedation how would you manage this patient?

Keypoint: Despite adequate analgesia and sedation, the occurring of hypertension is a common postoperative problem and should be treated promptly, so as not to exacerbate bleeding or myocardial ischemia. Nitroprusside, nitroglycerin, clevidipine or nicardipine is generally used. β blockade may be particularly useful for patients recovering from coronary artery surgery.

5. For this patient what you need to consider for extubation and how do you manage this patient's obesity with obstructed airway and COPD?

Key Point: Extubation should be considered only when muscle paralysis agent has worn off (or been reversed) and the patient is hemodynamically stable. Caution should be exercised in obese and those with underlying pulmonary disease. Cardiothoracic procedures are typically associated with marked decreases in functional residual capacity (FRC) and postoperative diaphragmatic dysfunction. Immediate after extubation, CPAP or BiPAP may be employed to maintain her airway patency and support respiration.

**Post-CPB hypotension differentiation: hemodynamic subgroups**

| | Group Ⅰ: Vigorous | Group Ⅱ: Hypovolemic | Group ⅢA: LV Pump Failure | Group ⅢB: RV Failure | Group Ⅳ: Vasodilated (Hyperdynamic) |
|---|---|---|---|---|---|
| BP | Normal | Low | Low | Low | Low |
| CVP | Normal | Low | Normal or high | High | Normal or low |
| PAWP | Normal | Low | High | Normal or high | Normal or low |
| TEE findings | Normal | Underfilled RV/LV | Reduced LV performance | Dilated RV | Normal or underfilled RV/LV |
| CO | Normal | Low | Low | Low | High |
| Systemic vascular resistance | Normal | Low, normal, or high | Low, normal or high | Normal or high | Low |
| Treatment | None | Volume | Inotrope; IABP, LVAD | Inotrope, pulmonary vasodilator RVAD | Vasoconstrictor, volume |

BP, blood pressure; CVP, central venous pressure; PAWP, pulmonary artery wedge pressure; CO, cardiac output; CPB, cardiopulmonary bypass; LV, left ventricular; RV, right ventricular; IABP, intraaortic balloon pump; LVAD, left ventricular assist device; RVAD, right ventricular assist device; TEE, transesophageal echocardiography.

## > 术 后 管 理 <

1. 运送患者到 ICU,你如何准备?

要点:危重患者从手术室运送到重症监护室,是个复杂的过程,应考虑各种可能,例如运送途中监护测仪失灵、用药过量或中断输药、血流动力学不稳定等。手术结束之前准备好:便携式监护仪、输液泵、充满的氧气瓶与简易呼吸器用于通气。运送过程中至少监测心电图、有创血压、脉搏氧饱和度。运送患者中,气管导管、喉镜、琥珀胆碱和紧急抢救药物应随时备用。

2. 运送途中和在 ICU 时,你如何为患者提供镇静?

要点:心脏病患者术后最常用的镇静方法为静脉输注丙泊酚或右美托咪定。

3. 如果在第一个 2 个小时的胸腔引流量＞250～300 mL/h[10 mL(kg·h)],你怎样判断病情,需要准备什么?

要点:在第一个 2 小时超过 250～300 mL/h 胸腔引流量[10 mL(kg·h)],对于无凝血缺陷的患者来说引流量过多,可能需要再次手术探查。随后的引流量超过 100 mL/h 也令人担忧。胸腔出血引流不充分可引起心包填塞,需要立即再次开胸。

4. 尽管镇痛和镇静适当,患者仍出现高血压,你将如何处理?

要点:尽管镇痛镇静适当,高血压仍是术后常见的问题。应及时治疗,以免加重出血或心肌缺血。硝普钠、硝酸甘油、氯维地平或尼卡地平为常用药,β受体阻滞剂尤其适用于冠状动脉手术的患者。

5. 对于这个患者,拔管前需要考虑哪些问题? 该患者肥胖并伴有 OSA 和 COPD,你如何处理?

要点:只有当肌松作用完全消失(或已拮抗),患者血流动力学稳定才考虑拔管。处理肥胖和有肺部疾病患者应高度慎重。心胸手术均会明显降低功能残气量和导致术后膈肌功能显著下降。拔管后应立即使用持续呼吸道正压(CPAP)或双压持续呼吸道正压(BiPAP)以保持呼吸道通畅及辅助支持患者自主呼吸。

表 17-1 心肺转流后低血压鉴别诊断:血流动力学亚组

| | Ⅰ组肌力正常 | Ⅱ组低血容量 | ⅢA组左室衰竭 | ⅢB组右室衰竭 | Ⅳ组血管扩张心室过度收缩 |
|---|---|---|---|---|---|
| 血压 | 正常 | 低 | 低 | 低 | 低 |
| 中心静脉压 | 正常 | 低 | 正常或高 | 高 | 正常或偏低 |
| 肺动脉楔压 | 正常 | 低 | 高 | 正常或高 | 正常或偏低 |

（续表）

| | Ⅰ组肌力正常 | Ⅱ组低血容量 | ⅢA组左室衰竭 | ⅢB组右室衰竭 | Ⅳ组血管扩张心室过度收缩 |
|---|---|---|---|---|---|
| 经食道超声心动图 | 正常 | 左/右心室充盈不足 | 左室功能降低 | 右室扩张 | 正常或左/右心室充盈不足 |
| 心输出量 | 正常 | 低 | 低 | 低 | 高 |
| 全身血管阻力 | 正常 | 低、正常或高 | 低、正常或高 | 正常或高 | 低 |
| 治疗 | 不需要 | 补充容量 | 正性肌力药；主动脉球囊反搏；左心室辅助装置 | 正性肌力药；肺血管扩张剂；右心室辅助装置 | 血管收缩剂；补充容量 |

BP（blood pressure）：血压；CVP（central venous pressure）：中心静脉压；PAWP（pulmonary artery wedge pressure）：肺动脉楔压；CO（cardiac output）：心输出量；CPB（cardiopulmonary bypass）：心肺转流；LV（left ventricular）：左心室；RV（right ventricular）：右心室；TEE（transesophageal echocardiography）：经食道超声心动图；IABP（intraaortic balloon pump）：主动脉球囊反搏；LVAD（left ventricular assist device）：右心室辅助装置；RVAD（right ventricular assist device）：右心室辅助装置。

**Reference**

Morgan & Mikhai's Clinical Anesthesiology，5th Edition，Chapter 22：Anesthesia for Cardiovascular Surgery. 2013 by The McGaw-hill Companies，Inc.

Yanfu Shao

邵燕夫

# 19 Pediatric anesthesia — anesthesia for tonsillectomy

## 小儿手术麻醉——扁桃体切除术的麻醉

> **Basic information** <

A 5 years old boy with chronic tonsillitis and snore was scheduled for an elective tonsillectomy in outpatient surgical center. He has history of asthma, worsening during spring, which requires albuterol and atrovent inhaler. He weighs 42 kg, otherwise active and healthy. Normal vital in PAC（anesthesia clinic）.

> **基 本 信 息** <

5岁男性患儿,因慢性扁桃体炎伴打鼾,拟于日间手术中心接受择期扁桃体切除术。该患儿既往有哮喘病史,春季加重,应用万托林(沙丁胺醇)及爱全乐(异丙托溴铵)可缓解。患儿体重42 kg,除哮喘病史,既往体健,发育正常。麻醉门诊所示生命体征正常。

> **Preoperative management** <

1. Laboratory test: Would you need to obtain any laboratory tests? If so, list the lab items you wanted, and explain?

Keypoint: This question tests the ability to make a thorough, yet cost-effective preoperative assessment. A valuable preoperative test should help with clinical decision making, either an abnormal result implicates increased perioperative risk, or a normal result indicates a reduced risk.

No additional preoperative tests are needed for a healthy child undergoing minor procedures.

If felt strongly, a preoperative consultation with a pediatric pulmonologist might be helpful. The goal is to assess the recent course of asthma, to ascertain the patient is in an optimal condition for elective surgery. Further information, like upper respiratory tract infection within 2 weeks, which will increase the risk for perioperative respiratory adverse events should be gathered.

2. Recent cold: The patient had a cold 5 days ago, no fever, no need for antibiotics, did treat with albuterol and OCT (over the counter) Robitussin Cough syrup, concerned? Postponed the surgery, why/why not? How it might affect the surgery and anesthesia? How long should the patient be waiting?

Keypoint: Recent upper respiratory infection and its clinical implications on elective surgery.

The greatest concern is that a recent upper respiratory infection would put a patient at greater risk for perioperative respiratory complications (e. g. laryngospasm, bronchospasm, airway obstruction, desaturation, atelectasis). This also leads to unplanned hospital admission, prolonged length of stay, and increased medical expense. However, this child may never be totally "clean" for 4 weeks before the surgery.

It would be ideal to postpone any elective surgery until 4~6 weeks before subject the patient to general anesthesia and airway instrumentation.

3. Transfusion: Do you think a blood type & cross necessary? What would be your transfusion threshold? What if the patient has a von Willebrand disease? If so, explain your preparations? If intraoperative bleeding is associated with von Willebrand disease, what would be your first choice of treatment?

Keypoint: This question is for pediatric transfusion, for children with or without co-morbidities, undergoing different types of procedures.

For healthy children undergoing minor procedures, type and crossmatch the blood preoperatively is not indicated.

A hematocrit of 20%~26% is generally well tolerated in healthy older children.

Only when the benefit of transfusion outweighs its risk in which the transfusion is considered necessary. Different medical centers have different transfusion thresholds. Patients' age, preoperative hemoglobin level, comorbidities, estimated blood loss, physical condition, etc. should all be taken into consideration.

Normally in healthy children, consider transfusion when estimated blood loss exceeds 15% of blood volume.

Patients with any inherited or acquired coagulopathy (e.g. von Willebrand disease) are at great risk for intraoperative hemorrhage. Crossmatch would be safer.

If intraoperative bleeding is associated with von willebrand disease, one could consider first to treat with desmopressin (DDAVP), it could raise vWF levels in some patients with mild von Willebrand's disease (as well as normal individuals). DDAVP could be administered at a dose of 0.3 mcg/kg 30 min before surgery. For patients not responding to DDAVP, then treat with cryoprecipitate or factor Ⅷ concentrates, both of which are rich in vWF.

4. Pediatric airway assessment: What are difference of the anatomy airway in child and adult? Explain how would you assess his airway?

Keypoint: Be familiar with the anatomical differences between a child's and an adult's airway, and their clinical implications.

Compared to adults, the children have relatively larger heads and tongue, narrower nasal passages, anterior and cephalad larynx, relatively larger epiglottis, shorter trachea and neck, and more prominent adenoids and tonsils.

Airway assessment for children is similar to the adult including history of snoring, facial abnormality, mouth opening, Mallampati classification, thyromental distance. Pay attention to loosen teeth. Because children have smaller FRC compared to adults, and increased metabolic rate, they would have a more rapid decrease in $SpO_2$ at induction.

Please note that this is an obese child (assume that his height is 114 cm, and his BMI would be 32 kg/m$^2$), thus he is susceptible for OSA. Special attention should be paid to possible upper airway obstruction.

5. Perioperative risks: You met the mother in PAC (pre-anesthesia clinic), how would explain the anesthesia risks to his mother?

Keypoint: The ability to provide risk-versus-benefit discussion for a procedure.

Considering the patient's history of asthma and recent upper respiratory infection, emphasis should be put on perioperative respiratory risks in this child using lay term-non-medical language.

6. Pain management: They would like to hear from you the plan for postoperative pain management? After heard from you, the mother wanted you to ensure that the child would wake up no pain at all, would you?

Keypoint: The understanding of pediatric pain management. The ability to communicate and console the parent.

Acetaminophen could be given orally or rectally to children undergoing minor procedure. Patient controlled analgesia with low dose narcotics will further facilitate the effect of pain management. May ask the surgeon to infiltrate with local anesthetics.

Ensure the mother that we would try to achieve optimal postoperative pain management. But some degree of discomfort should be expected.

## > 术 前 管 理 <

1. 实验室检查：你需要什么化验检查，请依次列出并给出理由？

要点：考察选择全面的、成本效益好的术前检查的能力。术前检查应具有临床指导意义。异常的化验应提示围术期风险增加，或者正常的化验结果提示某项临床风的降低。

不需要。对于拟行中小手术既往体健的患儿，一般不需要进行额外的术前检查。

若认为十分有必要，术前可请儿科呼吸专科会诊，目的是评估哮喘控制情况，确定患儿术前肺功能处于最佳状况，适宜接受择期手术。此外，还应了解是否有其他增加围术期呼吸系统并发症风险的情况，例如近2周内是否有上呼吸道感染。

2. 近期感冒：患儿5天前感冒，不伴发热，未使用抗生素。自用沙丁胺醇及非处方药诺比舒（Robitussin）咳嗽糖浆治疗。你的担心是什么？是否需要推迟手术并简述理由。感冒会对手术及麻醉产生什么影响？你建议推迟手术多长时间？

要点：考察近期上呼吸道感染对择期手术风险的影响。

最大顾虑是近期上呼吸道感染增加患儿围术期呼吸系统并发症（例如喉痉挛、支气管痉挛、气道梗阻、低氧血症、肺不张）的风险。同时可能导致日间手术患儿意外收入院，延长住院时间，增加住院费用。值得注意的是，很难保证此类患儿在术前4周完全不表现出任何上呼吸道感染的症状。

理想状况下，应在上呼吸道感染痊愈4～6周后再行需要全麻和使用气道辅助装置的择期手术。

3. 输血：你是否认为有必要进行术前交叉配血？你的输血阈值是多少？如果患儿伴有 vW 因子缺乏症你的诊疗计划是否会改变，并简述理由。若伴有 vW 因子缺乏症的患儿出现明确的术中出血，首选治疗措施是？

要点：掌握儿童围术期输血指征，充分考虑手术类型及患儿是否有并发症。

对于拟行中小手术既往体健的患儿，术前交叉配血没有必要。

多数健康大孩子可以耐受 20%～26% 的血细胞比容。

只有当输血获益大于输血风险时，才考虑输血。不同医院有不同的输血阈值。需要综合评估患儿年龄、术前血红蛋白水平、是否有并发症，手术预计出血量和患儿身体状况等。

通常情况下，对于既往体健的患儿，当估计出血量超过全身血容量的 15% 时，考虑输血。

当伴有先天性或获得性出凝血异常时（如 vW 因子缺乏症），预计术中出血风险较大，术前交叉配血更安全。

若术中出血考虑与 vW 因子缺乏症相关，可采用静脉输注去氨加压素（DDAVP）以提高部分轻度 vW 因子缺乏者。vW 因子浓度（DDAVP 同样可以提高正常人体内 vW 因子浓度），给药剂量为 $0.3\ \mu g/kg$，于术前 30 min 给药。对于 DDAVP 反应欠佳的患者，可输入冷沉淀或Ⅷ因子，这两种药物中同样富含 vW 因子。

4. 小儿气道评估：儿童与成人气道解剖方面有何不同？简述你准备如何评估患儿的气道？

要点：熟悉儿童与成人气道解剖学差异及其临床意义。

与成人相比，儿童的头和舌体更大、鼻腔狭窄、喉腔更靠近身体的前方及头侧，会厌相对较大，气管及脖颈更短，有些患儿伴有明显的腺样体及扁桃体肥大。

患儿气道评估大致同成人患者：主要询问是否有打鼾病史，是否有颜面部发育异常，评估张口度、Mallampati 分级和甲颏距。注意是否有活动牙齿。由于儿童功能残气量低于成人，而基础代谢率又较高，麻醉诱导时血氧饱和度的降低更为快速而明显。

注意他是肥胖患儿（假设身高 114 cm，则他的 BMI 是 $32\ kg/m^2$），因此是阻塞性睡眠呼吸暂停低通气综合征的高危人群，气道评估应特别注意是否存在上呼吸道梗阻。

5. 围术期风险：在术前麻醉门诊，你准备如何向患儿母亲解释麻醉风险？

要点：考察沟通临床获益及风险的能力。

考虑到患者支气管哮喘及近期上呼吸道感染病史，麻醉术前门诊应充分向患儿家长交代围术期呼吸系并发症的风险，并注意使用患儿家长可以理解的非医学术语进行解释。

6. 术后镇痛：患儿家属想了解你的术后镇痛计划。患儿母亲希望你能保证患儿术后醒来不会有任何疼痛及不适，你会如何应答？

要点：考察对小儿术后镇痛要点的理解以及与患儿父母沟通的能力。

小手术的术后镇痛可以采用对乙酰氨基酚口服或纳肛。使用小剂量阿片类药物术后患者自控镇痛可以提供更为完善的镇痛效果。同时还可以请外科医师在手术时进行局麻药的局部浸润。

宽慰患儿家长，麻醉医师会尽最大努力保证术后镇痛效果，然而患儿在术后仍有可能会经历一定程度的不适。

## Intraoperative management

1. Premedication：Would you pre-medicated this patient，why/why not? If you decided to do so，list the agents，doses，and route? Would you wait till the medication worked?

Keypoint：Understand the clinical implication of premedication. Be familiar with each drug's pharmacology and pediatric usage.

Bronchodilators（either by mouth or inhalation）should be continued till the day of surgery at its usual dose.

Premedication in anesthesia practice should be justified by individual needs， the types of surgery, and the anesthetic agents and techniques used.

Anticholinergics could decrease pharyngeal secretion, thus lower the risk of laryngospasm or bronchospasm.

Sedatives may help children with separation anxiety: Oral midazolam (0.3~0.5 mg/kg, maximum 15 mg); intramuscular midazolam (0.1~0.15 mg/kg); intramuscular ketamine (2~3 mg/kg) with atropine (0.01 mg/kg); rectal midazolam (0.5~1 mg/kg, maximum 20 mg); intranasal dexmedetomidine (1~2 $\mu$g/kg). Sedatives should be given under closely monitoring, especially in obese children.

Onset of sedation will usually be achieved within 15~30 minutes.


2. Parents presenting at the induction, the mother requests to go back to OR with the child, agree or not agree? How would you respond? The mother said last time her another child here for the same surgery, the anesthesiologist allowed her to carry the patient to the OR? It is common in most places, agree?

Keypoint: This question tests the interpersonal and communication skills. One should be able to provide effective information exchange with the patient as well as the families.

Whether or not to have the mother present for induction depends on several factors: the regulation of different medical centers, the preoperative interview with the patient and the parent (to gather information on patient's past experience, mental maturity and cooperativeness).

To allow someone the child trusts presenting for induction may provide a calming effect. That person could either be a parent, a nurse or a training physician children trusted. But significant debate still surrounds this issue, and parental state of anxiety might affect with children's preoperative anxiety. In addition, the anesthesia team should be prepared to management the unanticipated accident could happen in the parents.

3. Induction: How would you induce anesthesia to this patient, inhalational or intravenous? Describe your techniques on inhalation induction? Explain how to prevent the incidence of laryngospasm?

Keypoint: Be familiar with both the pros and cons of inhalational and intravenous inductions for pediatric patients. Understand the risk factors and preventions of laryngospasm.

If the patient has a history of airway obstruction or apnea, and the patient is overweight with anticipated difficult airway, inhaled induction is more appropriate. Withhold paralytics until the ability to ventilate with positive pressure is established.

There are several techniques to make an inhalation induction smooth for a child. ① A 5 years old child mostly would listen and cooperative, I will describe the procedure to him, so he knows and follow the command. ② Premedication, choice of p.o. versed, intranasal dexmedetomidine, till the child sleepy enough. ③ Put the child preferred fruit flavored drops inside the mask so he will more likely accept it. ④ Coaching a cooperative child to breath while turn on the odorless mixture of $O_2$ (30%) and $N_2O$ (70%), then increasing sevoflurane in 0.5% incrementally every few breaths. ⑤ Single breath induction (7% ~ 8% sevoflurane in 60% $N_2O$ 40% $O_2$ mixture) would be more appropriate for a uncooperative child who could take vital capacity breath. ⑥ Allow the child to sit starting inhalation induction in some young uncooperative child. ⑦ Obtain the iv access after adequate depth of anesthesia has been achieved, then give iv propofol and opioids for adjunction.

Approaches to prevent laryngospasm: the most important thing is to ensure an adequate anesthesia, and avoid becoming light; other including premedication with anticholinergics to decrease secretion (especially when ketamine is used), avoid crying, wait for adequate depth of anesthesia before any airway instrumentation, choose volatile agents less likely to irritate the airway (sevoflurane).

4. ETT: Would you place a cuffed or uncuffed ETT? Does it matter? The ENT surgeon came to you that there were studies reported using LMA to minimized waking up agitation, your response?

Keypoint: This question tests the distinctive features of cuffed ETT and uncuffed ETT. One should understand their advantages and disadvantages in different clinical scenario. Also one should know the advantages of a supraglottic airway device and its limitations. Interpersonal communications skills with other medical staff.

Uncuffed ETTs are traditionally used for children under the age of $5\sim8$. Because the cricoid cartilage is the narrowest point of the airway, uncuffed ETTs are supposed to decrease the risk of post-extubation tracheal injury (croup). But they require precise sizing, and have a higher risk of air leak and aspiration.

It is common practice now for most practitioners using a downsized cuffed ETT with the cuff completely deflated before intubation. Minimal inflation of the cuff can stop air leak and decrease the risk of aspiration. They are more appropriate for cases like tonsillectomy and adenoidectomy.

LMA could minimize emergence agitation. However, whether or not LMA can be used safely for tonsillectomy depends on the experience of the surgical and anesthetic teams. The supraglottic airway instrument offers less protection against aspiration and should be used with great caution in high-risk surgeries. There are many reports of successfully used for tonsillectomy, I would refer this is to individual anesthesiologist based on his or her own clinical preference.

5. Ventilator setting: Explain your intraoperative ventilation set up, VC (volume control) or PC (pressure control), explain your preference and why? How about allow the patient breathing spontaneously?

Keypoint: Basic understanding of pediatric respiratory setting.

Pressure control is the preferred ventilation mode for small children. It could avoid unintentional delivery of large tidal volume, which could lead to pulmonary barotrauma. For smaller children ($<$ 10 kg), peak inspiratory pressure could be set around $15 \sim 18$ cmH$_2$O. For larger children ($>$10 kg), volume ventilation with tidal volume set at $6 \sim 8$ mL/kg may be enough.

If the patient is intubated, spontaneous breathing on a closed circuit will slightly increase the work of breathing (normal child should be able to breath without problem), and hypoventilation could lead to hypercapnia. Spontaneous breathing on an open circuit maintained by volatile agents will produce air pollution. So spontaneous breathing could only be considered in anesthesia maintained total intravenously, otherwise controlled ventilation is more appropriate.

Usually, the surgery will be done under general anesthesia with ETT and controlled ventilation, pressure control ventilation is the most common ventilator mode for pediatric patient; however, maintaining spontaneous respiration is acceptable at the anesthesia provider's preference, however extra attention should be payed to ETT, etCO$_2$, and SpO$_2$.

6. Airway issues: the procedure started uneventful, shortly you noticed there was dramatic increase in PIP (peak inspiratory pressure), from 12 to 30 cmH$_2$O and the PIP$>$35 cmH$_2$O now, your differential, approach to figure out the causes? Could this be caused by the surgeon?

Keypoint: Trouble shooting for intraoperative mechanical ventilation.

Kinking of the ETT: which is the most common cause when the surgeon place the retractor to open the mouth, which could be confirmed by direct visualizing the surgical field, or have the surgeon inspect the surgical field. Feel under surgical drapes. Could be cause by the surgeon.

Accidental bronchial intubation caused by a change in head position: no breath sound or diminished breath sound on one side.

Bronchospasm: Bilateral wheezing, increased peak inspiratory pressure, decreased exhaled tidal volume，slowly rising waveform on capnography.

Obstruction of the ETT by secretion：Rales.

Pneumothorax：Diminished breath sound on the affected side. It could be confirmed by chest x-ray.

Anaphylaxis：Other clinical signs might be present，like hives，flushing，edema，hemodynamic instability，wheezing as well as increase peak inspiratory pressure.

7. Blood loss：How could you accurately assess the amount of blood loss? How to assess his volume status intraoperatively? At what point you would check his hematocrit and made a decision for transfusion? Assuming you were planning to give iv fluid to replace the volume，choice of crystalloid or colloid? How would you know the replacement was adequate?

Keypoint：Strategies of intraoperative fluid management in pediatric patients.

**Blood loss assessment：**

Accurate blood loss is difficult to assess in this type of surgery，because some blood could be drained into stomach.

Measurement of blood in the surgical suction container.

Visual estimation of blood loss on surgical sponges or pads is less accurate. To measure the weight of surgical sponges and pads before and after use is more appropriate for pediatric patients.

Monitor the hemodynamic changes although it usually is a later sign but indicate the amount is significant，will draw blood to check the Hgb/Hct.

**Intraoperative volume status assessment：**

The fullness of a peripheral pulse.

Response of blood pressure to positive ventilation and to the vasodilating or negative inotropic effects of anesthetics.

**Intraoperative fluid requirement：**

Maintenance fluid requirement：the "4：2：1" rule.

Deficits: related to preoperative fasting. Balanced salt solution like lactate Ringer could be the choice of fluid.

**Replacement requirement:**

Blood loss.

Non-glucose-containing crystalloid 3 : 1.

Colloid (e.g. 5% albumin, packed red blood cell) 1 : 1.

Third space loss: lactate Ringer.

0~2 mL/kg/h for relative atraumatic surgery.

6~10 mL/kg/h for traumatic procedure.

When the estimated blood loss exceeds 15% of total blood volume, a hematocrit should be checked and consider transfusion. Assessment of fluid replacement: the same as intraoperative volume status assessment.

8. Deep anesthesia extubation: The surgeon requested no coughing during extubation, reasonable? If so, how would you do it in steps?

Keypoint: Basic skills on extubation: two elements, depth of anesthesia and adequate spontaneous breath.

It is reasonable. A smooth extubation could decrease postoperative bleeding and prevent blood clot dislodgement from coughing or straining.

To ensure a smooth extubation doesn't mean to extubate under deep anesthesia.

Awake extubation: signify by the opening of the eyes.

Deeply anesthetized extubation: spontaneous breathing but no swallowing or coughing (before the return of airway reflex). Although deep extubation reduces laryngospasm or bronchospasm on emergence, it carries the risk for aspiration and upper airway obstruction. Not suitable for patients with a history of snoring or procedures like tonsillectomy.

Oropharyngeal spray of 2% lidocaine would decrease the coughing response to secretion and other stimulations.

**To ensure a smooth extubation, certain techniques could be applied:**

Gentle inspection and suction of the pharynx before extubation.

Adequate analgesia.

Lidocaine as bolus (1.5~2 mg/kg) to help decrease airway reflex (This is more commonly used to prevent bronchospasm).

9. Laryngospasm: Shortly after extubation, the patient's respiration became labored along with progressive desaturation, your response and action? What would you do if this was a laryngospasm? How would you differentiate a laryngospasm from bronchospasm? Is laryngospasm more common in pediatric, why/why not? Explain your management options? When would you give Sux (succinylcholine), if so, the dose and route? What if the iv catheter was out? What if you have administered the reversals, the pharmacology of Sux?

Keypoint: This question tests the ability to recognize and differentiate laryngospasm. Be familiar with its risk factors and management. The pharmacology and clinical applications of Sux.

This is a very obese child, and he is in a high risk for OSA. The first thing is to rule out the presence of upper airway obstruction, if confirmed, nasal and/ or oral airway, and will discuss with the surgeon if he agrees with the oral airway.

Other differentials include: laryngospasm, bronchospasm, breath-holding, and foreign body aspiration, most likely this could be laryngospasm.

Laryngospasm: stridor and retraction.

Bronchospasm: wheezing.

**Treatment for laryngospasm:**

Positive pressure ventilation by close the APL (adjustable pressure valve) with a mask.

Forward jaw thrust.

Deepening the anesthesia by intravenous lidocaine or propofol or turn on the volatile anesthetic（sevoflurane）.

Paralyze with intravenous Sux（0.5～1 mg/kg）or intravenous rocuronium（0.4 mg/kg）would be my last solution; intramuscular Sux（4 mg/kg）. Apply paralytics only when all conservative measures have failed. To give intramuscularly when iv is out.

Controlled ventilation.

Laryngospasm is more common in children. Young age is one of the most important risk factors for laryngospasm. The central regulation system of upper airway reflex is not well developed in small children.

**Pharmacology of Sux：**

Depolarizing muscle relaxant act as acetylcholine receptor agonist.

Not metabolized by acetylcholinesterase. Cleared from neuromuscular junction and hydrolyzed in the plasma by pseudocholinesterase.

10. Suspected airway foreign body：What if you suspect his emergence acute respiratory distress was caused by a packing sponge, it migrated to the throat? How would you confirm it? If you indeed saw it, would you try to pull it out or push it down?

Keypoint：Trouble shooting for airway foreign body.

Inspect with direct or indirect laryngoscope to confirm.

Try to pull it out. When the upper airway obstruction is suspected, the trying to pull out not successful while oxygenation is in jeopardy, I would push it down to esophagus under direct laryngoscope to ensure the delivery oxygen.

## > 术 中 管 理 <

1. 麻醉前用药：你是否会给患儿麻醉前用药，请简述理由。若你准备进行麻醉前用药，请列出拟用药物名称、剂量以及给药方式。你是否会等待药物起效后再行麻醉诱导?

要点:了解麻醉前用药的意义,熟悉各种麻醉用药的药理作用及儿科应用。

支气管扩张剂(口服或吸入)需要维持常规治疗剂量,应用至手术当日。

使用术前药取决于患儿个体需求、手术种类以及所使用的麻醉药物和方法。

抗胆碱能药物可以减少口腔分泌物,因此降低喉痉挛及支气管痉挛的风险。

对于和家长有分离焦虑的患儿,适当术前镇静可以缓解患儿的焦虑。口服咪达唑仑(0.3~0.5 mg/kg,最大剂量 15 mg);肌注咪达唑仑(0.1~0.15 m/kg);联合肌注氯胺酮(2~3 mg/kg)和阿托品(0.01 mg/kg);咪达唑仑纳肛(0.5~1 mg/kg,最大剂量 20 mg);右美托咪定滴鼻(1~2 μg/kg)。需在严密监测下方可使用镇静药,特别是肥胖患儿。

术前用药通常可在 15~30 min 达到镇静效果。

2. 是否允许患儿麻醉诱导时母亲在场:患儿母亲要求陪同孩子进入手术室,你是否同意? 对于患儿母亲的要求你如何应对? 患儿母亲讲述,上次她的另一个孩子在这里接受相同手术,麻醉医师允许她将孩子抱入手术室,这种情况是否司空见惯?

要点:考察临床医患沟通能力。应有效的为患儿及家长解惑。

是否允许患儿母亲进入手术室陪同麻醉诱导取决于多种因素:医院的诊疗常规,在麻醉术前访视时与患儿及母亲的交流(了解此前就医经历,患儿的心理年龄及配合程度)。

邀请患儿比较信任的人员陪同诱导可以使患儿更加平静,这些人员可以是患儿家长,也可以是患儿信任的护士或医师。但这一问题目前还存在争议,家长的焦虑程度可能与孩子的术前焦虑相关。此外,麻醉团队还需做好应对陪同的患儿家长突发意外的准备。

3. 麻醉诱导:请简述你对该患儿的麻醉诱导计划,采用静脉诱导还是吸入诱导? 请简述吸入诱导的技术要点,并阐述应如何预防喉痉挛的发生。

要点:熟悉小儿麻醉静脉诱导与吸入诱导的优缺点。了解喉痉挛的危险因素及预防措施。

如果患儿有明确上呼吸道梗阻及呼吸暂停病史,并且过度肥胖,存在可预计的困难气道,则宜采用吸入诱导。在确保能建立有效正压通气之前,暂不使用肌松药。

如下措施可以使得患儿的吸入诱导更加平稳。① 5 岁的患儿一般已有较好的沟通理解能力,可在诱导前向患儿详细描述麻醉诱导过程,使患儿能更好地配合麻醉。② 术前应用口服咪达唑仑,右美托咪定等滴鼻镇静药物使患儿困倦。③ 在面罩里滴入有水果香味的香精减少患儿对面罩的抗拒。④ 鼓励患儿采用面罩吸入无刺激味道的笑气(70%)及氧气(30%)混合气体,并随着每一口呼吸,逐渐增加七氟醚的吸入浓度(每次增加 0.5%)。⑤ 对于不配合的患儿,采用 60%氧化亚氮及40%氧气的高新鲜气体流量吸入高浓度七氟醚(7%~8%),通常 1 次呼吸患儿即可意识消失。⑥ 对于年龄较小的不配合患儿,允许其在坐位时开始吸入诱导。⑦ 待吸入诱导麻醉深度足够时建立静脉通路,给予丙泊酚及阿片类药物。

预防喉痉挛的方法:最重要的是需要保证麻醉深度,防止麻醉过浅。其他方法还包括麻醉前预先给予抗胆碱能药物(尤其在氯胺酮诱导时),避免哭闹,避免在麻醉深度不够时进行任何气道操作,选用呼吸道刺激性小的挥发性麻醉药(如七氟醚)。

4. 气管导管:请简述你会选用有套囊还是无套囊的气管导管? 两种气管导管是否有区别? 耳鼻喉科医师提出,有文献报道喉罩(LMA)的使用可以减少麻醉复苏时躁动的发生率,你该如何回答?

要点:考察有套囊及无套囊气管导管的特点,了解不同临床情况两者的优缺点。了解声门上通气装置的优势和应用局限性。与医护人员的沟通能力。

无套囊气管导管通常可用于 5~8 岁以下的患儿,该年龄段患儿气管最狭窄处位于环状软骨水平。无套囊气管导管理论上可以减少插管后的气道损伤,然而需要非常精确地选择合适大小,且有相对较高的漏气和误吸风险。

目前,多数麻醉医师采用相对患儿气道略小一点的有套囊气管插管,在插管前抽瘪套囊,插管后向套囊内充入尽可能少的气体以满足不漏气,同时可降低误吸的风险。对于口咽腔手术如扁桃体切除术和腺样体切除术更为合适。

喉罩可以减少拔管时的躁动。然而实际情况下喉罩是否可以安全地用于扁桃体切除术取决于手术及麻醉团队对于喉罩使用的经验。作为一种声门上通气工具，喉罩的误吸风险相对于更大，需要谨慎使用。目前有很多喉罩成功用于扁桃体切除的报道，具体应用还需依赖每个麻醉医师的临床偏好。

5. 呼吸机设置：简述术中呼吸机参数的设置，是选用容量控制(VC)还是压力控制(PC)并阐述理由。是否可以让患者保留自主呼吸？

要点：了解小儿麻醉呼吸参数设置基本要素。

对于年龄较小患儿，压力控制通气的模式更好，可以避免意外大潮气量对肺部造成气压伤。体重<10 kg的患儿，吸气峰压设定在15～18 cmH_2O。对于较大的患儿(体重超过10 kg)，可以采用容量控制方式通气，潮气量设置为6～8 mL/kg。

若患儿已行气管插管，闭合呼吸回路保留自主呼吸将轻度增加呼吸做功(通常对于发育正常的患儿并不存在太大影响)，可能导致通气不足，高碳酸血症。开放呼吸回路保留自主呼吸，并采用挥发性吸入麻醉药可导致空气污染。所以，仅在全凭静脉麻醉时方可考虑保留自主呼吸，否则，控制通气更为恰当。

通常此类手术会在全身麻醉气管插管控制通气的条件下进行。对于儿科患者通常选用压力控制的通气模式。然而，依据麻醉医师的偏好也可以选择保留自主呼吸的全身麻醉，此时更应注意气管插管位置、呼气末二氧化碳及血氧饱和度的监测。

6. 气道管理：手术顺利开始，不久你发现呼吸机PIP(吸气峰压)突然升高，从12 cmH_2O升高至30 cmH_2O，压力持续升高超过35 cmH_2O，你的鉴别诊断是什么？是否可能是手术医师操作造成的？

要点：解决术中机械通气异常的能力。

气管导管打折：是最常见的原因，通常发生在外科医师放置开口器时，直接查看手术视野，或者建议外科医师检查口腔术野。排除手术铺巾所遮挡的管路打折。此类情况可能与手术操作相关。

气管导管误入一侧支气管，可能由手术期间头部位置改变导致：双肺听诊一侧呼吸音减弱或消失。

支气管痉挛:双肺听诊哮鸣音,吸气峰压上升,呼气容量降低,呼气末二氧化碳曲线上升缓慢。

气管导管被分泌物堵塞:听诊闻及痰鸣音。

气胸:患侧呼吸音小时,可经胸部 X 线检查证实。

过敏反应:可能伴有其他临床征象,如皮肤风团、潮红、肿胀、血流动力学不稳定、双肺哮鸣音以及吸气峰压上升。

7. 术中失血:你如何精确评估术中失血? 如何评估患儿术中容量状态? 何种情况下你会检测血细胞比容并考虑输血? 假如你准备通过静脉输液补充容量,是选用晶体液还是胶体液? 你如何判断补液已经充分?

要点:掌握小儿麻醉术中液体管理基本原则。

**判断失血量:**

此类手术准确判断失血量比较困难,因为部分失血可能直接流入胃里。

吸引器瓶中的吸引血量。

通过纱布纱垫数量初步计算失血量不够准确;对于小儿患者,应在纱布纱垫使用前后称重以精确估计失血量。

不要忘记密切监测血流动力学变化,虽然血流动力学指标通常不能非常及时反应患儿容量状况,但明确的血流动力学改变通常预示着已存在显著的出血。建议及时检查血红蛋白/血细胞比容。

**术中容量状态的评估:**

外周动脉搏动的强弱。

患儿血压对正压通气的反应,患儿血压对麻醉药的扩血管作用和心肌抑制作用的反应。

**术中液体管理:**

生理需要量:按照"4∶2∶1"原则计算。

术前累计丢失量:与术前禁食水时间有关。一般补充平衡盐溶液,如乳酸林格氏液。

**补充量:**

失血量。

不含糖晶体液：按照 3∶1 补充。

胶体（如 5% 白蛋白或浓缩红细胞）：按照 1∶1 补充。

第三间隙丢失量：乳酸林格氏液。

小手术：0～2 mL/kg/h。

大手术：6～10 mL/kg/h。

当预计失血量超过全身血容量的 15% 时，测量红细胞压积并考虑输血。评估补液是否充足：大致同术中容量评估的方法。

8. 深麻醉状态下拔管：手术医师要求麻醉拔管时无呛咳，是否合理？若合理，请一步步阐述你的拔管计划。

要点：掌握拔管的基本策略：两个要点，麻醉深度和自主呼吸恢复。

外科医师的要求基本合理。平稳拔管可以减少术后出血，防止呛咳导致的伤口血块脱落。

平稳拔管并不意味着深麻醉状态下拔管。

清醒拔管：一般伴有患儿自主睁眼。

深麻醉状态下拔管：自主呼吸恢复但无吞咽反射或呛咳（即在气道反射恢复之前）。虽然深麻醉状态下拔管可以降低苏醒期喉痉挛和支气管痉挛的风险，但同时增加误吸及上呼吸道梗阻的风险。对于有明确打鼾病史及接受扁桃体切除术的患儿并不适合。

以 2% 利多卡因对口咽腔行局部麻醉可有效减少呼吸道分泌物或其他刺激所致的呛咳反射。

**为确保平稳拔管，可采取如下措施：**

拔管前轻柔吸净口咽腔中的积血和分泌物。

充分镇痛。

必要时静脉应用利多卡因（1～1.5 mg/kg）减轻气道反应（此方法通常用于减少支气管痉挛）。

9. 喉痉挛：拔管后不久，患儿表现出呼吸费力并伴有脉搏氧饱和度进行性下降，你采取何种措施应对？如果是喉痉挛你将如何应对？如何鉴别喉痉挛与支气管痉挛？喉痉挛是否更容易在儿科患者中发生？为什么？阐述你的诊疗计划。你准备何时应用琥珀胆碱,剂量和给药途径？如果静脉通路脱落了该怎么办？如果你已经使用过肌松拮抗剂怎么办？琥珀胆碱的药理学特性？

要点：本题考察喉痉挛的诊断和鉴别诊断。熟悉喉痉挛的危险因素及处理方法。熟悉琥珀胆碱的药理学特性及临床应用。

考虑到该患儿肥胖,具备阻塞性睡眠呼吸暂停低通气综合征的危险因素,故应首先排除上呼吸道梗阻的可能。若已明确存在上呼吸道梗阻,应迅速置入口咽或鼻咽通气道,并进一步与外科医师沟通。

其他鉴别诊断包括：喉痉挛、支气管痉挛、屏气,以及呼吸道异物。其中喉痉挛可能性最大。

喉痉挛：喘鸣,吸气三凹症。

支气管痉挛：哮鸣音。

**喉痉挛的治疗措施：**

关闭可调压力阀,采用面罩正压通气。

托下颌。

加深麻醉：静注利多卡因或丙泊酚,或吸入挥发性麻醉气体(如七氟醚)。

使用肌松药：当以上措施无效时,应用肌松药。静注琥珀胆碱(0.5～1 mg/kg),或静注罗库溴铵(0.4 mg/kg)。肌注琥珀胆碱(4 mg/kg)。只有当常规方法无效时才用肌松药。如果静脉通路脱落,则肌注给药。

控制通气。

喉痉挛在儿童中更为常见。低龄是喉痉挛的重要危险因素之一,由于幼儿控制咽喉反射的中枢发育尚不完善。

**琥珀胆碱的药理学：**

去极化肌松药,乙酰胆碱受体激动剂。

不能被乙酰胆碱酯酶所分解。通过肌肉神经接头清除,继而被血浆中假性胆碱酯酶所分解。

10. 可疑气道异物：若怀疑该患儿苏醒期急性呼吸窘迫是由于止血海绵误入咽喉腔所造成的,你将如何确定诊断？若诊断确立,你会选择将海绵取出还是推下去？

要点：可疑异物的处理措施。

采用直接或间接喉镜检查口咽腔是否有异物。

尝试取出异物。如未能取出异物，且患儿氧饱和度已难以维持，可以考虑在喉镜直视下将咽腔异物推入食管以尽快开放气道恢复通气。

## > **Postoperative management** <

1. Delirium/agitation：The child was agitated in the PACU，crying and struggling，would you consider to treat? If so，which agent? What if the intravenous line was pulled out? Is emergence delirium more common in pediatric patient? Why? Would you consider pre-medication to prevent this happened，is so，the choice of a drug?

Common cause and management of pediatric postoperative delirium/agitation.

Keypoint：Emergence delirium is a complex of perceptual disturbances and psychomotor agitation that occurs most commonly in preschool-aged children in the early post-anesthetic period. Emergence delirium should be treated since it can increase the risk of self-injury and delayed discharge，require additional nursing staff and can increase medical care costs.

Before any specific treatment for his delirium，I would like to rule out the common causes，such as uncontrolled pain，airway obstruction，urinary retention，etc.，which is easier to treat.

The prevalence of emergence delirium has increased with growing use of low-solubility inhalational anesthetics such as sevoflurane. Physiological factors，pharmacological factors，the type of procedure，the anesthetic agent administered，painful stimuli，and various patient factors can all contribute to emergence delirium.

Adjunctive agents can be rated in the following order of most effective to least effective interventions: dexmedetomidine, fentanyl, ketamine, clonidine, and propofol bolus at the end of sevoflurane-based anesthesia.

Inadequate pain control could be corrected with morphine $10\sim15$ $\mu$g/kg iv bolus, or fentanyl $0.5\sim1$ $\mu$g iv bolus. If the iv was pulled out, opioids or ketamine can be given intramuscularly (should emphasis a low dose opioid, the goal is to discharge the patient home shortly).

Premedication with iv or intranasal dexmedetomidine might help.


2. Persistent bronchospasm: A bilateral wheezing was heard in the PACU, would you treat it, if so how? List the choice of medications? Would you consider to use steroid? If so, by inhaler or iv, does it matter? How long would take the steroid to start work? Did the occurring of severe bronchospasm surprise you? Anything could be done to prevent it?

Keypoint: This question is on basic skill for bronchospasm management.

Treatment of persistent bronchospasm: supplemental $O_2$, aerosolized beta2-agonists, anticholinergics.

By personal experience, steroid would better be given by inhaler when it's possible. Iv steroids (hydrocortisone or methylprednisolone) takes hours to work. However, there is no evidence that inhaling steroids works faster than iv form.

A child with history of asthma and recent upper respiratory infection is at greater risk for bronchospasm. The most proper approach to prevent it is to postpone any elective surgery involving general anesthesia and airway instrumentation until $4\sim6$ weeks after recovery from upper respiratory infection.


3. Discharge: The original plan was going home the same day, would you discharge him after these? You and the surgeon decided to admit him, where

would be the best place, day-hospital, in-patient floor, pediatric ICU?

Keypoint: Postoperative considerations for pediatric cases.

Admit to day-hospital for further monitoring.

4. Re-bleeding: Five days after the surgery, the mom brought the child to ER (emergency department). After a bag of potato chips, the child started coughing and spitted out some blood. The ENT surgeon posted an emergent surgery to stop the bleeding. The child was agitated, not cooperative, won't let you start an iv. Explain your anesthesia plan? Would you consider inhalation induction? How do you assess his volume status? Would you insist to T & C before the surgery?

Keypoint: Basic concepts on emergent pediatric cases: preoperative evaluation, airway assessment and management, intravascular volume status, risk-versus-benefit on different induction techniques, intraoperative fluid management. It also requires the ability to communicate with the surgical team to achieve optimal perioperative management.

Premedication with anticholinergic. Inhaled induction. Establish iv for propofol and opioids. Adequate suction before endotracheal intubation.

Assess volume status, start with physical exam, exam the mucosa/tongue dryness, the color of finger and eye conjunctive membrane, peripheral capillary refill time; ask the mom when was the last the child urinated; vital signs, BP and HR, mental status, etc. Also assume there is a significant of blood in the stomach. Check hematocrit only if there were iv access. Stop bleeding as soon as possible and communicate with surgical team to decide whether to T & C.

At this point, insist to obtain the iv access if the child does not have one, and iv induction with (ketamine 1 mg/kg) would be my preference which would be the least affect his blood pressure and sux to facilitate the intubation; if volume status is suspected to be low, would give fluid bolus 10 mL/kg right before the induction. Also will a colleague or experienced nurse to apply cricoid pressure to prevent the risk of aspiration.

## 〉 术 后 管 理 〈

1. 术后谵妄/躁动：该患儿术后在恢复室出现躁动，哭闹挣扎，你认为是否需要处理？使用何种药物？若此时静脉通路已意外脱落怎么办？苏醒期躁动是否在儿科患者中更为常见？为什么？你是否会选择麻醉前用药以减少术后躁动的发生，你的用药选择是什么？

要点：儿童常见术后谵妄及躁动的原因及处理。

苏醒期躁动是麻醉后早期出现的一种感知和精神运动障碍，最常见于学龄前儿童。苏醒期躁动可能增加患儿自我伤害的风险、延长住院时间、增加护理人员投入，从而提高医疗费用，所以应该积极治疗。

在开始苏醒躁动针对性治疗之前，首先排除或积极纠正如下几种情况：术后疼痛、呼吸道梗阻、尿潴留等。

苏醒期躁动的发生率随着低溶解度吸入麻醉药（如七氟醚）的推广而增加。其他影响因素还包括患儿生理特点、药理学特性、手术种类、麻醉用药、疼痛刺激及其他患儿本身因素等。

七氟醚吸入麻醉结束之前单次给予以下药物可从强到弱减轻苏醒期躁动：右美托咪定、芬太尼、氯胺酮、可乐定和丙泊酚。

若为镇痛不足导致疼痛，可加强镇痛：吗啡 $10\sim15\ \mu g/kg$ 静注或芬太尼 $0.5\sim1\ \mu g/kg$ 静注。如果静脉脱出，可肌注阿片类药物或氯胺酮（注意应采用小剂量阿片类药物进行术后镇痛，以免延误早期出院）。

术前应用右美托咪定静注或滴鼻可减轻苏醒期躁动。

2. 持续性支气管痉挛：在恢复室，患儿双肺可闻及哮鸣音，你将如何处理？列出你的药物选择。你是否会考虑采用激素治疗，若准备应用激素，吸入还是静脉应用，两种给药方式是否有区别？激素的起效时间是多久？对于该患儿发生的严重支气管痉挛你是否感到意外？术前是否有预防策略？

本题考察支气管痉挛的基本诊疗策略。

持续性支气管痉挛的治疗：吸氧、雾化吸入 $\beta_2$ 受体激动剂或抗胆碱能药物。

个人经验认为，若使用激素，最好采用雾化吸入，静脉激素（琥珀酸氢化可的松或甲泼尼龙）通常需要若干小时才能起效。然而目前尚无临床证据显示吸入激素起效时间快于静脉激素。

伴有支气管哮喘及近期上呼吸道感染病史的患儿围术期发生支气管痉挛风险升高。为避免上述情况，最安全的方法是待上呼吸道感染痊愈4～6周以后再行需要气道操作的全麻手术。

3. 出院计划：原定计划为手术当日出院，你是否还考虑患儿当日出院？你和手术医师决定收患儿入院观察，请问是收入日间病房、住院部普通病房，还是儿科 ICU？

要点：儿童全麻手术后管理要点。

收入日间病房继续观察。

4. 术后出血：术后5天，患儿食用薯片后开始咳嗽伴吐血，由母亲陪同入医院急诊。耳鼻喉科医师提交急诊手术申请拟行止血。患儿躁动明显，不配合，无法建立静脉通路。简述你的麻醉计划。你是否考虑采用吸入诱导？如何评估患儿容量状态？你是否会在术前坚持行交叉配血？

要点：儿科急诊手术的基本概念：术前评估、气道评估及管理、容量状态评估，不同麻醉诱导的利弊及技术要点，术中液体管理。同时考察与外科医师的沟通协调及团队合作能力。

麻醉前使用抗胆碱能药物。吸入诱导。足够麻醉深度后建立静脉通路给予丙泊酚及阿片类药物。气管插管前充分吸引。

评估患儿容量状态应首先从体格检查开始，检查患儿口唇黏膜/舌头是否干燥，检查肢端、睑结膜是否苍白，检查外周毛细血管再充盈时间；询问患儿母亲患儿最后一次小便是多久以前；检查患儿血压、心率等生命体征，检查患儿意识状态等。时刻谨记患儿胃里可能存有大量吞咽下去的血液。在已建立静脉通路的情况下检查血细胞比容。快速止血，与此同时，与外科医师沟通，决定是否交叉配血。

结合此患儿情况,一定尽快建立静脉通路,静脉诱导可采用氯胺酮(1 mg/kg),以确保最小的血流动力学改变,并采用琥珀胆碱协助气管内插管。若患儿存在容量不足,可在诱导前给予 10 mg/kg 的补液治疗。麻醉诱导时请有经验的护士或另一位麻醉医师采取环状软骨压迫以减少误吸的风险。

## Reference

[1] Marinella Astuto, Pablo M. Perioperative Medicine in Pediatric Anesthesia. New Delhi: Springer, 2016.

[2] John F, Butterworth IV, David C, et al. Morgan & Mikhail's Clinical Anesthesiology. (5th edition), Pediatric Anesthesia. New York: McGraw-Hill Education, 2013.

[3] Cao JL, Pei YP, Wei JQ, et al. Effects of intraoperative dexmedetomidine with intravenous anesthesia on postoperative emergence agitation/delirium in pediatric patients undergoing tonsillectomy with or without adenoidectomy: A CONSORT-prospective, randomized, controlled clinical trial. Medicine (Baltimore). 2016; 95(49): e5566.

[4] Dahmani S, Michelet D, Abback PS, et al. Ketamine for perioperative pain management in children: a meta-analysis of published studies. Paediatr Anaesth. 2011; 21(6): 636-652.

[5] Collins CE. Anesthesia for pediatric airway surgery: recommendations and review from a pediatric referral center. Anesthesiol Clin. 2010; 28(3): 505-517.

[6] Li X, Zhou M, Xia Q, Li J. Parecoxib sodium reduces the need for opioids after tonsillectomy in children: a double-blind placebo-controlled randomized clinical trial. Can J Anaesth. 2016; 63(3): 268-274.

[7] Coté CJ. Anesthesiological considerations for children with obstructive sleep apnea. Curr Opin Anaesthesiol. 2015; 28(3): 327-332.

[8] von Ungern-Sternberg BS. Respiratory complications in the pediatric postanesthesia care unit. Anesthesiol Clin. 2014; 32(1): 45-61.

[9] Goel R, Cushing MM, Tobian AA. Pediatric Patient Blood Management Programs: Not Just Transfusing Little Adults. Transfus Med Rev. 2016; 30(4): 235-241.

Bo Zhu, Wenjuan Guo, Jing Zhao

朱波,郭文娟,赵晶

# 20 Anesthesia management for MVA trauma victim

## 车祸/多发伤手术麻醉

·········· > **Basic information** < ··········

A level one trauma code went off，a 38 years old male was brought to ER (emergency room) due to a high speed MVC (motor vehicle collision，110 km/h)，the EMS reported he was a restrained driver.The victim had a brief episode of LOC (loss of consciousness) at scene. He complains severe left leg pain in ED (emergency department).

Arrived ER with C-collar on，he was confused and combative. DPL (diagnostic peritoneal lavage) test is positive，the patient's blood pressure is trending down. The trauma surgeon decided to bring him straight to OR emergent exploratory laparotomy for possible spleen，liver，and/or bowel injury. Other positive findings were open fracture of the left tibia and fibula bones，the anterior rim of pelvic fracture with slight displacement.

PE：Weight 125 kg，BP 110/98，HR 132，SaO$_2$ 88% on FSO$_2$ 40%.

The patient takes no medication and no allergy.

Lab test：pending for CBC and BMT，and T&C (blood type and cross match).

## > 基 本 信 息 <

一级创伤警报响起，一名 38 岁的男性由于机动车高速碰撞事故（110 km/h）被送到急诊室。急救中心报告他开车时系保险带。受害者在现场有短暂的意识丧失。患者在急诊科抱怨严重的左腿疼痛。

到急诊手术室时已行颈托固定，思维混乱并且行为冲动。诊断性腹膜灌洗检查为阳性，患者的血压有下降趋势。创伤外科医师决定直接把患者送至手术室，对可能存在的脾、肝和/或肠损伤行急症剖腹探查术。其他阳性发现有左胫腓骨开放性骨折、骨盆前缘骨折伴轻度移位。

体检：体重 125 kg，血压 110/98 mmHg，心率 132 次/min，吸入氧浓度 40%时氧饱和度 88%。

患者没有用药史及过敏史。

实验室检查：全血细胞计数（CBC）和肝肾功能、出凝血时间报告还没有出来，交叉配血也没有完成。

## > Preoperative management <

1. Anesthesia set up: What would you do the anesthesia set up for such a major trauma surgery? List the lines, drugs, monitors, airway, etc., which you might needed for the anesthesia and resuscitation management?

Keypoint: want to know the anesthesia preparation for a major trauma surgery, a lot extra, drugs, blood products, fluid and fluid warmer, even the OR room should be pre-warmed, etc.

2. Communication: What would be the most efficient way to find out 1) the patient's information? Does that matter? Assuming; 2) you are the attending anesthesiologist, how would you communicate with your team, they are

resident，CRNA，anesthesia techs? 3）How would you recruit more helpers? Explain how would you find out the patient's conditions from the surgeon? 4）How do you communicate with other OR staffs，why/why not?

Keypoint：communication，clear communication so all team members could understand each role is the paramount，it is an acquired skill，learn from practice.

3. Blood products：Will you start the case without blood products ready? Will you accept "O" Rh negative blood if the type and cross specific not ready? Why/why not? How long would you be willing to wait for FFP and platelet?

Keypoint：to test whether the candidate could foresee the needs of large amount RBC，FFP，and platelet to save this patient's life，and understand the related policy on transfusion.

4. Consent：How do you obtain the consent? What if the patient is not able to give the consent（comatose，intoxicated）and the family members are not available? What if this is a child victim and no parents present?

Keypoint：This is a moral and ethical issue，when encounter a life and death situation which is the most important，also known the hospital policy，how to be able to defend your action.

5. IV access：what would be your minimal iv access? Your colleague suggested his role of thumb is 18 G × 2 for adult and 22 G × 2 for child< 5 years old，agree? Options for alternative if you just could not get the peripheral access?

Keypoint：Known the minimal need for iv access，known the alternative iv route，e.g.，IO（intraosseous），extra jugular vein，known when to demand a central line.

> **术 前 管 理** <

1. 麻醉方法:对这样一个重大的急症创伤手术你怎样做好麻醉的准备? 陈述你在麻醉和抢救复苏时的液体通路、药物、监测和气道管理等。

要点:想知道考生对于重大创伤性手术的麻醉准备的思考,包括药品、血液制品、液体和液体加温,甚至手术室应预热等。

2. 沟通:什么是了解患者信息的最有效的方式? 这个重要吗? 假设你是一位麻醉主治医师,你将如何与你的团队成员沟通,他们分别是住院医师、麻醉护士及麻醉技师? 你如何在很短时间里招募更多的帮手? 解释你如何从外科医师那里了解患者的状况? 以及如何与其他手术室工作人员沟通?

要点:沟通,确切的沟通可以让所有团队成员认识到每个工作都是至关重要的,这是一个可以从实践中学习而获得的技能。

3. 血液制品:你会在血制品没有准备好的情况下开始手术吗? 在血型和交叉配型未完成的情况下你会给患者输"O"型阴性血吗? 为什么/为什么不? 你可以等待 FFP 和血小板的时间多久?

要点:测试考生能否预见为了挽救患者的生命,可能需要大量的红细胞、新鲜冰冻血浆和血小板,以及是否了解输血的相关规定。

4. 知情同意:你如何获得知情同意? 如果患者不能签知情同意书(昏迷,醉酒),又没有家人,怎么办? 如果这是一个儿童患者,父母并不在场,又该怎么办?

要点:这是在遭遇生死抉择时面临的一个道德和伦理问题,也是最重要的问题,考生应该了解医院的相关政策,能够为你的行为辩护。

5. 静脉通路:这样的手术,对于静脉通路你的最低要求是什么? 你的同事说他的经验是成人至少开放两个 18 G,而<5 岁的儿童至少是两根 22 G 的静脉针,你同意吗? 如果没有外周静脉通路,你有什么其他选择?

要点：知道静脉通路的最低要求，知道可以选择的开放静脉的途径，例如髓内针注射、颈外静脉，知道何时需要开放中心静脉通路。

> **Intraoperative management** <

1. Induction：the choice of agents and dose? What is the main factor affecting your decision? Age，co-morbidity，or hemodynamic status，etc. explain?

Keypoint：knowledge of the pharmacology changes in hypovolemic patient，the goal is to prevent the circulatory collapse during induction，while ensure amnesia and no memory of surgery.

2. Cervical spine protection：does this patient have a cervical spine injury? What is MISL（manual inline stabilization）? How would prevent the potential c-spine injury during endotracheal intubation?

Keypoint：the candidate should be aware of potential cervical spine injury，and known the protocol of protecting c-spine during intubation guided by ATLS（adult trauma life saving）.

3. Would you perform the RSI（rapid sequence intubation），why/why not? Describe the steps? What if this is a difficult intubation，your approach? Would you ever consider a fiberoptic intubation on this patient，why/why not?

Keypoint：question for the concept of RSI and understand all trauma patients are full stomach.

4. Arterial line：Would you place it before or after introduction，why/why not?

Keypoint：surely an arterial line would be wonderful to monitor the instant BP changes and drawing blood for checking Hgb and electrolytes，but it won't be easy and should be balanced for the priority of the patient's care, it is not just for monitoring.

5. The patient has been prepared and draped, the surgeon is ready with a knife in hand and insists, he is rushing you to start induction even before the RBCs are brought and ready in room, agree? Explain your reason?

Keypoint: in most circumstance, the principle is RBC must be in room and ready then the surgeon can make the incision, the closed abdomen has a tamponade effect to slow down the bleeding.

6. ETT is placed in and confirmed by positive etCO$_2$, the surgeon start splenectomy and repairing the liver laceration, you noticed progressive increase in PIP (peak inspiratory pressure), and decrease in SpO$_2$, explain your differential (causes) and management? Tension pneumothorax? Aspiration? Bronchospasm?

Keypoint: ATLS requires ABCDE (airway, breath, circulation, drug/ differentiation, exam) at the scene, ER, at OR, each time reconfirm the diagnosis and may have new findings; in the case, the anesthesia care team should make a quick diagnosis of pneumothorax/tension pneumothorax, which is a life-threatening condition.

7. Transfusion threshold: When would consider RBC transfusion? Would it be the same for an elective surgery, why/why not? What is MTP (massive transfusion protocol)? When would it trigger the MTP code for this patient?

Keypoint: the guideline for transfusion of Hgb 6~8 g/dL is for an elective surgery with/without other comorbidities, however, for this trauma victim, there is an ongoing blood lose for trauma victim during surgery, in general the preferred Hgb is 8 - 10 g/dL; evidence support to transfusion RBC with FFP and platelet together, while could stable the blood pressure earlier and to reduce the total amount product-a concept of MTP (massive transfusion protocol).

8. Transfusion reaction: while the RBC and FFP were hanging, the patient blood pressure was not rising rather trending down, why? Could this be a transfusion reaction? Your diagnosis and management approach? Any tests you may want to order? What is the most complication associated with transfusion? What does TRALI stands for?

Keypoint: the candidate should be able to recognize the transfusion reaction, the mechanisms, and management options, know other transfusion related complications.

9. The spleen is out, the several places of liver laceration have been repaired, still there was lot oozing in the surgical field, any test and treatment could you offer?

Keypoint: coagulopathy commonly occurs in trauma surgery, the candidate should be able to explain difference causes, such as dilutional, consumption, dysfunctional, and able to apply different lab test.

10. The patient is now on Neo (phenylephrine) infusion 150 mcg/min and IV fluid wide open to maintain MAP around 70 mmHg, the orthopedic surgeon would like to perform an ORIF for the tibia and fibial fractures, your response? Remember this is an open fracture?

Keypoint: "damage control" is an important concept in trauma medicine, the goal is control the life-threatening condition rather treat the injury/disease; in this case, once the major bleeding has been stopped, the next step is to stabilized the patient in ICU. In this case, the patient was unstable from various bleeding, as for the open fracture, the option would be either splint the leg or external quick fixation the fracture, take the patient to ICU for volume, reassessment, while ORIF (open reduction and internal fixation) is not recommended in unstable patient.

## > 术 中 管 理 <

1. 诱导：药物的选择及剂量？影响你做决定的主要因素是什么？年龄、并发症，或是血流动力学状态等，请解释？

要点：了解低血容量患者的药理学变化，目的是防止诱导期间的循环衰竭，同时确保没有意识和对手术的记忆。

2. 颈椎保护：这个患者是否有颈椎损伤的危险？什么是 MISL(手法原位固定)？如何在行气管插管时预防潜在的颈椎损伤？

要点：考生应该意识到潜在的颈椎损伤，并且知道在 ATLS(成人生命创伤救治)的指导原则下进行插管期间保护颈椎的策略。

3. 你会进行 RSI(快速诱导插管)吗，为什么/为什么不？描述一下具体的步骤？如果这是一个预期的困难插管，你的插管方法是什么？你会考虑纤维支气管镜插管吗？为什么/为什么不？

要点：RSI 概念的问题，并且知道所有创伤患者都是饱腹状态。

4. 动脉监测：你会在诱导前还是诱导后置入动脉导管，为什么/为什么不？

要点：开放有创动脉的确对监测瞬时血压变化和抽血化验 Hgb 和电解质很有用，但有时这并不容易，应该首先是抢救患者的生命，而不是仅仅为了监测。

5. 患者已消毒和铺单，外科医师已拿好手术刀准备切皮，催促你快点开始麻醉诱导，但此时患者的血还未准备好且并没拿到手术室，你会诱导吗？解释你的理由？

要点：一般情况下，原则是必须在红细胞已备好并拿到手术室，然后外科医师才可以开始手术，因为闭合的腹部有压迫作用可以减缓出血。

6. etCO$_2$证实气管导管在位,外科医师开始脾切除术,并修复肝脏,您注意到PIP(吸气峰值压力)进行性增加,同时氧饱和度下降,造成这些变化的原因有哪些,怎么处理?张力性气胸、误吸,还是支气管痉挛?

要点:创伤高级生命支持 ATLS 在现场、急诊室、手术室都需要 ABCDE(气道、呼吸、循环、药物/鉴别诊断和检查),需要不断地重新确认诊断,可能会有新的发现;在这种情况下,麻醉团队应该快速做出气胸/张力性气胸诊断,这是危及生命的状况。

7. 输血阈值:何时需要考虑输注 RBC?与择期手术的标准是否一致,为什么/为什么不?什么是 MTP(大量输血方案)?什么时候应该对该患者启动 MTP?

要点:输血指南中对于择期手术伴/不伴其他并发症时,在 Hgb 60~80 g/L 时给予输血,然而对于创伤患者,在手术期间存在持续的血液丢失,通常推荐当 Hgb 为 100 g/L 时予输血;有证据支持输注红细胞的同时给予 FFP 和血小板,可以提早稳定血压,并减少最后输血的总量-这是 MTP(大量输血方案)的一个概念。

8. 输血反应:输注 RBC 和 FFP 后,患者的血压不但没有上升而是趋向下降,为什么?这是输血反应吗?你的诊断和治疗是?你需要进一步做什么检查?与输血相关的最常见的并发症是什么?什么是 TRALI(输血相关性肺损伤)?

要点:考生应该能够识别输血反应、机制及治疗手段,知道其他输血相关并发症。

9. 脾脏切除后,肝脏的几处裂伤也已经修复,但手术区域还有很多渗血,什么检查能帮助明确原因和治疗?

要点:在创伤手术中凝血障碍经常会发生,考生应该能够解释各种不同的原因,如凝血因子的稀释、消耗、功能障碍,并能够应用不同的实验室检查。

10. 患者现在需要静脉输注 Neo(去氧肾上腺素)150 $\mu$g/min 和快速补液来维持平均动脉压 MAP 在 70 mmHg 左右,骨科医师这时想要为他进行胫腓骨折切开复位内固定术,你的反应是什么?请记住这是一个开放性骨折损伤?

要点:"创伤控制"是创伤医学中的一个重要概念,目标是控制危及生命的状况而不是治疗损伤/疾病；在这种情况下，一旦主要的出血止住以后，下一步是到 ICU 进一步稳定患者状况。这一病例，患者由于多处出血病情不稳定，至于开放性骨折，可以考虑用夹板固定或行外部固定折，尽早将患者送至 ICU 进行容量复苏和重新评估。而此时，对于此类不稳定的患者不建议进行 ORIF（开放性骨折复位内固定术）。

-------------------- > **Postoperative management** < --------------------

1. Extubation criteria: Would you extubate the patient at the end of surgery in OR? Explain the criteria, would it be different from an elective surgery?

Keypoint: knowledge of extubation criteria and the application to elective vs. trauma patient, remember the patient also has ribs fracture.

2. ICU ventilator set up: the patient was left intubated and the respiratory therapist want you give the ventilator set up order? What is difference between VCV and PCV? Would you consider to use SIMV or PSPro (pressure support), why/why not?

Keypoint: knowledge of ventilator, difference mode, the application for different stage of respiratory failure or ventilator dependent patient; the ability to assess the clinical condition and apply the concept well.

3. ARDS: two days later, you saw a critical care colleague in the hall way, he told you that your patient now is in ARDS (acute respiratory distress syndrome), explain what is ARDS, are you surprise to hear this? Should his ventilator setting be changed, if so, explain?

Keypoint: understand the concept of ARDS, the principle of protective ventilation.

4. Explain the difference between sepsis and SIRS (systemic inflammatory

response syndrome)？ Would it be avoidable in this patient？ Could you do anything in OR to prevent？

Keypoint：knowledge of clinically common terminology regarding systemic inflammatory，their similarity and difference.

5. One week later，the hospital risk manager called you that patient complained for missing his front upper incisors tooth，your response？

Keypoint：to test the candidate's ability to defend for himself. Sometime，despite the best practice，mistake do happen，it should be handle different from negligence；also the candidate should be able to demonstrate his vigilance in early recognition and action，proper treatment，etc.

6. Six months later，the patient filed a complaint against you and your hospital for the transfusion reaction during which he said was the main cause of his complicated ICU course and mounting medical fees，your response？

Keypoint：again，this is to test whether the candidate can defend his/her medical practice，have the knowledge and be able to project the outcome of such a major trauma condition，after the successful resuscitation，the rough hospital course is related to the original injury and secondary systemic inflammation，which is total expected. Now，he should be able to defend and help the patient and his family member to understand this，as well as the hospital administrators.

## 〉 术 后 管 理 〈

1. 拔管标准：您在手术结束时拔除气管导管吗？解释你的拔管标准,这与择期手术有区别吗？

要点：知道拔管标准,及其在择期手术和创伤患者的应用,需要记住患者还有肋骨骨折。

2.ICU 呼吸机设置:患者送入时留置气管导管,呼吸治疗师要求你给呼吸机设置参数? 容量控制和压力控制这两种通气模式有什么区别? 你会考虑使用 SIMV 或 PSPro(压力支持)模式吗,为什么/为什么不?

要点:知道有关呼吸机、不同的模式、呼吸衰竭不同阶段或呼吸机依赖患者的应用;评估临床状况并把概念很好地应用于临床的能力。

3.急性呼吸窘迫综合征(ARDS):2 天后,你在大厅里看到一名重症监护同事,他告诉你,你的患者现在并发 ARDS,解释一下 ARDS 的定义? 你觉得这患者发生 ARDS 惊奇吗? 他的呼吸机设置需要改变吗,如果是,请解释。

要点:了解 ARDS 的概念,保护性通气的原理。

4.解释败血症和全身炎症反应综合征(SIRS)之间的差异? 这个患者可以避免吗? 在手术室你能预防吗?

要点:知道有关全身性炎症的临床常见术语,它们的相似性和差异。

5.1 周后,医院风险管理者打电话给你,患者抱怨他的前上门牙没有了,你的反应是?

要点:测试考生为自己辩护的能力。有时,尽管已做到最好,还是会有错误发生,这应该与疏忽大意区别对待;同时,考生也应该能够证明其早期识别和行动的警觉性。

6.6 个月后,患者因输血原因向你和你的医院发文提出投诉,他说这是造成他复杂的 ICU 治疗过程和医疗费用增加的主要原因,你的回答是?

要点:再一次测试考生能否为自己辩护的能力,具有扎实的医学知识,能够预知这样的严重创伤患者,在抢救他的生命成功后,其凶险的住院过程与最初的损伤和继发的全身炎症反应有关,这一切都在预料之中的。需要能把这一切向患者和家属,甚至医院的管理人员解释清楚。

Chuanyao Tong

童传耀